Quick Reference Dictionary for
Occupational Therapy

Sixth Edition

Quick Reference Dictionary for
Occupational Therapy

Edited by

Karen Jacobs, EdD, OTR/L, CPE, FAOTA
Clinical Professor
Program Director
Online Post-Professional Doctorate in
Occupational Therapy Program
Boston University
Boston, Massachusetts

Laela Simon, OTR/L
School-Based Occupational Therapist
Middletown, Connecticut

SLACK
INCORPORATED

www.Healio.com/books
ISBN: 978-1-61711-646-9

The procedures and practices described in this publication should be implemented in a manner consistent with the professional standards set for the circumstances that apply in each specific situation. Every effort has been made to confirm the accuracy of the information presented and to correctly relate generally accepted practices. The authors, editors, and publisher cannot accept responsibility for errors or exclusions or for the outcome of the material presented herein. There is no expressed or implied warranty of this book or information imparted by it. Care has been taken to ensure that drug selection and dosages are in accordance with currently accepted/recommended practice. Off-label uses of drugs may be discussed. Due to continuing research, changes in government policy and regulations, and various effects of drug reactions and interactions, it is recommended that the reader carefully review all materials and literature provided for each drug, especially those that are new or not frequently used. Some drugs or devices in this publication have clearance for use in a restricted research setting by the Food and Drug and Administration or FDA. Each professional should determine the FDA status of any drug or device prior to use in their practice.

Any review or mention of specific companies or products is not intended as an endorsement by the author or publisher.

SLACK Incorporated uses a review process to evaluate submitted material. Prior to publication, educators or clinicians provide important feedback on the content that we publish. We welcome feedback on this work.

Published by: SLACK Incorporated
                       6900 Grove Road
                       Thorofare, NJ 08086 USA
                       Telephone: 856-848-1000
                       Fax: 856-848-6091
                       www.Healio.com/books

Contact SLACK Incorporated for more information about other books in this field or about the availability of our books from distributors outside the United States.

Library of Congress Cataloging-in-Publication Data
Quick reference dictionary for occupational therapy / edited by Karen Jacobs, Laela Simon.
-- Sixth edition.
    p. ; cm.
  Includes bibliographical references.
  ISBN 978-1-61711-646-9 (paperback : alk. paper)
  I. Jacobs, Karen, 1951- editor. II. Simon, Laela, editor.
    [DNLM: 1. Occupational Therapy--Dictionary--English. 2. Occupational Therapy--Terminology--English. WB 15]
  RM735
  615.8'51503--dc23

                              2014017037

Printed in the United States of America.

Last digit is print number: 10 9   8   7   6   5

Dedication

To Sophie, Zachary, Liberty, and Zane.

Contents

**Additional appendices are located at
www.healio.com/books/qrdappendices6th**

Acknowledgments

Thank you to the contributors to past editions of the *Quick Reference Dictionary for Occupational Therapy* and to the new contributors to this Sixth Edition. Our gratitude is extended to Boston University occupational therapy graduate student Flora Cole, who provided invaluable support in making this Sixth Edition a reality, and to SLACK Incorporated for all their support.

About the Editors

Karen Jacobs, EdD, OTR/L, CPE, FAOTA is a past president and vice president of the American Occupational Therapy Association, received the 2011 Eleanor Clarke Slagle Lectureship, and was a 2005 recipient of a Fulbright Scholarship to the University of Akureyri in Akureyri, Iceland. Karen is a clinical professor and the program director of the On-Line Post-Professional Doctorate in Occupational Therapy (OTD) program at Boston University, Boston, Massachusetts. She earned a doctoral degree at the University of Massachusetts, a Master of Science in occupational therapy at Boston University, and a Bachelor of Arts at Washington University in St. Louis, Missouri.

Karen's research examines the interface between the environment and human capabilities. In particular, she examines the individual factors and environmental demands associated with increased risk of functional limitations among populations of university and middle school-aged students, particularly in notebook computing, use of tablets, and backpack use. She is also part of a 5-year study entitled, Project Career: Development of an Interprofessional Demonstration to Support the Transition of Students With Traumatic Brain Injuries From Postsecondary Education to Employment.

In addition to being an occupational therapist, Karen is also a certified professional ergonomist and the founding editor of the international, interprofessional journal *WORK: A Journal of Prevention, Assessment and Rehabilitation* (http://blogs.bu.edu/kjacobs/).

Karen is a faculty-in-residence and lives in an apartment in one of the dormitories at Boston University. She is the mother of three children—Laela, Joshua, and Ariel—and the amma (grandma in Icelandic) to Sophie, Zachary, Liberty, and Zane. She balances work with occupations such as cross-country skiing, kayaking, photography, and travel.

Laela Simon, OTR/L received her degree in occupational therapy from Florida Agricultural and Mechanical University, Tallahassee, Florida. She practiced for more than 10 years as a rehabilitation coordinator/manager with expertise in vestibular, neurological, and orthopedic rehabilitation. Currently, Laela is a school-based occupational therapist in Connecticut, where she provides services to children with a variety of different diagnoses; she also has a consulting practice.

Laela is passionate about teaching handwriting to children and spends time volunteering her expertise at local preschools and elementary schools.

Laela and her husband, Craig, are the proud parents of Sophie and Zachary. Laela balances work with occupations such as music, art, travel, and spending time with her family.

Introduction

U.S. President Barack Obama said, "Change will not come if we wait for some other person or some other time. We are the ones we've been waiting for. We are the change that we seek."

These inspirational words have helped to continue to guide this Sixth Edition of the *Quick Reference Dictionary for Occupational Therapy*. We have made changes based on thoughtful feedback from occupational therapy and occupational therapy assistant students and faculty. Terminology and new definitions have been updated to reflect technology and new documents both internal and external to the profession. New appendices have been added, such as Energy Conservation Techniques; Evidence-Based Practice, Levels of Evidence, and Qualitative Research; Glasgow Coma Scale; Grip Development and Stages of Writing; Health Literacy; Safe Patient Handling and Movement Skills for Occupational Therapy Practitioners and Students; Stages of Alzheimer's Disease: Seven Stages From the Alzheimer's Foundation; and Thoracic Outlet Syndrome.

We hope that you find the *Quick Reference Dictionary for Occupational Therapy, Sixth Edition,* a helpful resource during academic study, when on Level I and II Fieldwork, and in practice.

Karen Jacobs, EdD, OTR/L, CPE, FAOTA
Laela Simon, OTR/L

The following resources are noted throughout the
*Quick Reference Dictionary for Occupational Therapy,
Sixth Edition.*

OTPF 2014: American Occupational Therapy Association. (2014). Occupational therapy practice framework: Domain and process (3rd ed.). *American Journal of Occupational Therapy, 68*(Suppl. 1), S1-S48. http://dx.doi.org/10.5014/ajot.2014.682006

OTPF 2008: American Occupational Therapy Association. (2008). Occupational therapy practice framework: Domain and process (2nd ed.). *American Journal of Occupational Therapy, 62*, 625-668.

AOTA Framework: American Occupational Therapy Association. (2002). Occupational therapy practice framework: Domain and process. *American Journal of Occupational Therapy, 56*, 609-639.

UTIII: American Occupational Therapy Association. (1994). Uniform terminology for occupational therapy (3rd ed.). *American Journal of Occupational Therapy, 48*, 1047-1054.

CAOT: Townsend, E., & Polatajko, H. (2007). *Enabling occupation II: Advancing an occupational therapy vision for health, well-being & justice through occupation.* Ottawa, Ontario, Canada: Canadian Association of Occupational Therapists.

ICF: World Health Organization. (2001). *The international classification of functioning, disability and health—Towards a common language for functioning, disability and health.* Geneva, Switzerland: Author.

C: BCPR Consulting, Inc. and Center for Psychiatric Rehabilitation, Boston University, Sargent College of Health and Rehabilitation Sciences, 2001.

Small Business Administration: www.sba.gov

A

abbreviation expansion program: Software that allows a person to rapidly enter a few defined characters (abbreviation) to print out an expanded long string of characters (expansion) on a computer or communication aid. This system saves the user typing time and effort.

abduction (ABD): Movement of a body part (usually the limbs) away from the midline of the body.

abductive reasoning: To find the best explanation in a complex situation; it is "a matter of utilizing the principle of maximum likelihood in order to formalize a pattern of reasoning known as the 'inference to the best explanation'" (Fetzer, 1990, p. 103); to advance already existing conceptual ideas or theoretical understandings; or create new concepts that broaden current descriptions of phenomena (Aliseda, 2006).[CAOT]

abscess: A swollen, inflamed area in body tissues in which pus gathers.

absence: An epileptic seizure characterized by an abrupt loss of consciousness for a few seconds, followed by a rapid, complete recovery.

absolute endurance: Muscular endurance when force of contraction tested does not consider individual differences in strength.

absorption: Process by which a substance is made available to the body fluids for distribution.

abstinence: A period of alcohol- and drug-free living.

abstract thinking: Ability to derive meaning from an event or experience beyond the tangible aspects of the event itself.

abuse: Improper or excessive use, injury, or mistreatment of individuals.

Jacobs, K., & Simon, L. (Eds.). *Quick Reference Dictionary for Occupational Therapy, Sixth Edition* (pp. 1-27). © 2015 SLACK Incorporated.

academic fieldwork coordinator: A university's representative responsible for coordinating fieldwork, assigning students, and negotiating contracts and placements.

academic medical centers: Large complexes of buildings located in city centers that draw patients from all over their geographic region (and sometimes beyond), focused on teaching and research in addition to health care.

acalculia: Inability to do simple mathematical calculations.

acceleration: Increase in the speed or velocity of an object or reaction.

accessibility: Degree to which an exterior or interior environment is available for use in relation to an individual's physical and/or psychological abilities.

accessory movers: Muscles capable of performing a motion; assist prime movers.

accommodates: Modifies his or her actions or the location of objects within the workspace in anticipation of or response to problems that might arise. The client anticipates or responds to problems effectively by (a) changing the method with which he or she is performing an action sequence, (b) changing the manner in which he or she interacts with or handles tools and materials already in the workspace, and (c) asking for assistance when appropriate or needed.^AOTA Framework

accommodation (A): Process of adapting or adjusting one thing or set of things to another.

accreditation: Process used to evaluate educational programs against a set of standards that represent the knowledge, skills, and attitudes needed for competent practice. The Accreditation Council of Occupational Therapy Education accredits occupational therapy and occupational therapy assistant programs.

acculturation: When one assumes the attitudes, values, and behaviors of a culture different from his or her own to be accepted.

accuracy of response: Percentage of errors and correct responses recorded.

acetabulum: The cup-shaped depression on the hip bone where the head of the femur attaches.

achalasia: Failure of a circular sphincter or other muscle to relax and open (e.g., cardiac sphincter between the esophagus and stomach).

achievement behavior: Guided by societal standards, the behavior facilitates risk-taking ability and the development of a sense of competition.

achieving/maintaining valued roles: Psychiatric rehabilitation program that focuses on involving the consumer in assessing and developing the skills and supports needed and wanted for functioning in his or her chosen environmental role.[C]

achieving stage: Schai's early adulthood stage that involves the application of intelligence to situations that have profound consequences for achieving long-term goals (e.g., those involving careers and knowledge).

achromatopsia: Color blindness.

acquired amputation: Person is born with all limbs but, after injury or accident, has a limb removed in part or total.

acquired immunodeficiency syndrome (AIDS): Syndrome caused by the human immunodeficiency virus that renders immune cells ineffective, permitting opportunistic infections, malignancies, and neurologic diseases to develop; it is transmitted sexually or through exposure to contaminated blood.

acromion process: Outer projection of the spine of the scapula; considered to be the highest part of the shoulder, it connects laterally to the clavicle.

action: A set of voluntary movements or mental processes that form a recognizable and purposeful pattern, such as grasping, holding, pulling, pushing, turning, kneeling, standing, walking, thinking, remembering, smiling, chewing, and winking (adapted from Polatajko et al., 2004; Zimmerman, Purdie, Davis, & Polatajko, 2006).[CAOT]

action research: Research aimed at social change through self-reflective inquiry undertaken by participants within any shared situation to increase understanding of the ideologies and practices of their particular situation and to empower and improve them through action. It is usually described as a dynamic, spiraling process with ongoing observation, reflection, planning, and action and is aligned with critical research.

active assistive range of motion (AAROM): Amount of motion at a given joint achieved by the person using his or her own muscle strength with assistance.

active listening: Skills that allow a person to hear, understand, and indicate that the message has been communicated.

active play therapy: Therapy in which the therapist uses toys and particular play to advance a child's treatment or development.

active range of motion (AROM): Amount of motion at a given joint achieved by the person using his or her own muscle strength.

active stretch: Stretch produced by internal muscular force.

activin: Hormone releasing factor that assists production of follicular-stimulating hormone at the pituitary.

activities: Actions designed and selected to support the development of performance skills and performance patterns to enhance occupational engagement.[OTPF 2014]

activities of daily living (ADLs): Activities oriented toward taking care of one's own body (adapted from Rogers & Holm, 1994). ADLs also are referred to as basic activities of daily living (BADLs) and personal activities of daily living (PADLs). These activities are "fundamental to living in a social world; they enable basic survival and well-being" (Christiansen & Hammecker, 2001, p. 156).[OTPF 2014]

activity: The execution of a task or action by an individual.[ICF] A set of tasks with a specific endpoint or outcome that is greater than that of any constituent task, such as writing a report (adapted from Polatajko et al., 2004; Zimmerman et al., 2006).[CAOT] Productive action required for the development, maturation, and use of sensory, motor, social, psychological, and cognitive functions.

activity analysis: Analysis of "the typical demands of an activity, the range of skills involved in its performance, and the various cultural meanings that might be ascribed to it" (Crepeau, 2003, p. 192).[OTPF 2014] Breaking down the activity into components to determine the human functions needed to complete the activity.

activity configuration: An evaluative tool that identifies one's use of time, the value of one's daily activities, and the changes one would like to make in time management and routines.

activity demands: Aspects of an activity or occupation needed to carry it out, including relevance and importance to the client, objects used and their properties, space demands, social demands, sequencing and timing, required actions and performance skills, and required underlying body functions and body structures.[OTPF 2014]

activity limitations: Problems in health functioning when an individual has difficulty executing activities.[ICF]

activity pattern analysis: Any method for determining the type, amount, and organization of activities individuals engage in on a recurring basis.

activity theory of aging: Psychosocial theory of aging suggesting that successful aging occurs when the older person continues to participate in the satisfying activities of his or her earlier adulthood.

activity therapies: Therapies in which doing, rather than talking, is the primary mode of intervention.

activity tolerance: The ability to sustain engagement in an activity over a period of time.

acuity: Ability of the sensory organ to receive information.

acupressure: Use of touch at specific points along the meridians of the body to release the tensions that cause various physical symptoms.

acupuncture: Chinese practice of inserting needles into specific points along the meridians of the body to relieve pain and induce anesthesia. It is used for preventive and therapeutic purposes.

acute: Of a short and intense duration.

adapt: A key occupational therapy enablement skill to make suitable to or fit for a specific use or situation (Answers.com) and to respond to occupational challenges (Schkade & Schultz, 1992) with all clients, from individuals to populations, given that "individuals continuously adapt their occupations" (Meltzer, 2001, p. 17). In the *Profile of Occupational Therapy Practice in*

Canada (CAOT, in press), this skill is part of the occupational therapy competency role as change agent.[CAOT]

adaptation: Occupational therapy practitioners enable participation by modifying a task, the method of accomplishing the task, and the environment to promote engagement in occupation (James, 2008).[OTPF 2014] Satisfactory adjustment of individuals within their environment over time. Successful adaptation equates with quality of life.

adaptation (as used as an outcome): "A change a person makes in his or her response approach when that person encounters an occupational challenge. This change is implemented when the individual's customary response approaches are found inadequate for producing some degree of mastery over the challenge" (Christiansen & Baum, 1997, p. 591).[AOTA Framework]

adaptation (as used as a performance skill): Relates to the ability to anticipate, correct for, and benefit by learning from the consequences of errors that arise in the course of task performance (Fisher & Kielhofner, 1995).[AOTA Framework]

adaptive device: Special tool that is an adaptation of a common item designed to allow an easier completion of self-care, recreation, or work-related activities by a person.

adaptive equipment: Devices used to allow performance of a functional task.

adaptiveness: Capacity toward adaptation; adjustment to environmental conditions.

adaptive response: Behavior elicited by sensory stimulation that is of a more advanced, organized, flexible, or productive nature than that which occurred before stimulation.

Additive Activities Profile Test (ADAPT): Self-administered test that relates activities of daily living to physical fitness.

adduction (ADD): Movement toward the midline of the body.

adductor pads: Pads at the sides of a wheelchair to hold the hips and legs toward the midline of the body.

adenohypophysis: The anterior lobe of the pituitary gland.

adherence: Consistent behavior that is accomplished through an internalization of learning, enhanced by independent coping and problem-solving skills.

adhesion: Fibrous band holding parts together that are normally separated.

adhesive capsulitis: Inflammation of the joint capsule, which causes limitations of mobility or immobility of the joint.

adiadochokinesis: Inability to perform rapidly alternating movements, such as pronation and supination.

adjustment reaction disorder: Characterized by a reduced ability to function and adapt in response to a stressful life event. The disorder begins shortly after the event, and normal functioning is expected to return when the particular stressor is removed.

adjusts: Changes working environments in anticipation of or response to problems that might arise. The client anticipates or responds to problems effectively by making some change (a) between working environments by moving to a new workspace or bringing in or removing tools and materials from the present workspace or (b) in an environmental condition (e.g., turning on or off the tap, turning up or down the temperature).AOTA Framework

administration (ADM): Management of institutional activities.

Administration on Aging: U.S. federal agency designated to carry out the provisions of the Older Americans Act of 1965.

administrative controls: Decisions made by management intended to reduce the duration, frequency, and severity of exposure to existing workplace hazards. It leaves the hazards at the workplace but attempts to diminish the effects on the worker (e.g., job rotation or job enlargement).

advanced directives: Living wills and care instruction in which a competent adult expresses his or her wishes regarding medical management in the event of serious illness.

advanced level practice: Occupational therapist or occupational therapy assistant with 3 or more years of experience and advanced skills in specialty areas.

adverse effects: Undesired consequences of chemical agents resulting from toxic doses or allergies.

advocacy: Efforts directed toward promoting occupational justice and empowering clients to seek and obtain resources to fully participate in their daily life occupations. Efforts undertaken by the practitioner are considered advocacy, and those undertaken by the client are considered self-advocacy and can be promoted and supported by the practitioner.[OTPF 2014] Actively supporting a cause, idea, or policy (e.g., speaking in favor); recommending accommodations under the Americans with Disabilities Act.

advocate: A key occupational therapy enablement skill enacted with or for people to raise critical perspectives, prompt new forms of power sharing, or lobby or make new options known to key decision makers; to speak, plead, or argue in favour of (Houghton-Mifflin Company, 2004). In the *Profile of Occupational Therapy Practice in Canada* (CAOT, in press), advocacy contributes to the occupational therapy competency role of change agent.[CAOT]

aerobic capacity: A measure of the ability to perform work or participate in activity over time using the body's oxygen uptake and delivery and energy release mechanisms.

aerobic exercise: Any physical exercise that requires additional effort by the heart and lungs to meet the increased demand by the skeletal muscles for oxygen. Oxygen is present during exercise (as opposed to during anaerobic exercise).

aerobic metabolism: Energy production utilizing oxygen.

aerobic power: Maximal oxygen consumption; the maximal volume of oxygen consumed per unit of time.

aerobic training/exercise: Exercise of sufficient intensity, duration, and frequency to improve the efficiency of oxygen consumption during activity or work. Endurance-type exercise that relies on oxidative metabolism as the major source of energy production.

aesthesiometer: Tool used to apply and test two-point discrimination stimuli.

affect: Emotion or feelings conveyed in a person's face or body; the subjective experiencing of a feeling or emotion.

affection stage: Third stage in group development. The focus of this stage is on how group members feel about one another. *Synonym*: stage of group cohesiveness.

affective disorder: Marked disturbances of mood; typically characterized by disproportionately elevated mood (mania), extremely depressed mood (depression), or swings between the two (bipolar disorder/manic depressive disorder).

affective state: The emotional or mental state of an individual, which can range from unconscious to very agitated; sometimes referred to as behavioral state.

afferent: Conducting toward a structure.

afferent neuron: A nerve cell that sends nerve impulses from sensory receptors to the central nervous system.

Affordable Insurance Exchange: A new transparent, competitive insurance marketplace in which individuals and small businesses can purchase affordable and qualified health benefit plans.

Afolter technique: Treatment technique using nonverbal hand-over-hand guiding to facilitate cognitive perceptual development. Looking at the relationship between tactile kinesthetic input and problem solving skills.

age-appropriate activities: Activities and materials that are consistent with those used by nondisabled age mates in the same culture.

age-integrated housing: Communities that are for people of all ages.

ageism: Prejudice that one age is better than another.

age-segregated housing: Communities specifically for older adults.

age stratification model: Influential model in human development based on society's behavioral expectations, as expressed through age-specific statuses and roles to which societal participants are expected to conform.

agglutination: Act of blood cells clumping together.

aging: Passage of years in a person's life; the process of growing older.

aging in place: Where older adults remain in their own homes, retirement housing, or other familiar surroundings as they grow old.

agnosia: Inability to comprehend sensory information due to central nervous system damage.

agonist: Muscle that is capable of providing the power so a bone can move.

agoraphobia: An abnormal fear of being in an open space.

agraphia: Inability to write, caused by impairment of central nervous system processing (not by paralysis).

agrarian: A way of life centered on an agricultural economy.

airplane splint: Conforming positioning splint that is applied after skin graft surgery. It stabilizes and maintains the shoulder in approximately 90 degrees of horizontal abduction.

akathisia: Motor restlessness.

akinesia: Inability to initiate movement.

alarm reaction: The body's immediate response to imposed stress.

alcoholism: A chronic disease characterized by an uncontrollable urge to consume alcoholic beverages excessively to the point that it interferes with normal life activities.

aldosterone: A steroid hormone produced by the adrenal cortex glands and the chief regulator of sodium, potassium, and chloride metabolism, thus controlling the body's water and electrolyte balances.

alexia: Condition of being unable to read.

alienation: A state in which through historically created human possibilities a person, community, or society is estranged to an activity or its results or products, the nature in which it lives, other human beings, and to self.

alienist: Early term for psychiatrist.

aligns: Maintains an upright sitting or standing position without evidence of a need to persistently prop during the task performance.[AOTA Framework]

allele: Alternative form of a gene coded for a particular trait.

Allen Cognitive Levels: Six levels of cognitive ability with corresponding expectations for functional capabilities for daily living.

Allen Cognitive Level Test (ACL): Test that screens and assesses individual cognitive levels through the performance of set tasks. Developed by occupational therapist Claudia Allen.

allied health: Broad field of study encompassing diverse health professionals with special training in fields such as occupational therapy, physical therapy, respiratory therapy, speech pathology, and health information services, as well as laboratory, radiology, and dietetic services. It does not include physicians, nurses, dentists, or podiatrists.

allograft: Grafted skin from the same species; could be the skin from a cadaver.

ally: A heterosexual and/or individual whose gender expression matches biological sex who is an advocate and friend to the communities (E. Simpson, PhD, OTR/L, personal communication).

alogia: Inability to speak. *See* aphasia.

alopecia: Absence or loss of hair; baldness.

alpha error (or Type 1 error): When the null hypothesis is rejected, the probability of being wrong or the probability of rejecting it when it should have been accepted.

alternative delivery system (ADS): Generic term for new systems (e.g., managed care) seen as alternatives to traditional fee-for-service indemnity health insurance plans.

alternative keyboard: Matrix of shapes, sizes, and switches that is used to input data into a computer.

alternative therapies: Interventions to provide holistic approaches to the management of diseases and illnesses, such as acupuncture, massage, or nutrition.

altruism: Unselfish concern for the welfare of others.

alveolar: A general term used in anatomical nomenclature to designate a small sac-like dilatation, such as the sockets in the mandible and maxilla in which the roots of the teeth are held or the small outpocketings of the alveolar sacs in the lungs, through whose walls the gaseous exchange takes place.

Alzheimer's disease (AD): Disabling neurological disorder that may be characterized by memory loss; disorientation; paranoia; hallucinations; violent changes of mood; loss of ability to read, write, eat, or walk; and finally dementia. It usually affects people over the age of 65 years and has no known cause or cure.

ambulate: To walk from place to place.

ambulatory care: Care delivered on an outpatient basis.

amenorrhea: Absence of monthly menstruation.

American Journal of Occupational Therapy **(AJOT):** Official journal of the American Occupational Therapy Association. It provides literature on occupational therapy research, education, and practice.

American National Standards Institute (ANSI): Clearinghouse and coordinating body for voluntary standards activity on the national level.

American Occupational Therapy Association (AOTA): The American professional society that represents the field of occupational therapy and those who practice within that field. It monitors the quality of occupational therapy services through determining guidelines for occupational therapy training programs, setting standards for practice, and supporting regulations, legislation, and research. It also publishes several publications, such as the *American Journal of Occupational Therapy*, *OT Week*, *SIS Newsletters*, and *OT Practice*.

American Occupational Therapy Foundation (AOTF): Established in 1965, the AOTF fosters research in the field of occupational therapy.

American Sign Language (ASL): Nonverbal method of communication using the hands and fingers to represent letters, numbers, and concepts (see Appendix 8).

American Society of Hand Therapists (ASHT): Established in 1978, the ASHT is concerned with hand rehabilitation education and research among practitioners in this area. The *Journal of Hand Therapy* is a publication resulting from the work of the ASHT.

Americans with Disabilities Act (1990) (ADA): U.S. federal act that protects persons with disabilities from discrimination in employment, transportation, public accommodations, telecommunications, and activities of state and local government.

amnesia: Dissociative disorder characterized by memory loss during a certain time period or of personal identity.

amniocentesis: A low-risk prenatal diagnostic procedure of collecting amniotic fluid and fetal cells for examination through the use of a needle inserted into the abdomen.

amnion: Innermost membrane enclosing the developing fetus and the fluid in which the fetus is bathed (amniotic fluid).

amphetamines: Group of stimulating drugs that produce heightened levels of energy and, in large doses, nervousness, sleeplessness, and paranoid delusions.

amphiarthrodial joint: A nonsynovial joint; a direct connection of bony surfaces by cartilage, allowing for minimal movement (e.g., the hyaline cartilage connecting the ribs to the sternum).

amputation: Partial or complete removal of a limb; may be congenital or acquired.

amyotrophic lateral sclerosis (ALS): A progressive neurodegenerative disease of the nerve cells located in the brain and spinal cord that control voluntary movement. As motor neurons degenerate, they can no longer send impulses to the muscle fibers that normally result in muscle movement. Early symptoms of ALS often include increasing muscle weakness, especially involving the arms and legs, speech, swallowing, or breathing. Most commonly diagnosed between ages 40 to 70 years. *Synonym*: Lou Gehrig's disease.

anaerobic exercise: Exercise without oxygen; oxygen intake cannot keep up with amount of exercise, so oxygen debt occurs.

anakusis: Total hearing loss; deafness.

analgesic: Drug for reducing pain. Some mild analgesics are nonsteroidal anti-inflammatory drugs (e.g., ibuprofen), and some analgesics are narcotics (e.g., morphine).

analog: Continuous information system (e.g., a clock with dials that move continuously on a continuum, as opposed to a digital clock).

analogue: Contrived situation created in order to elicit specific client behaviors and allow for their observation.

analysis: An examination of the nature of something for the purpose of prediction or comparison.

analysis of covariance (ANCOVA): Controlling the effects of any variable(s) known to correlate with the dependent variable.

analysis of occupational performance: The step in the evaluation process in which the client's assets and problems or potential problems are more specifically identified through assessment tools designed to observe, measure, and inquire about factors that support or hinder occupational performance and in which targeted outcomes are identified.[OTPF 2014]

analysis of variance (or F ratio or ANOVA): Establishing whether a significant difference exists among the means of several samples.

anaphylactic shock: Condition in which the flow of blood throughout the body becomes suddenly inadequate due to dilation of the blood vessels as a result of an allergic reaction.

anaplasia: Reverting of a specialized cell to its primitive or embryonic state. *Synonym*: dedifferentiation.

anastomosis: Surgical formation of a passage between two open vessels.

anatomical position: Standing erect, arms at the sides, with palms facing outward.

anatomic focus: Title of the Splint Classification System category that delineates the major joints or body segments that the splint involves.

anatomy: Area of study concerned with the internal and external structures of the body and how these structures interrelate.

andragogical education: Stresses the unique and challenging needs of a mature learner and provides a more engaging and flexible experience of learning.

andragogy: Art and science of helping adults learn.

androgens: Substances that produce or stimulate the development of male characteristics.

anemia: A condition in which there is a reduction of the number or volume of red blood corpuscles or the total amount of hemoglobin in the bloodstream, resulting in paleness and generalized weakness.

anencephaly: Birth defect that characteristically leaves the child with little or no brain mass.

anesthetic: Drug that reduces or eliminates sensation. These can affect the whole body (e.g., nitrous oxide, a general anesthetic) or a particular part of the body (e.g., lidocaine, a local anesthetic).

aneurysm: Localized dilation of a blood vessel due to a congenital defect or weakness in the vessel wall.

Angelman syndrome (AS): This neurogenetic disorder is characterized by developmental delay, lack of speech, seizures, and walking and balance disorders. AS is often misdiagnosed as cerebral palsy or autism. The disorder occurs in 1 in 15,000 live births, and those individuals with AS will require life-long care (Angelman Syndrome Foundation, 2014).

angina: Chest pain due to insufficient flow of blood to the heart muscle.

angiography: Injection of a radioactive material so that the blood vessels can be visualized.

angioneurotic edema: Edema of an extremity due to any neurosis affecting primarily the blood vessels resulting from a disorder of the vasomotor system, such as angiospasm, angioparesis, or angioparalysis.

anhedonia: Inability to enjoy what is ordinarily pleasurable.

animal-assisted therapy (AAT): A type of therapeutic intervention that utilizes trained animals and handlers to achieve specific physical, social, cognitive, and emotional goals with patients. AAT can be administered in a variety of settings and may be given in a group or individual basis. *Synonym:* pet therapy.

ankylosis: Condition of the joints in which they become stiffened and nonfunctional.

anniversary reaction: Emotional feelings of sadness and loneliness on holidays, birthdays, and on the anniversary of the death of a significant other.

anomaly: Pronounced departure from the norm.

anomia: Loss of ability to name objects or to recognize or recall names; can be receptive or expressive.

anorexia nervosa: Eating disorder characterized by distortion of body image and fear of becoming fat, resulting in the refusal to eat enough to maintain appropriate weight (maintenance of weight 15% below normal for age, height, and body type is indicative of anorexia). Most often occurs in adolescent girls and young women.

anosmia: Loss of sense of smell.

anosognosia: Inability to perceive a deficit, especially paralysis on one side of the body, possibly caused by a lesion in the right parietal lobe of brain.

ANOVA (analysis of variance): Abbreviation for statistical method used in research to compare sample populations.

anoxemia: Absence or deficiency of oxygen in the blood.

anoxia: Absence or deficiency of oxygen in the tissues.

antacid: Drug that neutralizes hydrochloric acid in the stomach.

antagonist: Muscle that resists the action of a prime mover (agonist).

anterior (A, Ant): Toward the front of the body.

anterior cord syndrome: Usually the result of a flexion injury in the cervical region. Temperature and pain sensations are often impaired below the level of the lesion.

anterior fontanel: Region of the head that is found as a membrane-covered portion on the top of the head, generally closing by the time a child reaches 18 months. *Synonym*: the soft spot.

anterior spinothalamic tract: Pathway that conducts impulse related to poorly localized light touch and pressure.

anterolateral: In front and to one side.

anthropometry: Study of people in terms of their physical dimensions.

antianginal: Drug that prevents angina.

antiarrhythmic: Drug that helps restore heart rhythm to a regular cycle.

antibiotic: Chemical substance that has the ability to inhibit or kill foreign organisms in the body.

antibody: A protein belonging to a class of proteins called immunoglobins. A molecule produced by the immune system of the body in response to an antigen and which has the particular property of combining specifically with the antigen that induced its formation. Antibodies are produced by plasma cells to counteract specific antigens (infectious agents, such as viruses and bacteria). The antibodies combine with the antigen they are created to fight, often causing the death of that infectious agent.

anticholinergic drug: Drug that blocks parasympathetic nerve impulses.

anticoagulant: Agent that delays or inhibits blood clotting.

antidepressants: Drugs used for relief of symptoms of depression (e.g., Prozac, Zoloft).

antigen: A substance foreign to the body. An antigen stimulates the formation of antibodies to combat its presence.

anti-inflammatory: Counteracting or suppressing inflammation.

antimicrobial: Designed to destroy or inhibit the growth of bacterial, fungal, or viral organisms.

antineoplastic agents: Substances, procedures, or measures used in treating cancer, administered with the purpose of inhibiting the production of malignant cells.

antioxidant: A substance that slows down the oxidation of hydrocarbon, oils, fats, etc., and helps to check deterioration of tissues.

antisocial personality disorder: Personality disorder resulting in a chronic pattern of disregard for socially acceptable behavior, impulsiveness, irresponsibility, and lack of remorseful feelings. *Synonyms*: sociopathy, psychopathy, or antisocial reaction.

anuria: Absence of urine excretion.

anxiety: Characterized by an overwhelming sense of apprehension; the expectation that something bad is happening or will happen; class of mental disorders characterized by chronic and debilitating anxiety (e.g., generalized anxiety disorder, panic disorder, phobias, and post-traumatic stress disorder).

anxiolytic: Anxiety-reducing drugs formerly called tranquilizers.

aortic aneurysm: Aneurysm of the aorta.

aortic heart disease: A disease affecting the main artery of the body, carrying blood from the left ventricle of the heart to the main arteries of the body.

Apert syndrome: This is a genetic craniofacial/limb anomaly characterized by specific malformations of the skull, midface, hands, and feet. The skull is prematurely fused and cannot grow normally, the midface (i.e., middle of the eye socket to the upper jaw) appears sunken in, and the fingers and toes are fused together (*see* syndactyly). Apert syndrome occurs in approximately 1 per 160,000 to 200,000 live births (Apert International, 2014).

aphakia: Absence of the crystalline lens of the eye.

aphasia: Absence of cognitive language processing ability which results in deficits in speech, writing, or sign communication. Can be receptive, expressive, or both.

aphonia: Inability to produce speech sounds from the larynx.

apnea: Temporary cessation of breathing.

aponeurosis: Fibrous or membranous tissue that connects a muscle to the part that the muscle moves.

appearance-reality distinction: Person's ability to make an inference about underlying reality rather than merely translating perceived appearances into a judgment.

appendicular skeleton: Bones forming the limbs, pectoral girdle, and pelvic girdle of the body.

application: Putting something to use; administering; a form used to make a request.

Applied Behavior Analysis (ABA): A type of behavior analysis used to modify behaviors as part of a learning or treatment process. Based on the traditional theory of behaviorism, analysts focus on the observable relationship of behavior to environmental stimuli. Previously known as behavior modification, ABA is increasingly used with children with autism.

apprenticeship: Learning process in which novices advance their skills and understanding through active participation with a more skilled person.

apraxia: Inability to motor plan, execute purposeful movement, manipulate objects, or use objects appropriately.

apraxia of speech: Disruption of speech motor planning.

aquatherapy: The use of water as a therapeutic measure (e.g., hydrotherapy, whirlpools, pools for exercise).

archetypal places: Settings in the physical environment that support fundamental human functions, including taking shelter, sleeping, mating, grooming, feeding, excreting, storing, establishing territory, playing, routing, meeting, competing, and working.

architectural barrier: Structural impediment to the approach, mobility, and functional use of an interior or exterior environment.

Architectural Barriers Act (1969): U.S. federal legislation that requires accessibility to certain facilities.

areas of occupations: Various kinds of life activities in which people engage, including the following categories: ADL, IADL, rest and sleep, education, work, play, leisure, and social participation.[OTPF 2008]

arm sling: Orthosis used to provide support to the proximal upper extremity.

arousal: Internal state of the individual characterized by increased responsiveness to environmental stimuli.

arrhythmia: Variation from the normal rhythm, especially of the heartbeat.

art: A skilled way of decorating or illustrating.

arterial embolism/thrombosis: The obstruction of an arterial blood vessel by an embolus too large to pass through it or a thrombosis caused by the coagulation and fibrosis of blood at a particular site.

arteriosclerosis: Thickening and hardening of the arteries.

arteriovenous: Designating arteries or veins or arterioles and venules.

arteriovenous fistula: An abnormal passage between the artery and the vein caused by an abscess at the junction of these vessels.

arteriovenous oxygen difference: The difference between the oxygen content of blood in the arterial system and the amount in the mixed venous blood.

arteritis: Inflammation of an artery.

arthritis: Inflammation of the joints, which may be chronic or acute.

arthroclasia: Artificial breaking of an ankylosed joint to provide movement.

arthrography: Injection of dye or air into a joint cavity to image the contours of the joint.

arthrogryposis: Congenital disease in which a child is born with stiff joints and weak muscles.

arthrokinematics: Movement of joint surfaces.

arthroplasty: Surgical replacement; formation or reformation of a joint; surgical reconstruction of a joint.

arthroscopy: Procedure in which visual equipment can be inserted into a joint so that its internal parts can be viewed.

articular cartilage: The tough, elastic tissue that separates the bones in a joint.

articulates: Produces clear, understandable speech.^{AOTA Framework}

articulation: The joining or juncture between two or more bones.

artifact: A purposefully formed object; any object used, modified, or made by humans.

arts and crafts movement: Social philosophy, beginning around 1860, that grew as a reaction to the physically unhealthy and psychologically alienating effects of the growing industrial age. Proponents suggested that people leave their factory jobs and return to work in small villages as independent farmers and crafts people. Founded by William Morris and his Pre-Raphaelite associates.

ASCII (American Standard Code for Information Interchange): Standardized coding scheme that uses numeric values to represent letters, numbers, symbols, etc. ASCII is widely used in coding information for computers (e.g., the letter "A" is "65" in ASCII).

ascribed status: A position in society that one acquires by being born into it.

asks: Requests factual or personal information.^{AOTA Framework}

asociality: Refers to the lack of a strong motivation to engage in social interaction or the preference for solitary activities.

Asperger's syndrome: Severe and sustained impairment in social interaction and development of restricted, repetitive patterns of behavior, interest, and activities.

asphyxia: Condition of insufficient oxygen.

aspirate: To inhale vomitus, mucus, or food into the respiratory tract.

aspiration: Inhaling fluids or substances into the lungs.

assent: Affirmative agreement to participate in research.

assertiveness: Behavior aimed at claiming rights without denying the rights of others.

asserts: Directly expresses desires, refusals, and requests.[AOTA Framework]

assessing readiness: An interactive process involving the practitioner, consumer, and significant others that focuses on developing an understanding of the consumer's confidence and motivation to actively participate in choosing and/or preparing to function in a valued community role.[C]

assessment: Process by which data are gathered, hypotheses are formulated, and decisions are made for further action; a subsection of the problem-oriented medical record.

Assessment of Living Skills and Resources (ALSR): Combines more complex daily living activities, called instrumental activities of daily living, with available resources in order to determine the client's level of risk.

Assessment of Motor and Process Skills (AMPS): Performance-based evaluation, assessing complex activities of daily living tasks and their underlying motor and organizational components.

Assessment of Older People's Self-Maintenance and Instrumental Activities of Daily Living: Assessment containing a physical self-maintenance scale and an instrumental activities of daily living scale. Used with older adults to gather information.

assessments: "Specific tools or instruments that are used during the evaluation process" (AOTA, 2010, p. S107).[OTPF 2014]

asset approach: A research approach in which the researcher assumes that all individuals have dignity and worth and that they do everything for the most meaningful reason possible.

assimilation: Expansion of data within a given category or subcategory of a schema by incorporation of new information within the existing representational structure without requiring any reorganization or modification of prior knowledge.

assisted living facility: Medium- to large-sized facilities that offer housing, meals, and personal care, plus extras such as housekeeping, transportation, and recreation. Small-sized facilities are known as board and care homes.

assistive devices: A variety of implements or equipment used to aid patients/clients in performing tasks or movements. Assistive devices include crutches, canes, walkers, wheelchairs, power devices, long-handled reachers, and static and dynamic splints.

assistive equipment: Any object or tool that maximizes a person's independence in activities of daily living; assistive devices.

assistive technology (AT): Any item, piece of equipment, or product system, whether acquired commercially off the shelf, modified, or customized, that is used to increase, maintain, or improve functional capabilities of individuals with disabilities.

assistive technology services: Any service that assists an individual with a disability in the selection, acquisition, or use of an assistive technology device.

associated movements: Synchronous muscle or muscle group movements, not necessary for the function initiated.

associated reactions: Involuntary movements or reflexive increase of tone of the affected side of a person with hemiplegia or other central nervous system involvement.

association learning: Form of learning in which particular items or ideas are connected.

associative intrusions: Inappropriate associations that interfere with normal thought processes.

associative network theory of memory: Theory that related memories are stored in networks and that the stimulation of a network will result in the recall of the memories in that network.

associative play: Play in which each child is participating in a separate activity but with the cooperation and assistance of the others.

assumption: Proposition or supposition; a statement that links or relates two or more concepts to one another.

astereognosis: Inability to discriminate shape, texture, weight, and size of objects.

asthma: Respiratory disease in which the muscles of the bronchial tubes tighten and give off excessive secretions. This combination causes obstruction of the airway and results in wheezing; characterized by recurring episodes.

asymmetrical: Lack of symmetry.

asymptomatic: Showing or causing no symptoms.

asynchronous: Occurring at predetermined or regular intervals. The term is usually used to describe communications in which data can be transmitted intermittently rather than in a steady stream.

asynergia: Lack of coordination among muscle groups; movements are jerky and uncoordinated; common in cerebellar diseases.

ataxia: Inability to coordinate movement. Poor balance and awkward movement, especially related to gait.

atelectasis: Collapse or airless condition of the lung.

atherosclerosis: Deposits of fatty substance in arteries, veins, and the lymphatic system.

athetosis: Type of cerebral palsy that involves involuntary purposeless movements that fall into one of two classes—nontension involves contorted movements and tension involves blocked movements and flailing. Slow, involuntary, worm-like, twisting motion.

atomistic societies: Societies such as many in the West that are based on individualism, external connections, causal and reductionistic explanations, rule orientation, and artificial frameworks.

atonic: Absence of muscle tone.

atopic dermatitis: A clinical hypersensitivity of the skin.

atrioventricular block: Disruption in the flow of electrical impulse through the atrium wall of the heart leading to arrhythmias, bradycardiac, or complete cardiac arrest.

atrophy: Decrease in size of a normally developed organ or tissue due to a lack of use or deficient nutrition.

atropine: Drug that inhibits the actions of the autonomic nervous system, relaxes smooth muscle, is used to treat biliary and renal colic, and reduces secretions of the bronchial tubes, salivary glands, stomach, and intestines.

attachment: Deep affective bond between individuals or a feeling that binds one to a thing, cause, ideal, etc.

attendant care: Services that provide individuals with nonmedical, personal health and hygiene care, such as preparing meals, bathing, going to the bathroom, getting in and out of bed, and walking.

attends: Maintains focused attention throughout the task such that the client is not distracted away from the task by extraneous auditory or visual stimuli.[AOTA Framework]

attention: Ability to focus on a specific stimulus without distraction.

attention deficit disorder (ADD): Characterized by an inability to focus attention and impulsiveness; often diagnosed in children.

attention deficit hyperactivity disorder (ADHD): Characterized by an inability to focus attention, impulsiveness, and hyperactivity; often diagnosed in children.

attention span: Focusing on a task over time.[UTIII]

attitude: The position or posture assumed by the body in connection with an action, feeling, or mood. One's disposition, opinion, or mental set.

attitude-centered: An approach to teaching cultural competence focused on valuing of all cultures.

auditory: Interpreting and localizing sounds, and discriminating background sounds[UTIII]; pertaining to the sense or organs of hearing.

auditory defensiveness: Oversensitivity to certain sounds (e.g., vacuum cleaners, fire alarms).

augmentative communication: Method or device that increases a person's ability to communicate (e.g., nonelectronic devices, such as communication boards, or electronic devices, such as portable communication systems, that allow the user to speak and print text).

aura: Subjective sensation preceding a paroxysmal attack; a subtly pervasive quality or atmosphere seen as coming from a person, place, or thing; often described as a glow or flash of light. Known to be a precursor for some people that warns them of impending seizures or migraines.

auscultation: Process of listening for sounds within the body as a method of diagnosis. A stethoscope or other instruments may be used.

Australopithecus: A genus of fossil primates that lived 1 to 5 million years ago in Southern and Eastern Africa, coexisting for some of this time with early forms of humans (*see Homo*). They walked erect and had teeth resembling those of modern humans, but the brain capacity was less than half that of modern *Homo sapiens*.

authoritarian style: Main assumption of this style is that goals are quotas for the people who work to achieve them.

autism: Autism is a complex developmental disability that typically appears during the first 3 years of life and affects a person's ability to communicate, read facial expressions, and interact with others. Autism is defined by a certain set of behaviors, including repetitive actions, self-stimulation (e.g., rocking, hand flapping, spinning), avoidance of eye contact, and echoalia. Autism is a spectrum disorder that affects individuals differently and to varying degrees.

autistic spectrum disorders (ASDs): ASDs are a group of developmental disabilities that can cause significant social, communication, and behavioral challenges. ASDs affect individuals differently, and the spectrum includes those who are severely affected and experience great difficulty in communicating and building relationships to those with more mild forms, such as Asperger's, who mainly have difficulty with obsessive interests and social situations.

autocosmic play: Idea developed by Erikson in which a child plays with his or her own body during the first year of life.

autogeneic facilitation: Ability to stimulate one's own muscle to contract.

autogeneic inhibition: Ability to inhibit action in one's own muscle.

autograft: Grafted skin taken from an unburned area of the same individual.

autoimmunity: Condition in which the body has developed a sensitivity to some of its own tissues.

automatic processes: Processes that occur without much attentional effort.

automatization: When a learned motor skill is performed with little conscious thought.

autonomic dysreflexia: A life-threatening phenomenon that occurs in persons with spinal cord injuries above T4 to T6 level. It is caused by a response from the autonomic nervous system to stimulus such as fecal mass, distended bladder, pain, or thermal stimuli. *See* dysreflexia.

autonomic nervous system (ANS): Part of the nervous system concerned with the control of involuntary bodily functions.

autonomy: State of independence and self-control.

autosomal dominant: Genetic trait carried on the autosome. A disorder appears when one of a pair of chromosomes contains the abnormal gene. Children born to an affected parent have a 50% chance of having the disorder.

autosomal recessive: Genetic trait carried on the autosome. Both asymptomatic parents must carry the trait for a disorder to appear.

autosome: Any chromosome other than the X and Y (sex) chromosomes.

avocational: Leisure pursuits.

avoidance: Psychological coping strategy whereby the source of stress is ignored or avoided.

avoidance learning: Form of learning through stimuli avoidance and cause and effect (e.g., negative reinforcement).

avoidant personality disorder: A personality disorder characterized by hypersensitivity to rejection, low self-esteem, and social discomfort.

avolition: Absence of interest or will to undertake activities.

Award of Excellence: Highest award bestowed on certified occupational therapy assistants by the American Occupational Therapy Association; recognizes the contributions of certified occupational therapy assistants to the advancement of occupational therapy.

awareness: Being conscious of something; informed.

axial skeleton: Bones forming the longitudinal axis of the body; consists of skull, vertebral column, thorax, and sternum.

axilla: Area located dorsal to the humerus and glenohumeral joint. It is the site where the cords of the brachial plexus pass through in order to innervate the muscles of the arm, superficial back, and superficial thoracic region.

axiology: Branch of philosophy concerned with the study of values related to ethics, aesthetics, or religion.

axis: A line, real or imaginary, running through the center of the body; the line about which a part revolves.

axon: Long part of a nerve cell that sends information away from the cell, across a synapse, to the dendrites of another cell.

axonotmesis: Interruption of the axon with subsequent Wallerian degeneration; connective tissues of the nerve, including the Schwann cell basement membrane, remain intact.

azotemia: Presence of nitrogenous bodies, especially urea, in the blood.

Babinski's reflex: Reflex in which touching the sole of the foot results in the big toe pointing up and the toes spreading out; normal in newborns, but abnormal in children and adults.

Baby Boom generation: People born between the years of 1946 and 1964.

back injury: Injury to or diseases of the lower lumbar, lumbosacral, or sacroiliac region of the back.

balance: Ability to maintain a functional posture through motor actions that distribute weight evenly around the body's center of gravity.

balanced bill: The portion of a health care provider's charge exceeding the Medicare-approved amount, which is billed to the client.

balanced muscle tone: Muscle tone that is satisfactory for normal movement.

balance of power: Complementary functions of brain regions that result in well-modulated behavioral responses to environmental stimuli.

ballistic stretch: Repeated rhythmic movements at the outer limits of range of motion.

Baltimore Therapeutic Equipment (BTE) work simulator: Computerized equipment used to simulate various tasks developed by BTE.

banded scissors: Scissors that open with the help of a spring connecting the two handles.

barbiturate: Sedative that can cause both physiological and psychological dependence. *Trade/Generic names*: Seconal/secobarbital, Nembutal/pentobarbital.

Jacobs, K., & Simon, L. (Eds.). *Quick Reference Dictionary for Occupational Therapy, Sixth Edition* (pp. 28-38).
© 2015 SLACK Incorporated.

barrier: Something immaterial that impedes or obstructs.

barriers: The physical impediments that keep patients/clients from functioning optimally in their surroundings, including safety hazards (e.g., throw rugs, slippery surfaces), access problems (e.g., narrow doors, high steps), and home or office design difficulties (e.g., excessive distance to negotiate, multistory environment).

Barthel Self-Care Index: Moderately sensitive screening assessment used mainly in geriatrics. Includes 10 self-care tasks and a 1- to 10-point scale for each.

basal ganglia: A collection of nuclei at the base of the cortex, including the caudate nucleus, putamen, globus pallidus, and functionally includes the substantia nigra and subthalamic nucleus.

baseline: Known value or quantity representing the normal background level against which a response to intervention can be measured.

base of support (BOS): The body surfaces, such as the plantar surface of the feet, around which the center of gravity is maintained via postural responses.

basic activities of daily living (BADL): Activities of daily living tasks that pertain to self-care, mobility, and communication.

basic anxiety: Feelings of insecurity and helplessness due to the indifference displayed by a child's parents.

basic support services: Focus on maintaining or gaining the things required for survival.[C]

bathing/showering: Obtaining and using supplies; soaping, rinsing, and drying body parts; maintaining bathing position; and transferring to and from bathing positions.[AOTA Framework]

battery: Assessment approach or instrument with several parts.

Bay Area Functional Performance Evaluation (BaFPE): Standardized test designed to evaluate how a client may function in task-oriented and social interactional settings. Used to evaluate adults and adolescents who have brain injuries or developmental disabilities.

Bayley Scales of Infant Development (BSID-II): Mental, motor, and behavioral evaluation of a child's development in relation to other children of the same age. Often not preferred by occupational therapists who work in pediatrics because it neglects quality of movement, improvement in children who change slowly, and measurement of functional skills.

behavioral assessment: Systematic and quantitative method for observing and assessing behaviors.

behavioral/cognitive continuum: Balance of the influences of cognition (thoughts and understanding) and observable behavior on development. Part of the Cognitive/Behavior theory.

Behavioral Inattention Test (BIT): Assessment used to determine negligence in areas representing activities of daily living. Subsets include eating a meal, dialing a phone, reading a menu, telling time, setting a clock, sorting coins, copying an address, and following a map.

behavioral modification: Process of reinforcing desirable responses; food, praise, and tokens may be used.

behavioral setting: Milieu in which the specific environment dictates the kinds of behaviors that occur there independent of the particular individuals who inhabit the setting at the moment.

behavioral theory: Developmental theory suggesting that learning is a relationship between certain stimuli and their subsequent responses. This learning theory regards the individual as a result of present and past environments. Behaviorists believe that learning occurs through the processes of classical or operant conditioning.

behaviorism: Theory of behavior and intervention that holds that behavior is learned, that behaviors that are reinforced tend to recur, and that behaviors that are not reinforced tend to disappear.

being in becoming orientation: A value orientation found in some cultures that emphasizes activities that have the goal of developing the self.

being orientation: A value orientation found in some cultures in which the preference is for the kind of activity that is a spontaneous expression of the individual human's essence.

belief: Any cognitive content held as true by the client (Moyers & Dale, 2007).OTPF 2008

Bell's palsy: Facial paralysis due to a functional disorder of the seventh cranial nerve.

belly: Bulging part of a muscle between its two ends.

benchmark: Standard against which something else is judged.

Bender Visual-Motor Gestalt Test: Perceptual motor test developed by Bender that consists of geometric shapes.

bends: Actively flexes, rotates, or twists the trunk in a manner and direction appropriate to the task.[AOTA Framework]

beneficence: Concern of doing good for others.

benefit: Sum of money that an insurance policy pays for covered services under the terms of the policy.

benefit period: Time during which an insurance policy provides payments for covered benefits.

benefits: Anticipates and prevents undesirable circumstances or problems from recurring or persisting.[AOTA Framework]

Benton neuropsychological assessment: Includes a series of 12 neuropsychological tests designed specifically for screening for and specifying the nature of central nervous system damage.

Benzedrine: Amphetamine or stimulant. *Generic name*: amphetamine sulfate.

benzodiazepines: Group of pharmacologically active compounds used as minor tranquilizers and hypnotics.

bereavement: Normal grief or depression commonly associated with the death of a loved one.

best practice: Making and executing professional decisions and actions based on knowledge and evidence that reflect the newest, most innovative ideas available (Dunn, 2000a).

beta-blocker: Drug that blocks the action of epinephrine at sites on receptors of heart muscle cells, the muscle lining of blood vessels, and bronchial tubes.

beta error (or Type 2 error): When the null hypothesis is accepted, the probability of being wrong or the probability of accepting it when it should have been rejected.

biaxial joint: Movement occurs in two planes along two axes, allowing for two degrees of freedom (e.g., metacarpophalangeal joint of the index finger).

bicultural: Reflecting characteristics of two primary cultures.

bigender: A person whose gender identity encompasses both male and female genders. Some may feel that one identity is stronger, but both are present (Substance Abuse and Mental Health Services Administration, 2014).

bilateral integration: Ability to perform purposeful movement that requires interaction between both sides of the body in a smooth and refined manner.

bilingual: Used to describe a person who speaks two languages fluently.

bill mark-up: Process in which a legislative committee in the United States amends a bill by deleting, modifying, or adding to the bill according to the wishes of lobbyists, the public, or their own inclinations.

binocular: Pertaining to both eyes.

bioenergetic group: Therapeutic group that uses movement to express feelings.

bioethics: Application of ethics to health care.

biofeedback: Training program designed to enhance control of the autonomic (involuntary) nervous system by monitoring biological signals or responses and feeding them back to the individual in expanded signals.

biological age: Definition of age that focuses on the functional age of biological and physiological processes rather than on calendar time.

biology: The science of life and living things.

biomechanical approach: This approach concerns cardiopulmonary, integumentary, musculoskeletal, and nervous (except brain) system impairments. The goals of the biomechanical approach are increased endurance, joint range of motion, and strength and reduced edema.

biomechanics: Study of anatomy, physiology, and physics as applied to the human body.

biomedical model: A view of illness that holds that disease always has a definable (usually organic) cause and that medical treatment is the preferred intervention.

biopsychological assessment: Evaluation used to determine how the central nervous system influences behavior and to understand the relationship between the physical state and thoughts, emotions, and behavior.

biorhythm: Biological or cyclical occurrence or phenomenon (e.g., sleep cycle, menstrual cycle, or respiratory cycle).

biotope: The smallest subdivision of a habitat, characterized by a high degree of uniformity in its environmental conditions, plants, and animal life.

biperiden: Drug with effects similar to atropine that is used in the treatment of parkinsonism and certain forms of spasticity and to control the muscular incoordination that may result from the use of some tranquilizers. *Trade name:* Akineton.

bipolar disorder: A mood disorder marked by periods of mania alternating with longer periods of major depression.

bitemporal hemianopsia: Visual deficit of the temporal field (outside half) of both eyes.

bite reflex: Swift biting pathological reflex action produced by oral stimulation.

blepharorrhaphy: Suturing of an eyelid.

blindness: An inability to see.

blog: Self-published website that can focus on any subject matter and is often written as a journal or a first-person account. Blogs often use tags or categories to link subject matter and allow for easy referencing and usually allow comments from readers.

blogosphere: A word that describes the entire universe of blogs and conversations that happen within those websites.

blood-borne pathogen: Infectious disease spread by contact with blood (e.g., HIV, hepatitis B).

bloodless surgery: A surgical approach characterized by various procedures used to minimize blood loss, thereby reducing the need for transfusion.

blood pressure (BP): Pressure of the blood against the walls of the blood vessels. Normal in young adults is 120 mm Hg during systole and 70 mm Hg diastole.

Blue Cross/Blue Shield (BC/BS) Association: A nationwide federation of local, nonprofit insurance organizations that contract with hospitals and other health care providers to make payments for health care services to their subscribers.

boarding homes or board and care homes: Smaller sized housing for older adults that offer supervised housing, meals, and personal care, plus housekeeping, transportation, and recreational activities.

Bobath method: A neurodevelopmental approach used primarily with patients/clients with cerebral palsy but also applicable to dealing with patients who have had a stroke, using involuntary responses to movement of the head and body (e.g., postural reflexes and equilibrium reactions) for purposes of modifying muscle tone or eliciting desired movements. The utilization of associated reactions is avoided; such movements are hypothesized to hamper progress beyond the stage in which reflexes and reactions dominate toward performance of normal, discrete voluntary movements. Supplemental proprioceptive stimuli (muscle stretch and "tapping") are used to facilitate and direct the individual's emerging responses to the head, neck, and body movement stimuli that elicit equilibrium reactions.

body composition: Refers to the fat and nonfat elements of the body or to the relative leanness/fatness of the individual.

body functions: "Physiological functions of body systems (including psychological functions)" (WHO, 2001, p. 10).[OTPF 2014]

body image: Subjective picture people have of their physical appearance.

body mechanics (bm): The interrelationships of the muscles and joints as they maintain or adjust posture in response to environmental forces.

body righting reflex: Neuromuscular response aimed at restoring the body to its normal upright position when it is displaced.

body scheme: Acquiring an internal awareness of the body and the relationship of body parts to each other; perception of one's physical self through proprioceptive and interoceptive sensations.[UTIII]

body structures: "Anatomical parts of the body, such as organs, limbs, and their components" that support body functions (WHO, 2001, p. 10).[OTPF 2014]

boiler plates: Set paragraphs of narrative information available to modify and use repeatedly in letters or other manuscripts.

bolsters: Soft therapeutic equipment that provides support under a child's axilla when in the prone position.

bonding: The crucial attachment that develops between a mother, father, and their new baby after delivery.

bone grafts: Transplantation of bone.

bone marrow: Tissue filling the porous medullary cavity of the diaphysis of bones; site where blood formation occurs.

bone scan: Radiographic scan that evaluates skeletal involvement related to connective tissue disease.

bony prominence: Area where bone is close to the skin surface.

bookmarking: Saving the address of a website or item of content in a browser or app or on a social bookmarking site.

borborygmus: Rumbling and gurgling sound made by the movement of gas in the intestines.

borderline personality: Disorder characterized by abrupt shifts in mood; lack of coherent sense of self; and unpredictable, impulsive behavior.

botulism: Fatal toxemia caused by ingestion of botulinum neurotoxin, which causes muscle weakness and paralysis.

boutonniere deformity: Abnormality that results from interruption of the ulnar and median nerves at the wrist; it causes metacarpophalangeal joint hyperextension and interphalangeal joint flexion.

bowel and bladder management: Includes completing intentional control of bowel movements and urinary bladder and, if necessary, using equipment or agents for bladder control (Uniform Data System for Medical Rehabilitation, 1996, pp. III–20, III–24).[OTPF 2008]

brachial plexus: Network of nerves that originates as roots C5-C8 and T1, and terminates as nerves that innervate the upper extremity.

bradycardia: Slowness of heartbeat (e.g., less than 60 beats/minute).

bradykinesia: Slowness of body movement and speech.

Braille: Standardized system for communicating in writing with persons who are blind. Grade-II Braille is standard literary Braille.

brain death: Irreversible destruction of the cortex and brainstem. Ways to determine are lack of responsiveness, apnea, absence of reflexes, dilation of pupils, flatline electroencephalogram, and absence of cerebral blood flow for a given period of time.

brain impairment: Any loss or abnormality of brain structure or function.

brain lateralization: Refers to the differentiation of function with the brain's two hemispheres. The left hemisphere controls the right side of the body, as well as spoken and written language, numerical and scientific skills, and reasoning. The right hemisphere controls the left side of the body and influences musical and artistic awareness, space and pattern perception, insight, imagination, and generating mental images to compare spatial relationships.

brain scan: Nuclear medicine diagnostic procedure used to detect tumors, cerebrovascular accidents, or other lesions in the brain.

brain tumor (BT): Abnormal growth of cells within the cranium that may cause headaches, altered consciousness, seizures, vomiting, visual problems, cranial nerve abnormalities, personality changes, dementia, and sensory and motor deficits.

Brazleton Neonatal Assessment Scale: Scale that assesses the neurological condition of neonates, including reflexes, muscle tone, responsiveness to objects and people, motor capacities, and ability to control behavior and attention.

break-even point: The point, in any business, at which the volume of sales or revenues exactly equals total expenses—the point at which there is neither a profit nor loss. The break-even point tells the manager what level of output or activity is required before the firm can make a profit; reflects the relationship between costs, volume, and profits.Small Business Administration

break test: Form of muscle testing in which the therapist produces force against a muscle that is isometrically contracted at its greatest mechanical advantage. This test is used to determine the strength of that muscle.

Broca's area: Part of the human cerebral cortex involved in speech production. It is situated in the left frontal lobe and named after Paul Broca, a French surgeon.

bromides: Drugs administered to those with major motor and myoclonic seizures. They will cause drowsiness, mental dullness, toxic psychosis, and rashes. They are better tolerated by children.

bronchopneumonia: Inflammation of the bronchi accompanied by inflamed patches in the nearby lobules of the lungs. *Synonym*: bronchiolitis.

bronchopulmonary dysplasia: A disordered growth or faulty development of bronchial and lung tissue.

Brown-Séquard's syndrome: One side of the spinal cord is damaged. On the same side as the lesion, paralysis and deficits in kinesthesia and proprioception below the level of the lesion are observed. Contralateral to the lesion, there is a loss of temperature and pain sensation below the lesion.

browser: A computer program used to view websites and access Internet content. Well-known browsers include Chrome, Firefox, Internet Explorer, and Safari.

Bruininks-Oseretsky Test of Motor Proficiency (BOTMP): Norm-referenced test that measures gross and fine motor functioning in children ages 4½ to 14½.

bruit: Soft blowing sound heard upon auscultation.

Brunnstrom: Occupational therapy treatment approach based on the use of limb synergies and other available movement patterns in activities of daily living. Classified in six stages of recovery from hemiplegia.

bruxism: Grinding of teeth.

budget: Total amount of money allocated for a certain purpose.

budget neutrality: Provision of the Omnibus Budget Reconciliation Act of 1989, the legislation creating the Medicare Resource-Based Relative Value System payment system, that requires that expenditures resulting from changes in medical practice or payment methodology neither increase nor decrease from what they would have been under a continuation of the customary, prevailing, and reasonable charge system.

bulimia: Eating disorder that most often occurs in adolescent girls and young women, characterized by excessive eating binges followed by purging in the form of self-induced vomiting.

bulletin board: Online forum or website used for discussion, information seeking, networking, and collaboration between users.

burn: A lesion caused by the contact of heat; "tissue injury resulting from excessive exposure to thermal, chemical, electrical, or radioactive agents" (Thomas & Craven, 1997, p. 385).

burn hand splint: Splint used to prevent stress of the ligaments at the interphalangeal joints, to reduce edema, and to prevent burn claw deformity after a severe burn.

burnout: State of mental fatigue that results in the inability to generate energy from one's occupational performance areas.

bursa: Sac that contains synovial fluid. Bursae are located in superficial fascia, in areas where movement takes place, and aid in decreasing friction.

bursectomy: Excision of bursae.

bursitis: Inflammation of a bursa resulting from injury, infection, or rheumatoid synovitis. It produces pain and tenderness and may restrict movement at a nearby joint.

business plan: A comprehensive planning document which clearly describes the business developmental objective of an existing or proposed business. The plan outlines what, how, and from where the resources needed to accomplish the objective will be obtained and utilized.Small Business Administration

buttonhook: Small object attached to a cuff that is used to pull a button through the buttonhole.

byte: Unit of information in computer programming equal to one character.

C-Diff: *See Clostridium difficile.*

calcification: The deposition of calcium salts in body tissues. A calcified substance or structure.

calcium-channel blocker: Drug that blocks the entrance of calcium into the heart muscle and muscle lining of blood vessels; used in the treatment of hypertension, angina, and supraventricular tachycardia.

calendrical rituals: Rituals based on annual events, such as changes of season, commemoration of specific events, etc.

calibrates: Regulates or grades the force, speed, and extent of movement when interacting with task objects (e.g., not too much or too little).[AOTA Framework]

calibration: Determination of what the output of a measuring instrument means and then compared with known values.

callosities: Hardened, thickened places on the skin.

Calvinism: Christian doctrine as interpreted by John Calvin (1509-1564), a French-born Swiss Protestant church reformer and theologian. Its central doctrine is predestination.

Canadian Model of Client-Centred Enablement (CMCE): A visual metaphor for client-centred enablement, through occupation, illustrating occupational therapy's core competency in key and related enablement skills in a client-professional relationship (E. Townsend, H. Polatajko, G. Whiteford, J. Craik, & J. Davis, personal communication, July–December, 2006).[CAOT]

Canadian Model of Occupational Performance and Engagement (CMOP-E): An extension of the 1997/2002 conceptual framework that describes occupational therapy's view of the dynamic, interwoven relationship between persons, environment, and occupation; engagement signals occupational therapy interests

Jacobs, K., & Simon, L. (Eds.). *Quick Reference Dictionary for Occupational Therapy, Sixth Edition* (pp. 39-73). © 2015 SLACK Incorporated.

that include and extend beyond occupational performance over a person's lifespan (H. Polatajko, E. Townsend, & J. Craik, personal communication, July–December, 2006).CAOT

Canadian Occupational Performance Measure (COPM): Four-step process assessment tool used to determine a person's perception of his or her ability to satisfactorily perform meaningful daily activities.

Canadian Practice Process Framework (CPPF) (2007): A generic, occupational therapy framework that portrays the process of occupational enablement with clients from individuals to populations (J. Craik, J. Davis, H. Polatajko, & E. Townsend, personal communication, July–December, 2006).CAOT

cancer (Ca): Any malignant cellular tumor.

candidiasis: Infection by fungi of the genus *Candida*, most commonly involving the skin, oral mucosa, respiratory tract, and vagina.

cane: Stick or short staff used to assist one during walking; can have a narrow or broad base depending on the amount of support needed.

capacitance: Elastic capacity of vessels and organs of the body.

capacities: Innate and sometimes undeveloped potential, aptitude, ability, talent, trait, or power of individuals for anything in particular.

capacity: One's best, includes present abilities as well as potential to develop new abilities.

capacity for surprise: The ability to notice and accept that one's own interpretation is not the only one available.

capital: Assets less liabilities, representing the ownership interest in a business; a stock of accumulated goods, especially at a specified time and in contrast to income received during a specified time period; accumulated goods devoted to the production of goods; accumulated possessions calculated to bring income. Small Business Administration

capital expenses: Business spending on additional plant equipment and inventory.Small Business Administration

capitalized property: Personal property of the agency, which has an average dollar value of $300.00 or more and a life expectancy of one year or more. Capitalized property shall be depreciated annually over the expected useful life to the agency.^{Small Business Administration}

capitation: Method of payment for health services in which a provider receives a fixed, prepaid, per capita amount for each person enrolled in the health plan for whom the provider has responsibility for all necessary health care services.

capsular restriction: Limitation of mobility and range due to tightness or rigidity of the joint capsule.

carbamazepine: Anticonvulsant drug used in the treatment of epilepsy and to relieve the pain of trigeminal neuralgia. Common side effects include drowsiness, dizziness, and muscular incoordination; abnormalities of liver and bone marrow may occur with long-term treatment. *Trade name*: Tegretol.

carboxyhemoglobin: A compound formed from hemoglobin on exposure to carbon monoxide, with formation of a covalent bond with oxygen and without change of the charge of the ferrous state.

carbuncle: A painful bacterial infection deep beneath the skin having a network of pus-filled boils.

carcinogen: Any substance or agent that produces or increases the incidence of cancer.

carcinoma: A malignant new growth made of epithelial cells giving rise to metastases.

card holder: Plastic container with a slim opening and thin, wide base to allow a person to hold a handful of playing cards with a looser grip.

cardiac arrest: Cessation of effective heart action.

cardiac arrhythmia: Irregularity in the rhythm of the heartbeat.

cardiac contusion: Bruising of the heart due to direct trauma or injury to the myocardium.

cardiac output: Volume of blood pumped from the heart per unit of time. Cardiac output is the product of heart rate and stroke volume.

cardiac tamponade: Acute compression of the heart due to effusion of the fluid into the pericardium or the collection of blood in the pericardium from rupture of the heart or a coronary vessel.

cardiomyopathy: A subacute or chronic disorder of heart muscle of unknown or obscure etiology, often with associated endocardial, and sometimes with pericardial involvement, but not atherosclerotic in origin.

cardiopulmonary: Pertaining to the heart and lungs.

cardiorrhaphy: Suture of the heart muscle.

cardiotonic: Drug that promotes the force and efficiency of the heart.

cardiovascular (CV): Pertaining to heart and blood vessels.

cardiovascular insufficiency: Inability of the cardiovascular system to perform at a level necessary for basic homeostasis of the body.

cardiovascular pump: Structures responsible for maintaining cardiac output, including the cardiac muscle, valves, arterial smooth muscle, and venous smooth muscle.

cardiovascular pump dysfunction: Abnormalities of the cardiac muscles, valves, conduction, or circulation that interrupt or interfere with cardiac output or circulation.

card sort: Approach to gathering information that requires the person being evaluated to consider information contained on separate index cards, and to separate or sort the cards according to a specific set of instructions.

career breakpoint: A time of significant change in one's professional life.

caregiver: One who provides care and support to another person.

caregiver burnout: A state of physical, emotional, and mental exhaustion that may be accompanied by a change in attitude (from positive to negative). Burnout can occur when caregivers do not receive the help they need or if they try to do more than they are able to do, either physically or financially. Caregivers who are "burned out" may experience fatigue, stress, anxiety, and depression. Many caregivers also feel guilty if they spend time on themselves rather than on their ill or elderly loved ones.

caregiver stress syndrome (CSS): A syndrome seen in caregivers involving pathological, morbid changes in physiological and psychological function. This syndrome can be the result of acute or chronic stress directly as a result of caregiving activities.

care of others (including selecting and supervising caregivers): Arranging, supervising, or providing the care for others.^{AOTA Framework}

care of pets: Arranging, supervising, or providing the care for pets and service animals.^{AOTA Framework}

CARF: Commission on Accreditation of Rehabilitation Facilities.

carotid endarterectomy: Excision of the thickened, atheromatous tunica intima of the carotid artery.

carpals: Bones of the wrist; there are eight carpal bones in each wrist.

carpal tunnel syndrome: Compression of the median nerve as it enters the palm of the hand through the space between the carpal bones in the wrist (carpal tunnel). Common symptoms include pain and numbness in the index and middle fingers and weakness of the abductor muscle of the thumb.

carrier (Medicare): Private contractor to Health Care Financing Administration that administers claims processing and payment for Medicare B services.

Cartesian dualism: Separation of mind and soul from body and brain. The former can exist without the latter and withstand its corruption and death (term based on the work of René Descartes, *see* Descartian).

cascade effect: Ability of the blood to clot via multiple factors.

cascade system: Theoretical prototype used as a conceptual framework for providing educational services for children with disabilities. Children are placed into the class that best fits their needs and is as close as possible to an everyday classroom.

case conceptualization: A model or theory about a particular health situation based on the individual's assumptions, knowledge, and information gathered about the situation.

case history: Complete medical, family, social, and psychiatric history of a client up to time of admission.

case management: Uses a legally mandated case manager to oversee the coordination of services for a client. This manager, whose roles may include helper, teacher, planner, and advocate, assists in facilitating the needs of a client and his or her family.

case management services: Focus on negotiating for services that are needed and wanted.[C]

case manager: Individual who assumes responsibility for coordination and follow-up on a given client case.

cash flow: An accounting presentation showing how much of the cash generated by the business remains after both expenses (including interest) and principal repayment on financing are paid. A projected cash flow statement indicates whether the business will have cash to pay its expenses and loans and make a profit. Cash flows can be calculated for any given period of time and are normally done on a monthly basis.[Small Business Administration]

cataplexy: Sudden episodes of loss of muscle function.

cataract: Abnormal progressive condition of the lens of the eye characterized by loss of transparency.

catastrophic health insurance: A type of health insurance that provides protection against the high cost of treating severe or lengthy illnesses or disabilities.

catatonia: Motor abnormality usually characterized by immobility or rigidity, in which no organic base has been identified.

catecholamines: Active proteins epinephrine and norepinephrine.

categorization: Identifying similarities of and differences among pieces of environmental information[UTIII]; ability to classify; to describe by naming or labeling.

cathartic: Drug that relieves constipation and promotes defecation for diagnostic and operative procedures.

cauda equina: Spinal nerves descending in the spinal column below the level of L2.

caudal: Away from the head or toward the lower part of a structure.

causalgia: Painful, burning sensation often associated with reflex sympathetic dystrophy.

cause and effect: When something occurs as a result of a motion or activity.

celiac disease: An autoimmune illness of the small intestine that affects the digestive system when food containing gluten is ingested. The body's immune response causes inflammation in the small intestine, damaging the lining and reducing the intestine's ability to absorb dietary nutrients. Symptoms caused by nutritional, vitamin, and mineral deficiencies, including malnourishment, can occur.

cellulitis: An inflammation of connective tissue, especially subcutaneous tissue.

center of gravity: Point at which the downward force created by mass and gravity is equivalent or balanced on either side of a fulcrum.

center vision: The central part of what one sees when looking straight at an object.

central cord syndrome: Usually the result of a hyperextension injury in the cervical region. Because the cervical tracts for the upper extremities are more centrally located, the upper extremities are more severely involved.

central nervous system (CNS): Consists of all the neurons of the brain, brainstem, and spinal cord.

central tendency (measure of): The typical, middle, or central scores in a distribution.

centrifugal control: Brain's ability to regulate its own input.

centrifuge: Separates components of blood for further testing through high speed, rotational movement.

cephalad: Toward the head or upper portion of a part or structure. *Synonym*: superior.

cephalocaudal pattern: Sequence in which the greatest growth always occurs at the top (the head) with physical growth in size, weight, and feature differentiation, gradually working its way down from top to bottom.

cerebellar ataxia: Disorder of the brain that results in total or partial inability to coordinate voluntary bodily movements, as in walking.

cerebellar degeneration: Deterioration or loss of function or structure of brain tissue.

cerebral angioplasty: Injection of dye into the cerebrovascular system to observe its function.

cerebral atrophy: Deterioration of the cerebral tissue.

cerebral contusion: Bruising of brain tissue.

cerebral cyst: A sac-like structure filled with fluid or diseased matter in the tissue of the brain.

cerebral degeneration: Deterioration or loss of function or structure in the cerebral region of the brain.

cerebral embolism: The obstruction of a blood vessel by an embolus in the brain.

cerebral laceration: Torn or mangled cerebral tissue.

cerebral palsy (CP): Group of motor disorders resulting in muscular incoordination and loss of muscle control; caused by damage to the motor area of the brain during fetal life, birth, and infancy.

cerebrovascular accident (CVA): Diseases that result from changes in the blood vessels supplying the brain; may be characterized by hemiplegia, sensory dysfunction, aphasia and dysarthria, visual field defects, and mental and intellectual impairment. *Synonym*: stroke.

cerebrovascular insufficiency: A lack of oxygen in the brain due to restriction or blockage of cerebral vessels.

certification: Process developed to ensure that each practitioner has the knowledge, skills, and attitudes required for competent professional practice.

certified hand therapist (CHT): Individual who has been certified by the Hand Therapy Certification Commission to practice in the area of hand rehabilitation.

cervicalgia: Any disorder causing pain in the cervical region.

cervical spondylosis: Dissolution of the cervical vertebrae.

cervical vertebrae: Seven small neck bones between the skull and thoracic vertebrae that support the head and allow movement.

CHAMPUS (Civilian Health and Medical Program of the Uniformed Services): Program paid for by the Department of Defense that pays for care that civilian health providers deliver to retired members and dependents of active and retired military personnel. This program does not charge premiums but has cost-sharing provisions.

change: To take a different position, course, or direction (Merriam-Webster, 2003), or to experience a process of transition or transformation to a new, altered, or different state (Answers. com; Jonsson, in press) in order to maintain opportunities, to prevent losses, or to promote and develop opportunities (CAOT, 1991). CAOT

change of use: Varying the use of a building from private use to one that is open to and used by the public.

characteristic behavior: Behavior typical of one's performance under everyday conditions.

charge-off: An accounting transaction removing an uncollectible balance from the active receivable accounts.Small Business Administration

charged-off loan: An uncollectible loan for which the principal and accrued interest were removed from the receivable accounts.Small Business Administration

checklist: Type of assessment approach whereby a list of abilities, tasks, or interests is presented and those items meeting a designated criterion are checked. For example, an interest checklist might list a number of activities in varied categories and ask the respondent to check those that are viewed as most interesting.

chemotherapy: The use of drugs or pharmacologic agents that have a specific and toxic effect on a disease-causing pathogen.

chest pain: Angina resulting from ischemia of the heart tissue.

Cheyne-Stokes respiration: Breathing characterized by a fluctuation in the depth of breathing.

chickenpox: An acute communicable disease caused by a virus and marked by slight fever and an eruption of macular vesicles, which appears as a rash.

child abuse: Intentional physical or psychological injury inflicted upon children by caretaker(s).

child development play programs: Hospital play programs that include curricula ordinarily found in preschool or elementary school classrooms for children who have a long-term hospital stay.

Child Find: State organization for identifying children at risk for disabling conditions.

childhood disintegrative disorder: Marked regression in multiple areas of functioning following a period of at least 2 years of apparently normal development. Onset of disorder takes place before age 10 years. Loss of previously acquired skills in at least two of the following areas: expressive or receptive language, social skills or adaptive behavior, bowel or bladder control, play, or motor skills.

child neglect: Inadequate social, emotional, or physical nurturing of children.

child rearing: Providing the care and supervision to support the developmental needs of a child.[AOTA Framework]

chi-square (χ²): A statistical test used to establish whether frequency differences have occurred on the basis of chance.

chlorpromazine hydrochloride: Major tranquilizer and sedative used to treat anxiety, tension, and agitation and to control nausea and vomiting. It is used to enhance the effects of analgesics, especially in terminal illness, and in preparation for anesthesia. Common side effects are drowsiness and dry mouth. *Trade names*: Chloractil, Largactil.

cholecystectomy: Removal of the gallbladder.

choledocholithotomy: Incision into the bile duct for removal of gallstones.

cholestasis: Suppression or arrest of bile flow.

chondrocyte: Cartilage cell embedded in lacunae within the matrix of cartilage connective tissue.

chondromalacia: Softening of the articular cartilage.

chooses: Selects appropriate and necessary tools and materials for the task, including choosing the tools and materials that were specified for use prior to the initiation of the task.[AOTA Framework]

choosing valued role: Psychiatric rehabilitation program that focuses on providing opportunities and assistance that enable the consumer to make informed choices about the roles in which he/she wants to function.[C]

chorea: Abrupt irregular movements of short duration involving the fingers, hands, arms, face, tongue, or head.

choreoathetosis: Type of cerebral palsy characterized by uncontrollable, jerky, irregular twisting movements of the arms and legs.

chromosome: Thread-like structure made up of genes; there are 46 chromosomes in the nucleus of each human cell.

chronic bronchitis: Chronic inflammation of the bronchial tubes. A long-continued form, often with a more or less marked tendency to recurrence after stages of quiescence. Diagnosis is made when a chronic cough for up to 3 months in 2 consecutive years is present.

chronic disorders: Characterized by slow onset and long duration; rarely develop in early adulthood, increase in middle adulthood, and become common in late adulthood.

chronic obstructive lung disease (COLD): Family of age-related lung diseases that block the passage of air and cause abnormalities inside the lungs.

chronic obstructive pulmonary disease: "A disease process that decreases the ability of the lungs to perform ventilation. Diagnostic criteria include a history of persistent dyspnea on exertion, with or without chronic cough, and less than half of normal predicted maximum breathing capacity" (Thomas & Craven, 1997, p. 385).

chronic pain: A subjective response to distress that cannot be quantitatively measured, lasting 6 or more months and 3 to 4 weeks after "normal" healing should have occurred (Hansen & Atchison, 2000).

chronic renal failure: Progressive destruction of nephrons, leading to possible stoppage of kidney functions.

chronic respiratory disease: Lung disease resulting from constrictive or obstructive conditions of the airways.

chronological: Individual's age[UTIII]; definition of age that relies on the amount of calendar time that has passed since birth.

chronotropic: Affecting the time or rate, applied especially to nerves whose stimulation or agents whose administration affects the rate of contraction of the heart.

chylothorax: The presence of effused chyle (pockets of milky fluid) in the thoracic cavity.

cicatrix: Scar; the fibrous tissue replacing the normal tissue destroyed by injury or disease.

CINAHL (Cumulative Index to Nursing and Allied Health Literature): Provides access to virtually all major English-language nursing journal publications from the American Nursing Association and the National League for Nursing, and primary journals from 13 allied health professions, including occupational therapy.

circulation: Movement in a regular or circuitous course, as the movement of blood through the heart and blood vessels.

circumduction: Movement in which the distal end of a bone moves in a circle while the proximal end remains stable, acting like a pivot.

circumferential-pressure splints: Splint in which there is no middle reciprocal force present; forces involved in this type of splint are equally distributed on the opposing surfaces involved.

Civilian Industrial Rehabilitation Act (1920): First U.S. federal legislation to help occupational therapy. It commissioned federal aid for vocational rehabilitation for those disabled by accident or illness in industry.

claim: Request to an insurer for payment of benefits under an insurance policy.

claim adjudication: Determination of payment on a claim based on type of contract, type of coverage, and present use.

clang associations: Associations based on a rhyme. The result is often the intrusion of a new thought; occurs frequently in bipolar disorder.

class: Group containing members who share certain attributes, such as economic status, social identifications, or cultural identity.

class I lever system: Lever system in which the fulcrum is between the force and the resistance (e.g., seesaw). The mechanical advantage can be less than, more than, or equal to one.

class II lever system: Lever system in which the resistance is between the fulcrum and the force. The mechanical advantage is always greater than one.

class III lever system: Lever system in which the force is between the fulcrum and the resistance. The mechanical advantage is always less than one.

classical conditioning: Method of eliciting specific responses through the use of stimuli that occur within a period of time that permits an association to be made between them. *Also known as* Pavlovian conditioning, after the Russian scientist who made the technique famous.

classification: Arrangement according to some systematic division into classes or groups.

Classification of Jobs According to Worker Trait Factors (COJ): Lists the worker trait factors (e.g., environmental conditions, aptitudes) for those job titles listed in the *Dictionary of Occupational Titles* (DOT). Used in conjunction with the DOT.

claudication: Lameness, limping; usually caused by poor circulation of blood to the leg muscles.

clavicle: Bone that acts as a brace to hold the upper arm free from the thorax to allow free movement and serves as a place for muscle attachment. *Synonym*: collarbone.

cleaning: Obtaining and using supplies; picking up; putting away; vacuuming; sweeping and mopping floors; dusting; polishing; scrubbing; washing windows; cleaning mirrors; making beds; and removing trash and recyclables.[UTIII]

clear floor space: Minimum unobstructed floor or ground space required to accommodate a single, stationary wheelchair and occupant.

client: Person or persons (including those involved in the care of a client), group (collective of individuals, e.g., families, workers, students, or community members), or population (collective of groups or individuals living in a similar locale—e.g., city, state, or country—or sharing the same or like concerns).[OTPF 2014]

client-centered approach: An orientation that honors the desires and priorities of clients in designing and implementing interventions (adapted from Dunn, 2000a, p. 4).[AOTA Framework]

client-centered care (client-centered practice): Approach to service that incorporates respect for and partnership with clients as active participants in the therapy process. This approach emphasizes clients' knowledge and experience, strengths, capacity for choice, and overall autonomy (Boyt Schell et al., 2014a, p. 1230).[OTPF 2014]

client-centered rehabilitation: Therapeutic orientation in which the therapist guides and supports the client in problem solving and goal achievement.

client-centred enablement: Based on enablement foundations and employs enablement skills in a collaborative relationship with clients who may be individuals, families, groups, communities, organizations, populations to advance a vision of health, well-being, and justice through occupation.[CAOT]

client factors: Specific capacities, characteristics, or beliefs that reside within the person and that influence performance in occupations. Client factors include values, beliefs, and spirituality; body functions; and body structures.[OTPF 2014]

client participation: An active concept characterized by involvement and engagement and is driven in part by biological needs to act, find meaning, and connect with others through doing (Wilcock, 2006).[CAOT]

clients: In occupational therapy, may be individuals, families, groups, communities, organizations, or populations who participate in occupational therapy services by direct referral or contract or by other service and funding arrangements with a team, group, or agency that includes occupational therapy.[CAOT]

client satisfaction: The client's affective response to his or her perceptions of the process and benefits of receiving occupational therapy services (adapted from Maciejewski, Kawiecki, & Rockwood, 1997, pp. 67-89).[AOTA Framework]

climacteric: Major turning point in a woman's life from ability to reproduce to a state of nonreproductivity. Transitional phase of life leading to menopause.

clinical dementia rating: Staging instrument that categorizes the level of the disease experienced by the patient.

clinical guidelines: Systematically developed statements to assist practitioner and patient decisions about appropriate health care for specific clinical circumstances (e.g., *Guide to Physical Therapist Practice*).

clinical reasoning: "Process used by practitioners to plan, direct, perform, and reflect on client care" (Boyt Schell et al., 2014a, p. 1231). The term *professional reasoning* is sometimes used and is considered to be a broader term.[OTPF 2014] Thinking that directs and guides clinical decision making; reflective thinking.

clinical utility: Factors such as clarity of instruction, cost, and facileness in using the assessment to determine the amount of the assessment's utility.

clonus: Spasmodic alternation of contraction and relaxation of muscles.

closed-chain movements: The distal end of a kinematic chain is fixed or stabilized, and the proximal end (origin) moves (e.g., push-ups).

closed question: Question that asks for a specific response (e.g., one that may be answered with a "yes" or "no").

closed reduction: Situation in which a broken bone can be manipulated into its natural position without major surgery.

close-packed position: The point in a joint's range of motion where maximal stability exists due to the stretch placed on periarticular structures.

close supervision: Contact that is daily, direct, and given on the work premises.

Clostridium difficile: A species of bacteria of the genus *Clostridium* that causes diarrhea and other intestinal disease. Often occurs when competing healthy bacteria are wiped out by antibiotics. In severely affected patients, the inner lining of the colon becomes severely inflamed with the potential to perforate. *Synonym:* C-Diff.

clothing care: Obtaining and using supplies; sorting; laundering (hand, machine, and dry clean); folding; ironing; storing; and mending.[UTIII]

clubbing: A proliferative change in the soft tissues about the terminal phalanges of the fingers or toes with no osseous changes.

clubfoot: Birth defect in which the soles of the feet face medially and the toes point inferiorly; occurs in approximately 1 of 1,000 births and may be caused genetically or by the folding of the foot up against the chest during fetal development. *Synonym:* talipes.

clubhand: Medical condition seen in children in which the hand is radically displaced; the radius bone may be partially formed or may be absent.

cluster trait sample: Assesses a number of traits inherent in a job or various jobs, such as dexterity, strength, endurance, range of motion, and speed.

coach: A key occupational therapy enablement skill to develop and sustain ". . .an ongoing partnership designed to help clients produce fulfilling results in their personal and professional lives, improve their performance and enhance their quality of life" (International Coach Federation, 2006). In *Profile of Occupational Therapy Practice in Canada* (CAOT, in press), coaching is related to the competency roles of communicator and collaborator.[CAOT]

coagulation: The process of blood clot formation.

coagulopathy: A pathological defect in coagulation of the blood.

cocaine: Classified as a narcotic in 1914, cocaine is an alkaloid from the shrub *Erythroxylum coca*. The main pharmacological effect is the blocking of re-uptake of serotonin and the catecholamine neurotransmitters, particularly dopamine.

cochlear implants: Tiny transmitters implanted near the cochlea of a person with a hearing impairment to stimulate transmission of sound from the environment to the brain.

cocontraction: Simultaneous contraction of antagonistic muscle groups, which act to stabilize joints.

codeine: Narcotic derived from the opium family that is highly addictive.

code of ethics: Statement that a certain group follows; sets the guidelines so that a high standard of behavior is maintained.

codependence: Condition in which substance dependence is subtly supported by the codependent, who meets some need through the continued dependence of the individual.

Codman exercises: The use of gravity to facilitate relaxation and movement of the shoulder joint. With the trunk flexed at the waist and the arm hanging straight down and relaxed, pendulum-type movements in all planes are performed.

coefficient of contingency (C): A statistical test used on nominal data to determine correlation.

coefficient of determination (r^2): Determining what proportion of information about y is contained in x.

coercion: Constrain into obedience.

cognition: Mental processes that include thinking, perceiving, feeling, recognizing, remembering, problem solving, knowing, sensing, learning, judging, and metacognition.

cognitive appraisal: That part of the coping process during which one evaluates a stressor and chooses a strategy for dealing with it.

cognitive-behavioral framework: Focuses on how thought and information processing can become distorted and lead to maladaptive emotions and behavior.

cognitive complexity: Features of an environment that affect its information-processing demands, such as variety, familiarity, pace, complexity, and responsiveness potential of stimuli.

cognitive development: Process of thinking and knowing in the broadest sense, including perception, memory, and judgment.

cognitive disability: Physiologic or biochemical impairment in information-processing capacities, which produces observable and measurable limitations in routine task behavior.

cognitive disorder: A mental disorder characterized by significant loss of mental functioning, such as delirium or dementia.

cognitive domains: Levels of performance abilities delineated in a hierarchy related to knowing and understanding.

cognitive integration and cognitive components: The ability to use higher brain functions.[UTIII]

cognitive learning: Form of learning that encompasses the forming of mental plans of events and objects.

cognitive restructuring: Strategy for treating abnormal behavior in which the goal is to alter behavior by changing the way a person thinks about factors related to the behavior.

cognitive set: Predisposition to notice or interpret things in a specific way. Negative cognitive sets are associated with depression.

cognitive skills: Actions or behaviors a client uses to plan and manage the performance of an activity.[OTPF 2008]

cognitive stages in development: Jean Piaget's theory proposing that children's biological development is related to their environment, which enables children to progress through discrete, age-related stages in forming cognition.

cognitive theory: Theory that focuses on intelligence, reasoning, learning, problem solving, memory, information processing, and thinking as the tools that individuals use to understand environmental stimuli.

cognitive therapy: Approach to intervention that holds that emotional disturbance is the result of faulty belief systems.

cogwheel rigidity: During passive range of motion, a series of catches in the resistance.

cohesiveness: Growth of interpersonal harmony and intimacy within a group.

cohort effects: Effects due to an individual's time of birth or generation but not to his or her actual age.

coinsurance: Component of a health insurance plan that requires the insurer and client each to pay a percentage of covered costs.

co-leaders: Group members who assist the group leader in physical and emotional management of a group.

collaborate: Arguably the key enablement skill that involves power-sharing (Schaeffer, 2002) to work with clients versus doing things to or for them in a joint intellectual effort or toward a common end (Answers.com) by sharing talents and abilities in mutual respect with genuine interest, acknowledgement of others, empathy, altruism, trust, and creative communication to achieve results that are greater than the sum of individual efforts (Linden, 2003), with awareness that professions operate hierarchically in a top-down manner based on the priority given to professional expertise over client experience (Freidson, 1970, 1986, 1994, 2001). In *Profile of Occupational Therapy Practice in Canada* (CAOT, in press), collaborate is directly mirrored in the competency role of collaborator.[CAOT]

collaborates: Coordinates action with others toward a common end goal.[AOTA Framework]

collaborative approach: Orientation in which the occupational therapy practitioner and client work in the spirit of egalitarianism and mutual participation. Collaboration involves encouraging clients to describe their therapeutic concerns, identify their own goals, and contribute to decisions regarding therapeutic interventions (Boyt Schell et al., 2014a).^{OTPF 2014}

collapse in caregiving: A phrase that is used for the institutionalization of a client with dementia.

collateral: Something of value—securities, evidence of deposit or other property—pledged to support the repayment of an obligation.^{Small Business Administration}

collaterality: Social relationship structure defined by laterality.

collective variable: Fewest number of dimensions that describe a unit of behavior.

collectivist: Focused on group goals.

Colles' wrist fracture: Transverse fracture of the distal end of the radius (just above the wrist).

colloid osmotic pressure: The pressure exerted by substances capable of influencing osmosis of water across membranes.

color agnosia: Inability to recognize colors.

coma: Abnormally deep unconsciousness with the absence of voluntary response to stimuli.

combat exhaustion: Temporary neurotic or psychotic reactions to combat or war conditions due to the stress factors encountered in these environments.

coming out: To declare and affirm, both to oneself and to others, one's identity as lesbian, gay, bisexual, transgender, queer, etc. It is not just one event but rather a life-long process (International Spectrum, 2014).

Commission on Education (COE): Major commission of the American Occupational Therapy Association responsible for exploring ideas and sharing information regarding the improvement of occupational therapy teaching methods and curriculum.

commitment: Degree of importance attached to an event by an individual, based on his or her beliefs and values. The degree of commitment is an important element in motivation.

commitment procedures: Legal process by which persons are institutionalized.

communication: To impart information through verbal and non-verbal interactions. The act of transmitting thoughts or ideas. Giving or exchanging of information, signals, or messages by talk, gestures, or writing. A system of sending or receiving messages.

communication and social skills: Actions or behaviors a person uses to communicate and interact with others in an interactive environment (Fisher, 2006).^{OTPF 2008}

communication device use: Using equipment or systems such as writing equipment, telephones, typewriters, computers, communication boards, call lights, emergency systems, Braille writers, telecommunication devices for the deaf, and augmentative communication systems to send and receive information. ^{AOTA Framework}

communication management: Sending, receiving, and interpreting information using a variety of systems and equipment, including writing tools, telephones, typewriters, audiovisual recorders, computers, communication boards, call lights, emergency systems, Braille writers, telecommunication devices for the deaf, augmentative communication systems, and personal digital assistants.^{OTPF 2008}

communitarian: System in which the good of the group is dominant over the good of individuals.

community-based rehabilitation (CBR): Rehabilitation implemented through the combined efforts of people with disabilities, their families, and communities and the appropriate health, education, vocational, and social services.

community building: The process of recruiting participants to create or join a community or network that is based on shared interests and goals.

community development: Community consultation, deliberation, and action to promote individual, family, and community responsibility for self-sustaining development and well-being.

community forum: A needs assessment technique that invites residents/members of the target population to discuss their concerns at open "town hall"–type meetings.

community hospitals: Small health care facilities, usually with inpatient and other kinds of care, located within the community they serve and focused on direct care for relatively uncomplicated conditions.

Community Mental Health Act (1963): Under this act, the National Institute of Mental Health was mandated to establish community mental health centers as part of a national movement to take more responsibility for individuals with mental illness.

community mental health movement: During the 1960s, government, medical, and community organizations supported treatment approaches that would keep patients living in the community rather than confined in long-term hospitals.

community mobility: Moving oneself in the community and using public or private transportation, such as driving or accessing buses, taxicabs, or other public transportation systems.^{AOTA Framework}

community re-entry: Simulated or actual activities used to prepare a client for discharge into the public community.

community rehabilitation programs: Structured daily social alternatives, including daily, evening, and weekend programs; prevocational and vocational skills development; and leisure programs. They provide supported employment, work adjustment, and job placement.

comorbidity: Characterized by the presence of symptoms of more than one ailment (e.g., depression and anxiety).

compact fracture: Condition in which a broken bone pierces the skin so that it can be viewed.

compensatory action of the nervous system: Action that occurs when the central nervous system attempts to respond to stimuli without the usual full complement of information.

competence: Achievement of skill equal to the demands of the environment; also a legal term referring to the soundness of one's mind.

competent occupational therapist: Competent is the word that reflects the minimal and ongoing performance expectation of practitioners. In *Profile of Occupational Therapy Practice* *in Canada* (CAOT, in press), the performance expectations reflect the requisite knowledge, skills, and abilities to meet performance expectations throughout their career (i.e., newly registered and lifelong practice).[CAOT]

competition: Rivalry for objects, resources, facilities, or position in an organization.

complex society: A society that includes a large number of cultures.

compliance: Subservient behavior that implies following orders or directions without self-direction or choice. Also related to respiratory mechanics with change in respiratory volume over pressure gradient. Refers to the elasticity and expandability of the lungs.

components: Fundamental units; in relation to activities refers to processes, tools, materials, and purposefulness.

components of occupational performance: The affective, cognitive, and physical performance of individuals (CAOT, 1997a, 2002).[CAOT]

comprehensive battery: Battery of tests that measure different components of cognitive, perceptual, and motor functioning.

comprehensive child life play program: Intervention that allows children and their parents to use play as a means of anxiety reduction, emotional expression, and social and cognitive development during a child's prolonged hospital stay.

Comprehensive Evaluation of Basic Living Skills (CEBLS): Designed to assess the basic living skills of persons with chronic psychiatric illness through direct observation of performance and nursing report of basic self-care status. Personal care, higher level activities of daily living, and reading and writing are evaluated on a four-point rating scale.

Comprehensive Occupational Therapy Evaluation (COTE): Evaluation used in an acute care psychiatric setting for a single observation or a series of observations of a client performing a task; lists 25 behaviors and provides a rating scale for them.

compulsion: A repetitive, distressing act that is performed to relieve obsession-related fear.

computer-assisted tomography (CAT): Scanning procedure that combines x-rays with computer technology to show cross-sectional views of internal body structures.

computerized assessment: An assessment that includes the administration, scoring, and interpretation of test results done by a sophisticated computer program.

conative hypothesis: Theory that autistic children choose not to play and interact with other children rather than their being unintellectual.

concave/convex rule: If a concave joint surface moves on a convex surface, then the gliding movement is in the same direction. If a convex joint surface moves on a concave surface, then the movement occurs in the opposite direction.

concentration: Ability to maintain attention for longer periods of time in order to keep thoughts directed toward completing a given task.

concentric contraction: Muscular contraction during which the muscle fibers shorten in an attempt to overcome resistance.

concept: Mental image, abstract idea, or general notion.

concept formation: Organizing a variety of information to form thoughts and ideas.[UTIII]

concrete-operational stage: Term coined by Jean Piaget to denote development of a group of skills acquired in middle childhood, including decentration, class inclusion, and taking another's perspective. In this stage, such mental operations can only be applied to concrete objects.

concussion injury: Resulting from impact with an object (usually to the brain).

condign power: Power achieved by imposing an alternative to the unpleasant or painful preference of the individual or group so that such preferences are abandoned.

conditioned power: Power exercised by changing the belief of the individual through education or persuasion that causes the individual to submit to the will of others.

conditioning: Learning process that alters behavior through reinforcements or associating a reflex with a particular stimulus to trigger a desired response.

conditioning reasoning: One of three clinical reasoning styles used by occupational therapists.

conduct disorder: A childhood disorder characterized by a failure to conform to social norms, irresponsible behavior, aggression toward people or animals, lying, or theft. This is a common precursor to antisocial personality disorder.

conducting a functional assessment: Developing an understanding of the consumer's functioning in the critical skills needed to be successful and satisfied in his/her overall rehabilitation goal environment.[C]

conducting a resource assessment: Developing an understanding of the critical supports a person needs to be successful and satisfied in his/her environment of choice.[C]

conduction: Conveying energy (e.g., heat, sound, or electricity).

confabulation: Fabrication of facts that the individual cannot remember. The individual is not aware that he or she is fabricating them, and thus is not intentionally lying; often an indication of organically based cognitive disorder.

conference committee: Committee of legislators with one purpose of working out compromises between different versions of a bill.

confidence interval: Range of predicted values where it is presumed, with a stated degree of certainty, that the true limit will fall.

confidentiality: Maintenance of secrecy regarding information confided by a client.

conflict of interest: Situation in which a person may have hidden or other interests that conflict or are inconsistent with providing services to a client or agency.

conforms: Follows implicit and explicit social norms.[AOTA Framework]

congenital: Present or existing at birth.

congenital amputation: Child is born without part or all of a limb or limbs.

congenital anomalies: Structural abnormalities resulting from birth defects or genetic disorders.

congenital defects: Abnormalities or deformations of the skull or vertebrae where there is a failure to enclose the neural structures or a complete absence of different parts of the brain itself.

congregate housing: Housing for unrelated individuals, often older persons, that is usually sponsored by government or nonprofit organizations.

congregate meal site: Place where meals are provided to a group of older persons, located in a central setting, such as a senior center, housing site, or church.

conjunctivitis: Inflammation of the conjunctiva of the eye.

connective tissue: Structural material of the body that connects tissues and links anatomical structures together.

conscious use of self: Use of "planned interactions with another person in order to alleviate fear or anxiety, provide reassurances, obtain necessary information, provide information, give advice, and assist the other individual gain more appreciation, expression, and functional use of his or her latent inner resources" (Mosey, 1996).

consensual validation: Comparing one's personal perceptions with others in a group experience.

consensus: A common center or agreement.

consent: Agree to participate.

conservation: Cognitive skill that requires the realization that a quantity of a substance remains constant regardless of changes in form.

constrictive pericarditis: Inflammation of the pericardium that results in constriction. The pericardium is covered with fibrinous deposits.

construct: Conceptual structure used in science for thinking about the factors underlying observed phenomena.

constructional apraxia: Inability to reproduce geometric designs and figures.

construct validity: In research, the extent to which a test measures the construct (mental representation) variables that it was designed to identify.

consult: A key enablement skill to exchange views and confer (Answers.com) throughout the practice process with a wide range of clients or in management, education, or research, with team members, community support personnel, social agencies, government personnel, business representatives, nongovernmental organizations, consumer groups, special interest groups, and more. In *Profile of Occupational Therapy Practice in Canada* (CAOT, in press), consulting is part of the competency role of expert in enabling occupation.[CAOT]

consultation: Process of assisting a client, an agency, or other provider by identifying and analyzing issues, providing information and advice, and developing strategies for current and future actions.

consumer price index (CPI): Published by the U.S. Department of Labor, a measure of increases in the price of a market basket of goods and services by region of the country.

contacts: Makes physical contact with others.[AOTA Framework]

contact dermatitis: Inflammatory response of the skin due to contact with a toxic or caustic agent (e.g., chemical, poison ivy).

contact oriented approach to reasoning: Where a clinical problem is examined in terms of the problem, definition, and content.

content: Actual words spoken or used within a group.

content management systems (CMS): Software that offers the ability to create static webpages, document stores, blogs, wikis, and other online tools. Once content is developed, it can be uploaded to websites and updated as needed.

context: Variety of interrelated conditions within and surrounding the client that influence performance, including cultural, personal, temporal, and virtual contexts.[OTPF 2014]

contextual factors: The external environmental factors (e.g., social attitudes, architectural characteristics) and internal personal factors (e.g., gender, age) that influence how disability is experienced by a person (WHO, 2001).

contextual modifications: Cues from the therapist, task environment, and/or individual that affect task performance.

continues: Performs actions or action sequences of steps without unnecessary interruption so that once an action sequence is initiated, the individual continues on until the step is completed. [AOTA Framework]

continuing education: Educational programming that provides opportunities for certification or training to improve an individual's knowledge and practices.

continuing professional development: Planning, activities, and requirements to facilitate ongoing growth and development of occupational therapy professionals.

continuity theory of aging: Psychosocial theory of aging that focuses on the integration of the older person's past experiences, inner psyche, and the changes that occur with aging in such a way to preserve the individual's sense of self.

continuous passive motion machine (CPMM): Device used to passively move a joint through the full range of movement available. This device is usually used after joint surgery to prevent range of motion loss.

continuous reading: Reading long passages, such as a book or magazine.

contract: Agreement, usually written, between practitioner and agency that specifies the services to be provided and the responsibilities of each party.

contractual partnership: A formal agreement, promise, or undertaking that is shared jointly (Abate, 1996).

contracture: Static shortening of muscle and connective tissue that limits range of motion at a joint.

contraindication: Condition that deems a particular type of treatment undesirable or improper.

contralateral: Pertaining to, situated on, or affecting the opposite side.

contrast bath: The immersion of an extremity in alternating hot and cold water.

contrecoup injury: Usually more extensive damage on the opposite side of the brain from the point of impact during a strike to the head.

contributory insurance: Type of group insurance in which the employee pays for all or part of the premium, and the employer or union pays the remainder.

control group: Comparison group.

controls: The strategies used in ergonomics to eliminate or diminish the effects of hazards (problems). *Synonym:* abatement. There are three major controls: engineering, administrative, and work practice.

control stage: Second stage of group development; it includes a leadership struggle on a group and individual level.

contusion: Bruising of the brain caused by laceration of small arteries.

convergence: Ability of the brain to respond only after receiving input from multiple sources.

convergent problem solving: Developing one correct solution by the forming of separate pieces of information.

conversion disorder: Disorder characterized by the presence of physical symptoms or deficits that cannot be explained by medical findings.

convulsion: Paroxysms of involuntary muscular contractions and relaxation; spasm.

co-occupations: Occupation that implicitly involves two or more people (Boyt Schell et al., 2014a, p. 1232).[OTPF 2014]

cooperative group: Group in which the task is secondary to social aspects and goals.

cooperative play: Goal set form of play that involves two or more children striving for that goal.

cooptation: An organizational strategy for responding to change.

coordinate: A powerful and under-recognized key enablement skill through which occupational therapists integrate, synthesize and document information, link people with resources, manage teams with students and support personnel, facilitate interaction between government "silos" and otherwise harmonize and orchestrate initiatives by a broad range of stakeholders in a common action or effort (Houghton-Mifflin Company, 2004) in order to develop an accord, combine and adapt in order to attain a particular effect (Answers.com). In *Profile of Occupational Therapy Practice in Canada* (CAOT, in press), coordination is aligned with the leadership competency role to manage practice.[CAOT]

coordinated care: Term the Health Care Financing Administration often used, more or less generically, for managed care plans, particularly if they are gatekeepers.

coordinates: Uses two or more body parts together to stabilize and manipulate task objects during bilateral motor tasks.^AOTA Framework

coordination: Related to using more than one body part to interact with task objects in a manner that supports task performance.^AOTA Framework Property of movement characterized by the smooth and harmonious action of groups of muscles working together to produce a desired motion.

co-payment: Specified amount of money per visit or unit of time that the client pays, while the insurer pays the rest of the claim.

Copernicus, Nicolaus (1473-1543): Polish cleric and astronomer who formulated the heliocentric theory of the solar system. This theory, which replaced the Earth as the center of the universe against all established authorities of his time, caused a complete change of outlook in many spheres, known as the Copernican revolution.

coping: Process through which individuals adjust to the stressful demands of their daily environment.

coping skills: Identifying and managing stress and related factors.^UTIII

copying-fidelity: Reproduction of exact copies.

corporal potentiality: Ability to screen out vestibular and postural information at conscious levels in order to engage the cortex in higher order cognitive tasks.

cor pulmonale: Hypertrophy or failure of the right ventricle.

correlation coefficient: The relationship among two or more variables.

cortically programmed movements: Movements that are based on input from structure in the cortex (motor strip or basal ganglia).

corticorubrospinal pathway: Descending pathway that serves limb control; from the motor cortex through the red nucleus in the brainstem and on to the spinal cord.

corticospinal pathway: Oversees the finely tuned movements of the body by controlling finely tuned movements of the hands; this pathway travels from the motor cortex to the spinal neurons that serve the hand muscles.

cortisone: Hormone produced in the cortex of the adrenal gland that aids in the regulation of the metabolism of fats, carbohydrates, sodium, potassium, and proteins.

cosmesis: A concern in rehabilitation, especially regarding surgical operations or burns, for the appearance of the patient/client.

cost benefit analysis: Process used to evaluate the economic efficiency of new policies and programs by comparing an outcome and the costs required to achieve it.

cost containment: Approach to health care that emphasizes reduced costs.

cost-effective: Equipment that is worthwhile to make considering the therapist's time and materials involved.

cost effectiveness: Extent to which funds spent to improve health and well-being reduce overall cost of care.

cost sharing: Requirement in health insurance plans for the client to pay part of the cost of care.

costs: Money obligated for goods and services received during a given period of time, regardless of when ordered or whether paid for.Small Business Administration

counterculture: Subculture that rejects important values of the dominant society.

countertransference: A set of expectations, beliefs, and emotional responses that the therapist may bring into the therapist-client relationship. It may be an unconscious component based on conflict of which the professional is not aware; this may interfere with the therapist's ability to remain detached and objective.

country-club style: Manager who uses this style feels that attitudes and feelings of people are important, and it is assumed that production requirements are contrary to people's needs.

coup/contrecoup: Refers to points of actual contact made between the brain and the skull encasement in the event of trauma.

coup injury: Brain contusions and lacerations beneath the point of impact when the head is struck.

Cowan stabilizing pillow: An example of an adaptive device that assists a child's balance or stability when sitting.

coxa valgus: The angle of the neck of the femur to the shaft is greater than 120 degrees angled outward.

crackle: Abnormal respiratory sound heard upon listening.

craft: An object usually made by hand using tools and skill.

cranial nerve: Nerve extending from the brain.

cranial-sacral therapy (CST): A form of bodywork or alternative therapy focused primarily on the concept of primary respiration and regulating the flow of cerebrospinal fluid by using therapeutic touch to manipulate the synarthrodial joints of the cranium.

creative activities: Tasks that encourage expression.

credentialing: Process that gives title or approval to a person or program, such as certification, registration, or accreditation.

credit rating: A grade assigned to a business concern to denote the net worth and credit standing to which the concern is entitled in the opinion of the rating agency as a result of its investigation. Small Business Administration

creep: A measure of the deformation in a material as a result of a constant load applied over a specific time interval.

crepitation: Dry, crackling sound or sensation, such as that made by the ends of two bones grating together.

crisis intervention: Therapeutic goal aimed at supporting an individual through the crisis and assisting him or her in coping with the stress that led to the crisis.

crisis intervention services: Focus on resolving or stabilizing critical or dangerous problems, often with sudden onset due to trauma and/or deterioration.[C]

crisis interview: Following an emergency, an interview used to identify crisis problems and immediate interventions.

criterion: Particular standard or level of performance or expected outcome.

criterion-referenced tests: Goal of these tests is to evaluate specific skills or knowledge where the criterion is full mastery of them.

criterion validity: Test that measures and predicts the specific behaviors required to function in, meet the standards of, and be successful in daily life.

critical path: Optimal sequencing and timing of diagnosis or procedure-based intervention.

critical period: Fixed time period very early in development during which certain behaviors optimally emerge.

critical research: A research approach oriented toward advocacy and criticism in order to unmask the ideological roots in self-understanding that constrains equity and supports hegemony and to empower individuals/groups toward greater autonomy, social justice, and emancipation. It is openly ideological, political, and socially analytical.

critical social science: An interpretive critique of society, especially of the theoretical bases of its organization.

cross-addiction: Addiction to a variety of chemical substances.

cross-bridges: Portion of the myosin filaments that pulls the actin filaments during muscle contraction (Thomas & Craven, 1997, p. 462).

cross-cultural: Interaction between or among individuals of different cultural identities.

crossing the midline: Moving limbs and eyes across the midsagittal plane of the body.[UTIII]

cross-linking: Theory that aging is caused by a random interaction among proteins that produce molecules that make the body stiffer.

cross-sectional research: Nonexperimental research sometimes used to gather data on possible growth trends in a population.

cross slope: Slope that is perpendicular to the running slope and the direction of travel.

crowdsourcing: The process of using the skills and enthusiasm of those outside an organization to develop content, raise funds, or solve problems.

cry analysis: Acoustic measurement of an infant's crying in which research has shown those with hypoxic brain damage tend to have abnormal patterns.

cryotherapy (cold): The use of cold as a therapeutic agent. Used for post-traumatic edema and inflammation. It has been found to alter the conduction velocity and synaptic activity of the peripheral nerves, decreasing sensory and motor conduction velocities for the management of pain and muscle spasms. The use of cryotherapy is based on the physiologic responses to a decrease in tissue temperature. Cold decreases blood flow and tissue metabolism, thus decreasing bleeding and acute inflammation. Spasticity and muscle guarding spasms can be diminished, allowing for a greater ease of motion. Pain threshold is elevated, thus allowing exercises to be carried out with increased comfort. Application of cryotherapy can include ice packs, ice massage, ice towels, cold baths, vapocoolant sprays, or controlled cold-compression units.

crystal arthropathies: Diseases of the joints that result in crystallization, such as gout and pseudogout.

c-splint: Splint that maintains the thumb in abduction and partial rotation under the second metacarpal and maintains the first web space.

cue: Subjective and objective data.

cueing: Hints or suggestions that facilitate the appropriate response.

cultural: "Customs, beliefs, activity patterns, behavior standards, and expectations accepted by the society of which the [client] is a member. Includes ethnicity and values as well as political aspects, such as laws that affect access to resources and affirm personal rights. Also includes opportunities for education, employment, and economic support" (AOTA, 1994, p. 1054). OTPF 2008

cultural broker: A person who serves go-between functions at the edges of cultural groups in contact.

cultural competence: The ability to interact and intervene effectively with individuals from a wide array of cultures.

cultural context: Customs, beliefs, activity patterns, behavioral standards, and expectations accepted by the society of which a client is a member. The cultural context influences the client's identity and activity choices. OTPF 2014

cultural desert: A place devoid of culture and cultural events.

cultural development: Describes a child's increasing understanding of the system of meanings and customs shared by some identifiable group or subgroup and transmitted from one generation of that group to the next.

cultural exclusivity: The existence of a single culture in the absence of all others.

cultural interpreter: A person who is a member of the same group as a client but who is somewhat familiar with American health care procedures, systems, and values.

culturally competent: Understanding and attending to the total context of the individual's culture, including awareness of immigration, stress factors, and cultural differences.

culturally inclusive: Allowing for multiple cultural perspectives.

cultural relativism: Recognition that there is no way to compare cultures. A culture has to be looked at relative to itself and therefore cannot be judged as better or worse than another culture.

cultural sensitivity: Having respect for and sensitivity to other cultures.

cultural shift: Movement in response to societal forces that result in dynamic change.

cultural style: Collections of furnishings, objects, and decor with generally accepted cultural connotations of certain lifestyle behavior patterns.

cultural universals: Rules, concepts, and strategies for meeting needs that are found in every human group.

culture: A set of values, beliefs, traditions, norms, and customs that determine or define the behavior of a group of people (Wells, 1994); also "a shared system of meanings that involve ideas, concepts and knowledge and include the beliefs, values and norms that shape standards and rules of behaviour as people go about their everyday lives" (Dyck, 1998, p. 68) in a system of shared meanings and a dynamic process by which "meanings are ascribed to commonly experienced phenomena and objects" (Iwama, 2005, p. 8).[CAOT] Patterns of behavior learned through the socialization process, including anything acquired by humans as members of society (e.g., knowledge, values, beliefs, morals, customs, speech patterns, economics, production patterns). The system of meanings and customs shared by some identifiable group or subgroup and transmitted from one generation of that group to the next (Bottomley, 2003, p. 41).

culture-bound syndromes: Diseases that seem to be specific to a single culture or a group of related cultures.

culture emergent: A perspective on culture that emphasizes the dynamic, nuanced, and contextual nature of culture.

culture-specific expertise: Knowledge of the patterns of behavior learned through the socialization process, including anything acquired by humans as members of society (e.g., knowledge, values, beliefs, laws, morals, customs, speech patterns, economics, production patterns) of particular cultural groups.

cumulative trauma disorder: Musculoskeletal disorder in which chronic discomfort, pain, and functional impairment may develop over time as results of frequent, sustained movements. *Synonym:* repetitive strain injury.

curb cut: Short ramp cutting through a curb.

custom: Habitual practice that is adhered to by members of the same group or geographical region.

cyanosis: Blue discoloration of the skin and mucous membranes due to excessive concentration of reduced hemoglobin in the blood.

cybernetics: The study of communication and control between humans, machines, and organizations. The human ability to adapt and make decisions is imitated in the design of computer-controlled systems. Cybernetics has also been used as a link between the physical and life sciences, for instance in using information theory to explain how messages are transmitted in nervous systems and in genetic processes.

cyberspace: Another term for the Internet.

cyclodialysis: Formation of an opening between the anterior chamber and the suprachoroidal space for draining the aqueous humor.

cyst: Closed sac or pouch with a definite wall that contains fluid, semifluid, or solid material.

cystic fibrosis (CF): Hereditary, chronic, progressive disease characterized by abnormal mucus secretion in the glands of the pancreas and lungs; usually diagnosed early in life due to frequent respiratory infections or failure to thrive.

cytoarchitectonic maps: Maps of the brain in terms of the structure and function of cells.

D

dacryocystorhinostomy: Creation of an opening into the nose for draining of tears.

database: Collection of data organized in information fields in electronic format.

data glove: Gloves containing dual-axis sensors to detect wrist movements.

daytime splint: Splint used during the daytime that must be designed in such a way that it may be removed several times a day so that the client can prevent joint stiffening by moving the joint(s) to the full range of motion.

deaf: Complete or partial loss of the ability to hear.

death rate: Number of deaths occurring within a specific population during a particular time period, usually in terms of 1,000 persons per year.

debility: Weakness or feebleness of the body.

débridement: Removal of dead tissue and foreign matter from a wound.

decentration: Tendency to notice and take into account all or most of the relevant characteristics of an object when making an assessment (as opposed to toddlers' tendency toward centration, in which they attend only to one aspect of an object).

decision making: The process of making decisions (i.e., the choice of certain preferred courses of action over others).

declarative memory: The registration, retention, and recall of past experiences, sensations, ideas, thoughts, and knowledge through the hippocampal nuclear structures or the amygdala, which results in long-term memory.

Jacobs, K., & Simon, L. (Eds.). *Quick Reference Dictionary for Occupational Therapy, Sixth Edition* (pp. 74-89).
© 2015 SLACK Incorporated.

decorticate rigidity: Exaggerated extensor tone of the lower extremities and flexor tone of the upper extremities resulting in abnormal posturing due to damage to the brainstem.

decortication: Removal of portions of the cortical substance of a structure or organ, as of the brain, kidney, lung, etc.

decubitus ulcer: Open sore due to lowered circulation in a body part.

dedifferentiation: *See* anaplasia.

deductible: Amount of loss or expense that an insured or covered individual must incur before an insurer assumes any liability for all or part of the remaining cost of covered services.

deductive reasoning: A serial strategy where conclusions are drawn on the basis of premises that are assumed to be true.

deep venous thrombosis (DVT): A blood clot in the deep venous system of the lower or upper extremity, which can be extremely dangerous if the clot becomes dislodged; it could travel to the lungs and create a pulmonary embolism.

defense mechanisms: Unconscious processes that keep anxiety-producing information out of conscious awareness (e.g., compensation, denial, rationalization, sublimation, and projection).

defibrillation: The stoppage of fibrillation of the heart. The separation of the fibers of a tissue by blunt dissection.

defibrillator: An apparatus used to counteract fibrillation by application of electric impulses to the heart.

defibrination syndrome: A syndrome resulting from a deprival of fibrin.

deficiency: The quality or state of being deficient; absence of something essential; incompleteness; lacking; a shortage.

deficiency disease: A disease caused by a dietary lack of vitamins, minerals, etc., or by an inability to metabolize them.

deficit: Inadequate behavior or task performance.

Deficit Reduction Legislation Acts (1984, 1985, 1986): Extended U.S. federal coverage for health and social services through modification of Medicare legislation.

DeGangi-Berk Test of Sensory Integration: Criteria-referenced test for children 3 to 5 years that assesses gross motor, praxis, reflexes, fine motor, and vestibular.

deglutition: Act of swallowing.

degrees: In reference to the measurement of range of motion, the amount of movement from the beginning to the end of the action.

degrees of freedom: The options or directions available for movement from a given point.

dehydration: Absence of water. Removal of water from the body or a tissue. A condition that results from undue loss of water.

deinstitutionalization: Transfer to a community setting of patients who have been hospitalized for an extended period of time, usually years.

delayed return economies: Time investment in the future is part of daily life.

delay of gratification: Postponement of the satisfaction of one's needs.

delirium: Characterized by confused mental state with changes in attention, hallucinations, delusions, and incoherence.

delirium tremens (DT): Condition caused by acute alcohol withdrawal, characterized by trembling and visual hallucinations; may lead to convulsions.

delusion: Inaccurate, illogical beliefs that remain fixed in one's mind despite having no basis in reality.

delusional disorder: Psychosis characterized by the presence of persistent delusions often involving paranoid themes in an individual whose behavior otherwise appears normal.

dementia: State of deterioration of personality and intellectual abilities, including memory, problem-solving skills, language use, and thinking that interferes with daily functioning.

democratic community activities: Opportunities to participate in the development of the community as a whole.

demography: Scientific study of human populations particularly in relation to size, distribution, and characteristics of group members.

demyelinating disease: Disease that destroys or damages the myelin sheath of the nerves.

demyelination: The destruction of myelin, the "white lipid" covering of the nerve cell axons. The loss of myelin decreases conduction velocity of the neural impulse and destroys the "white matter" of the brain and spinal cord.

dendrite: Short processes found on the end of a nerve cell that send or receive information from another neurotransmitter.

dendritic growth: New evidence indicating growth (rather than the common descriptions of decline) in the brains of the elderly.

Denver Developmental Screening Test Revised (DDST-R): Criteria-referenced screening instrument for children 0 to 6 years that tests personal/social, communication, self-help, gross motor, and fine motor skills.

Department of Health and Human Services (DHHS): Department within the U.S. government that is responsible for administering health and social welfare programs.

dependence: Need to be influenced, nurtured, or controlled; relying on others for support.

dependent (Dep): Person who can be claimed on insurance.

dependent variable: Consequent variable.

depersonalization: Person often feels cut off from or unsure of his or her identity.

depolarization: The process or act of neutralizing polarity, such as in a heartbeat.

depression: Characterized by an overwhelming sense of sadness that may be brought on by an event or series of events but lasts far longer than a reasonable time.

depth perception: Determining the relative distance between objects, figures, or landmarks and the observer and changes in planes or surfaces[UTIII]; ability to determine the relative distance between the self and the objects and figures observed.

derailment: Sudden or gradual deviations in one's train of thought in which ideas change from one subject to another in a completely unrelated manner.

dermatome: Area on the surface of the skin that is served by one spinal segment.

dermatomyositis: Systemic connective tissue disease characterized by inflammatory and degenerative changes in the skin. Leads to symmetric weakness and some atrophy.

Descartian (link with Cartesian dualism): Theory named after René Descartes (1596–1650), French philosopher and mathematician. After a Jesuit education and military service, Descartes settled in Holland. His *Discourse on the Method* (1637) introduced themes that he developed in his greatest work, the *Meditations* (1641). Asking "How and what do I know?" he arrived at his famous statement "Cogito ergo sum" ("I think, therefore I am"). From this he proved to his own satisfaction God's existence (he was a Roman Catholic) and hence the existence of everything else. He believed that the world consisted of two different substances— mind and matter (the doctrine of Cartesian dualism).

descriptive approach: A method for representing a culture through the systematic identification of the particular traits and material goods of the group.

descriptive ethics: Ethics used to describe the moral systems of a culture.

descriptive statistics: An abbreviated description and summarizing of data.

desensitization: To deprive or lessen sensitivity.

design/build: A traditional key occupational therapy enablement skill that encompasses the design and/or building of products, such as assistive technology or orthotics (McKee & Morgan, 1998), designs to adapt the built and/or emotional environment (Clark et al., 2001), and the design and implementation of programs and services (Rebeiro, Day, Semeniuk, O'Brien, & Wilson, 2001) by formulating a plan or strategy (Answers.com) and in some situations actually building the technology, program, or service. In the *Profile of Occupational Therapy Practice in Canada* (CAOT, in press), design/build contributes to the competency role of change agent.[CAOT]

desquamation: Process by which old layers of skin cells (epidermis) are shed.

detectable warning: Standardized surface feature built in or applied to walking surfaces of other elements to give warning of hazards on a circulation path.

detoxification: Process of removing the substance from the person's system; frequently done under the management of a physician.

detrusor muscle: The muscular component of the bladder wall.

developing readiness: Psychiatric rehabilitation program focused on creating learning experiences that, when processed by the consumer, are likely to develop an individual's commitment to participate in rehabilitation services.[C]

developmental: Stage or phase of maturation.[UTIII]

developmental assessment: Evaluation of a child with disorders that should be repeated every 2 months until the child reaches age 2 years.

developmental delay: Wide range of childhood disorders and environmental situations where a child is unable to accomplish the developmental tasks typical of his or her chronological age.

Developmental Disabilities Act Amendments (1984): U.S. federal legislation that ensured that people with developmental disabilities receive necessary services and established a monitoring system.

Developmental Disabilities Services and Facilities Construction Act (1970): U.S. law giving the states broad responsibility for planning and implementing a comprehensive program of services to individuals with developmental delays, epilepsy, cerebral palsy, and other neurological impairments.

developmental disability (DD): Mental or physical impairment, or a combination of the two, that manifests itself before age 22 years and results in limitations.

developmental milestones: Key points or behaviors within our lives that help us to recognize that growth and development have taken place.

developmental skills: Skills that are developed in childhood, such as language or motor skills.

developmentally appropriate practice (DAP): An approach to teaching and working with children. Decisions about curriculum and plans for therapy are made based on knowledge of child development, taking into consideration individual learning differences and social and cultural influences. The goal of DAP is to develop a curriculum that meets the cognitive, emotional, and physical needs of children based on child development theories and observations of children's individual strengths and weaknesses.

deviance: Behavior that is in contrast to acceptable standards within a community or culture.

deviation score: Dissimilarity between a single score and the mean of the distribution.

Dexedrine: Stimulant of the amphetamine family that can cause psychological but not physiological dependence. *Generic name:* dextroamphetamine sulfate.

dexterity: Skill in using the hands or body, usually requiring both fine and gross motor coordination. *Synonym:* agility.

diabetes mellitus (DM): A metabolic disorder in which the pancreas is unable to produce insulin, a substance the body needs to metabolize glucose as an energy source. A chronic, systemic disorder characterized by hyperglycemia (excess glucose in the blood) and disruption of the metabolism of carbohydrates, fats, and proteins. Insufficient insulin is produced in the pancreas, resulting in high blood glucose levels. Over time, DM results in small- and large-vessel vascular complications and neuropathies.

diabetic retinopathy: Complication of diabetes in which small aneurysms form on retinal capillaries.

diagnosis (Dx): Technical identification of a disease or condition by scientific evaluation of history, physical signs, symptoms, laboratory tests, and procedures.

diagnosis-related groups (DRG): Classifications of illnesses and injuries that are used as the basis for prospective payments to hospitals under Medicare and other insurers.

***Diagnostic and Statistical Manual of Mental Disorders* (5th ed.) (DSM-5):** Text that defines and provides a standardized criteria for various mental illnesses; diagnosis, usually made by a psychiatrist, is made along a series of five axes.

diagnostic interview: Interview used by a professional to classify the nature of dysfunction in a person under care.

dialect: Variation of a language; particular to a certain geographical region.

dialysis: "The passage of a solute through a membrane. The process of diffusing blood across a semi-permeable membrane to remove toxic materials and to maintain fluid, electrolyte, and acid-base balance in cases of impaired kidney function or absence of the kidneys" (Thomas & Craven, 1997, p. 531); the process of separating crystalloids and colloids in solution by the difference in their rates of diffusion through a semipermeable membrane; crystalloids pass through readily, colloids very slowly or not at all.

diaphoresis: Perspiration, especially profuse perspiration.

diaphragmatic breathing: The use of the diaphragm to draw air into the bases of the lungs.

diarthrodial joint: A synovial joint; bones are indirectly connected via a joint capsule (e.g., knee, elbow).

diastole: Period of time between contractions of the atria or the ventricles during which blood enters the relaxed chambers from the systemic circulation and lungs; significant in blood pressure readings.

diazepam: Drug with muscle relaxant and anticonvulsant properties used to relieve anxiety and tension and in the treatment of epilepsy and muscular rheumatism. Common side effects are drowsiness and lethargy. *Trade name*: Valium.

***Dictionary of Occupational Titles* (DOT):** Text that provides information about the jobs that exist in the U.S. economy. It has an alphabetized list of all occupational job titles, a brief description of those jobs in the United States, a listing of those job titles arranged by industry, and an analysis of the requirements placed on the worker performing the job.

digital: Discreet form of information (e.g., a clock that displays only digits at given moment, as opposed to analog).

digital citizen: Someone who follows social and moral guidelines in his or her use of technology.

digital immigrant: An individual born before the existence of digital technology and adopted it to some extent later in life.

digitalis: Drug used to stop fibrillation of the heart; it reduces the heart rate and increases the strength of contraction.

digital native: An individual born during or after the general introduction of digital technologies and through interacting with digital technology from an early age has a good understanding of its concepts.

dignity: Importance of valuing the inherent worth and uniqueness of each person.

dilation and curettage (D&C): Widening of the cervical canal with a dilator and scraping the uterine endometrium with a curette.

dimethylglycine (DMG): Controversial substance used in the treatment of autism.

diminutive: Suffix added to a medical term to indicate a smaller size, number, or quantity of that term.

diplegia: Involvement of two extremities.

diplopia: Double vision.

direct selection: Any technique for choosing items that allows a person to point specifically to the desired choice without intermediate steps, generally allowing selections to be made more rapidly. Examples include pointing with a finger, pressing keys on a keyboard, or eye gaze.

direct service: Treatment or other services provided directly to one or more clients by a practitioner.

direct skills teaching: Leading the consumer through a systematic series of instructional activities resulting in the consumer's competent use of new behaviors.[C]

disability: An "umbrella term for impairment of body function or body structure, an activity limitation and/or a participation restriction" (WHO, 2001, p. 193).[CAOT] Any restriction or lack of ability (resulting from an injury) to perform an activity in a manner or within the range considered normal for a human being.

disability behavior: Ways in which people respond to bodily indications and conditions that they come to view as abnormal; how people monitor themselves, define and interpret symptoms, take remedial action, and use sources of help.

Disability Insurance Benefit Program (1956): U.S. federal legislation that provided benefits to qualified workers with disabilities.

disability status: Place in continuum of disability, such as acuteness of injury, chronicity of disability, or terminal nature of illness.[UTIII]

discharge (d/c): The process of discontinuing interventions included in a single episode of care, occurring when the anticipated goals and desired outcomes have been met. Other indicators for discharge include that the patient/client declines to continue care, the patient/client is unable to continue to progress toward goals because of medical or psychosocial complications, or the physical therapist determines that the patient/client will no longer benefit from physical therapy.

discharge documentation: Summary of treatment progress at the discontinuation of services.

discharge planning: To enhance continuity of care, plans are made to prepare the client for moving from one setting to another; usually a multidisciplinary process.

disclosure: In dealing with informed consent, the client has to be informed of what he or she is going to do for a study in which he or she participates.

disc prolapse: Displacement of intervertebral disc tissue from its normal position between vertebral bodies; also referred to as slipped, herniated, or protruded disc.

discrimination: Act of making distinctions based on differences in areas such as culture, race, gender, or religion.

disease (DZ): Deviation from the norm of measurable biological variables as defined by the biomedical system; refers to abnormalities of structure and function in body organs and systems.

disengagement theory of aging: Psychosocial theory of aging suggesting that successful aging occurs when both the elderly individual and society gradually withdraw from one another.

disinhibition: Inability to suppress a lower brain center or motor behavior, such as a reflex, indicating damage to higher structures of the brain.

dislocation: Displacement of bone from a joint with tearing of ligaments, tendons, and articular capsules. Symptoms include loss of joint motion, pain, swelling, temporary paralysis, and occasional shock.

disorder: Disruption or interference with normal functions or established systems.

disorganized speech: Phrases and ideas expressed that follow no theme or line of thought and may include perseveration (involuntary repetition of words or phrases), neologisms (newly coined words), or clanging (words are made to rhyme despite their meaning in the sentence).

disorientation: Inability to make accurate judgments about people, places, and things.

dissociative disorder: Group of mental disorders characterized by fragmentation of an individual's identity.

dissociative identity disorder: A disorder characterized by the presence of two or more distinct personalities that repeatedly take control of an individual's behavior. This disorder was formerly referred to as multiple personality disorder.

distal (D): From anatomical position, located further from the trunk.

distractibility: Level at which competing sensory input are able to draw attention away from tasks at hand.

distraction: Linear separation of joint surfaces without rupture of the binding ligaments and without displacement.

distress: The state of being in pain, uncomfortable, or suffering. Any affliction that is distressing.

distribution: Refers to manner through which a drug is transported by the circulating body fluids to the sites of action. Also, in statistical terminology, a collection of scores in order of magnitude.

distributive justice: Agent to discriminate the allocation of resources.

distributive practice: Spacing out practice sessions over time using small amounts of material. This increases the individual's memory of the material.

disuse atrophy: The wasting degeneration of muscle tissue that occurs as a result of inactivity or immobility.

diuresis: Increased secretion of urine.

diuretic: Drug that lowers blood pressure by increasing the production of urine and reducing the volume of fluid in the body.

divergence: Brain's ability to send information from one source to many parts of the central nervous system simultaneously.

diversion: Shifting from a course, action; something that distracts or amuses.

diversity: Diversity has not been defined in occupational therapy; rather a joint statement on diversity by the five national occupational therapy organizations states: "the profession is stimulating discussion to identify which definition or definitions of diversity most effectively move the profession forward" (ACOTRO, ACOTUP, CAOT, COTF, PAC, 2006, p. 1).[CAOT] Quality of being different or having variety.

division of labor: The separation of tasks. It may take several forms, such as social division of labor according to the economics of different societies and communities; division of labor by gender, which is a basic structural element in human social organizations that originates from differences in human physiology; and division of labor between workers who perform only a partial operation in production and what is produced is a social product of the collective workers.

DNA (deoxyribonucleic acid): The chief ingredient of chromosomes, DNA is necessary for the organization and functioning of living cells.

documentation: Process of recording and reporting the information gathered and intervention performed on a client. It ensures that the client receives adequate services and that the provider is reimbursed for them.

doing orientation: A value orientation found in some cultures that supports activity as the central focus of existence, with accomplishments measurable by external standards.

doll's eyes: When the head is turned in one direction eyes look in the opposite; this indicates damage to the higher brain centers.

domain: Profession's purview and areas in which its members have an established body of knowledge and expertise.[OTPF 2014] Specific occupational performance area of work (including education), self-care and self-maintenance, and play and leisure.

domain specificity: Term referring to the specific area of occupational performance to which a given assessment approach is directed.

dopamine: Neurotransmitter found in the brain; may be associated with Parkinson's disease, depression, and schizophrenia.

dormant: Time period when a disease remains inactive.

dorsal: From anatomical position, located toward the back.

dorsal column tracts: Afferent ipsilateral ascending tracts for fine discriminative touch, vibratory sense, and kinesthesia.

dorsal splint: "Splint fabricated on the dorsum of the hand to prevent full extension at one or more of the finger joints or wrist" (Trombly, 1995, p. 774).

dorsosacral position: *See* lithotomy position.

double-blind study: Strategy used in research that attempts to reduce one form of experimental error. Both the participants and the researchers are unaware of the treatments the participants are receiving.

double depression: Diagnosis of major depressive episode superimposed on a diagnosis of dysthymia.

down-aging: Refers to children who are using clothes, make-up, etc., that are typically used at an older age. *Synonym:* getting older younger.

Down syndrome: Congenital condition resulting from a chromosomal anomaly that causes physical and mental retardation with the distinct physical characteristics of a large tongue, poor muscle tone, a flat face, and heart problems.

doxepin: Drug used to relieve depression, especially when associated with anxiety. Side effects can include drowsiness, dry mouth, blurred vision, and digestive upsets. *Trade name:* Sinequan.

draw-a-person tests: Developed by Machover in 1949 to provide information about body image, self-esteem, and perceptual abilities.

dressing: Selecting clothing and accessories appropriate to time of day, weather, and occasion; obtaining clothing from storage area; dressing and undressing in a sequential fashion; fastening and adjusting clothing and shoes; and applying and removing personal devices, prostheses, or orthoses.[AOTA Framework]

dressing stick: Long rod with a clothes hook attached to one end used to pull on clothing.

drug abuse: The misuse or overuse of any drug that deviates from its intended prescription.

dual diagnosis: Presence of more than one diagnosis at the same time, most often a combination of a substance use disorder and some other condition but may include any situation in which comorbidity exists.

Duchenne's muscular dystrophy: Progressive fatal disorder of the skeletal muscles beginning in early childhood caused by a hereditary sex-linked gene on the X chromosome.

Dupuytren's contracture: Progressive fibrosis (increase in fibrous tissue) of the palmar aponeurosis, resulting in the shortening and thickening of the fibrous bands that extend from the aponeurosis to the bases of the phalanges. These fibrotic bands pull the digits into such marked flexion at the metacarpophalangeal joints that they cannot be straightened.

durable medical equipment, prosthetics, orthotics, and supplies (DMEPOS): Medically necessary equipment and supplies (e.g., oxygen equipment, wheelchairs, braces, or splints) that a health care provider prescribes for a patient's home use.

durable power of attorney: Legal instrument authorizing one to act as another's agent for specific purposes and/or length of time.

duration recording: Researcher's use of a device that keeps track of time and measures how long a given behavior lasts.

duty: Meeting one's responsibilities.

dyad: Relationship between two individuals in which interaction is significant.

dyadic activity: Activity involving another person.

Dycem: A nonslip plastic material that is used in food trays and mats. It enables a person to eat without worrying that the plate will slip away.

dynamic assessment: Describes a process used during intervention implementation for testing the hypotheses generated through the evaluation process. Allows for evaluation of change and intervention effectiveness during intervention. Assesses the interactions among the person, environment, and activity to understand how the client learns and approaches activities. May lead to adjustments in intervention plan (adapted from Primeau & Ferguson, 1999, p. 503). AOTA Framework

dynamic flexibility: Amount of resistance of a joint(s) to motion.

dynamics: Study of objects in motion.

dynamic sizing skills: Capability to compare commonly held views about a culture with the details of a particular situation to determine their relevance to that situation.

dynamic spatial reconstructor (DSR): Piece of equipment that transmits x-rays throughout the body to produce a full-sized three-dimensional image of an organ in motion on a television monitor.

dynamic splint: Orthosis that allows controlled movement at various joints; tension is applied to encourage particular movements.

dynamic strength: Force of a muscular contraction in which joint angle changes.

dynamic systems theory: Theory concerning movement organization that was derived from the study of chaotic systems. It theorizes that the order and pattern of movement performed to accomplish a goal comes from the interaction of multiple, nonhierarchical subsystems.

dynamometer: Device used to measure force produced from muscular contraction.

dysarthria: Group of speech disorders resulting from disturbances in muscular control.

dyscalculia: Learning disability in which there is a problem mastering basic arithmetic skills (e.g., addition, subtraction, multiplication, and division) and their application to daily living.

dysethesia: Sensation of "pins and needles," such as that experienced when one's extremity "goes to sleep."

dysfunction: Complete or partial impairment of function.

dysfunctional hierarchy: Levels of dysfunction including impairment, disability, and handicap.

dysgraphia: Imperfect ability to process and produce written language.

dyskinesia: Impairment of voluntary motion.

dyslexia: Impairment of the brain's ability to translate images received from the eyes into understandable language.

dysmetria: Condition seen in cerebellar disorders in which the patient overshoots a target because of an inability to control movement.

dyspareunia: Occurrence of pain during sexual intercourse.

dyspepsia: Poor digestion.

dysphagia: Difficulty swallowing.

dysplasia: Abnormal development in number, size, or organization of cells or tissue.

dyspnea: Difficulty breathing.

dyspraxia: Difficulty or inability to perform a planned motor activity when the muscles used in this activity are not paralyzed.

dysreflexia: A life-threatening uninhibited sympathetic response of the nervous system to a noxious stimulus, which is experienced by an individual with a spinal cord injury at T7 or above. *See* autonomic dysreflexia.

dysrhythmia: Disturbance in rhythm in speech, brain waves, or cardiac irregularity.

dyssomnia: Sleep disorder.

dystocia: A difficult childbirth; a fetal dystocia is difficult labor due to abnormalities of the fetus relative to size or position; a maternal dystocia is difficult labor due to abnormalities of the birth canal or uterine inertia.

dystonic: Distorted positioning of the limbs, neck, or trunk that is held for a few seconds and then released.

E

early childhood education: School or other educational program for children aged 3 to 5 years.

early intervention: Multidisciplinary, comprehensive, coordinated, community-based system for young children with developmental vulnerability or delay from birth to age 3 years and their families. Services are designed to enhance child development, minimize potential delays, remediate existing problems, prevent further deterioration, and promote adaptive family functioning.

eating: "The ability to keep and manipulate food or fluid in the mouth and swallow it; eating and swallowing are often used interchangeably" (AOTA, 2007b).[OTPF 2008]

eccentric contraction: Muscular contraction during which the length of muscle fibers is increased.

echodensities: Ultrasound changes that can be evidence of brain tissue damage.

echolalia: Uncontrollable repetitive verbalization of words spoken by another person that does not fit the situation.

echopraxia: Repetitive movement that does not fit the situation.

eclampsia toxemia: Toxic condition of pregnancy with symptoms of coma, seizures, high blood pressure, renal dysfunction, and proteinuria.

eclectic therapy: Therapist uses ideas and techniques from a variety of therapies in order to assist specific clients.

ecological sustainability: To uphold and support the ecology and ecosystems by practices that maintain, and continue to maintain, the natural environment and the relationships of different species.

Jacobs, K., & Simon, L. (Eds.). *Quick Reference Dictionary for Occupational Therapy, Sixth Edition* (pp. 90-107).
© 2015 SLACK Incorporated.

ecologic theory: Developmental theory that focuses on the process of development with all of the relevant variables (e.g., individual, contextual, mixed, cultural) of an individual's environment considered.

ecology: The scientific study of organisms in their natural environment, including the relationships of different species with each other and the environment.

Ecology of Human Performance Model (EHP): This framework provides a structure for thinking of context as a key variable in assessment and intervention planning, while taking into account the inherent dangers in examining performance out of context.

ecosystem: A biological community and the physical environment associated with it.

ectoderm: Layer of cells that develop from the inner cell mass of the blastocyst. Eventually, this layer develops into the outer surface of the skin, nails, part of teeth, lens of the eye, the inner ear, and central nervous system.

ectropion: Eversion of the edge of the eyelid.

eczema: An inflammatory skin disease characterized by lesions varying greatly in character, with vesiculation, infiltration, watery discharge, and the development of scales and crusts.

edema: Accumulation of large amounts of fluid in the tissues or body cavities.

educate: A key occupational therapy enablement skill and one of the historic knowledge foundations of occupational therapy, drawing on philosophies and practices of adult and childhood education, notably experiential and behavioral education that emphasize learning through doing (Dewey, 1900; Dewey & Bentley, 1949). In *Profile of Occupational Therapy Practice in Canada* (CAOT, in press), educate contributes to the competency role of change agent.[CAOT]

education: *As an occupation*—Activities involved in learning and participating in the educational environment. *As an intervention*—Activities that impart knowledge and information about occupation, health, well-being, and participation, resulting in acquisition by the client of helpful behaviors, habits, and routines that may or may not require application at the time of the intervention session.^OTPF 2014

educational activities: Participating in a learning environment through school, community, or work-sponsored activities, such as exploring educational interests, attending to instruction, managing assignments, and contributing to group experiences.

educational approaches: Interventions that make use of factual learning/teaching to change behaviors.

educational evaluator: Teacher who reports results of tests of academic, developmental, and readiness levels in number concepts, as well as the sequence of listening, speaking, reading, and writing.

Education of All Handicapped Children Act (1975): U.S. federal legislation that is intended to ensure that children with disabilities receive education in the least restrictive environment.

Education of the Handicapped Act Amendments (1986): Increase in U.S. federal funds for special education and other services provided to preschoolers ages 3 to 5 years.

effectiveness: Degree to which the desired result is produced.

effects of force: The effect that materials have upon bone and tissue.

efferent: Conducting away from a structure, such as a nerve or a blood vessel.

efferent neuron: Includes motor neurons.

efficacy: Having the desired influence or outcome.

effusion: Escape of fluid into a part or tissue.

ego: In psychoanalytic theory, one of three personality structures. It controls and directs one's actions after evaluating reality, monitoring one's impulses, and taking into consideration one's values and moral and ethical code. It is the executive structure of the personality.

egocentric-cooperative group: Group in which members select and complete a task. Social interaction is required to encourage members to respond to each other's emotional and social needs. The purpose of the task is to organize the group, using the therapist as a facilitator.

egophony: A bleating quality of voice observed in auscultation in certain cases of lung consolidation.

egress, means of: Continuous and unobstructed path of travel from any point in a building or structure to a public way and consisting of three separate and distinct parts: the exit access, the exit, and the exit discharge. A means of egress is composed of the vertical and horizontal means of travel and includes the intervening room spaces, doorways, hallways, corridors, passageways, balconies, ramps, stairs, enclosures, lobbies, horizontal exits, courts, and yards.

eHealth: A broad term encompassing health-related information and educational resources (e.g., health literacy websites and repositories, videos, blogs), commercial "products" (e.g., apps), and direct services delivered electronically (often through the Internet) by professionals, nonprofessionals, businesses, or consumers. May also be written as e-Health or E-Health; sometimes used interchangeably with health informatics (AOTA, 2014a).

ejection fraction: Percentage of blood emptied from the ventricles at the end of a contraction.

elastic traction: Splinting method often used for the correction of joint deformity. Materials used include rubber bands, elastic thread, and springs that are now available in varying degrees of strength.

elder: Term used to refer to individuals in the later years of the life span, arbitrarily set between age 65 to 70 years and older.

elder abuse: Intentional physical or psychological injury inflicted on older adults by caretakers.

electroconvulsive therapy (ECT): Treatment that involves the deliberate induction of a convulsion by passing electricity through one or both hemispheres of the brain.

electroencephalography: Study of the electrical activity of the brain.

electrogoniometer: Electronic device that measures the position of a joint or joints to which it is applied.

electrolytes: Mineral salts that conduct electricity in the body when in a solution.

electromyograph (EMG): Device used to record the electrical activity produced by a contracting muscle.

electrophoresis: A technique used for the analysis and separation of colloids; used extensively in studying mixtures of proteins, nucleic acids, carbohydrates, enzymes, etc. In clinical medicine, it is used for determining the protein content of body fluids.

embolism: Sudden blocking of artery by clot of foreign material (embolus) brought to the site of lodging via the bloodstream.

embryo: The fetus from conception to 8 weeks of gestation.

embryonic period: Prenatal period of development that occurs from 2 to 8 weeks after conception. During this period, cell differentiation intensifies, support systems for the cells form, and organs appear.

emergency response: Recognizing sudden, unexpected hazardous situations and initiating action to reduce the threat to health and safety.

emerging majority: "People of color—Black, Asian, or Pacific Islander; American Indian, Eskimo, or Aleut; and Hispanic origin, who it is expected will comprise a majority of the American population by the year 2020" (Rachel Spector, PhD, RN, CTN, FAAN, personal communication).

emetic: Drug that promotes vomiting.

emotional regulation skills: Actions or behaviors a client uses to identify, manage, and express feelings while engaging in activities or interacting with others.[OTPF 2008]

emotion-focused coping: Strategies that focus on managing the emotions associated with a stressful episode.

empathy: While maintaining one's sense of self, the ability to recognize and share the emotions and state of mind of another person.

emphysema: An abnormal swelling of the lung tissue due to the permanent loss of elasticity or the destruction of the alveoli, which seriously impairs respiration.

empirical base: Knowledge based on the observations and experience of master clinicians.

employee assistance program (EAP): Mental health services for workers through confidential counseling at work and outside referrals to appropriate professionals. EAPs attempt to treat employees in their current work and living settings. EAPs were originally established to decrease corporate costs resulting from problems such as alcoholism and drug abuse among workers.

employer shared responsibility: Although employers are not required to provide health coverage to their employees under the Affordable Care Act, employers of a certain size will be subject to the Employer Shared Responsibility provision of the law. Under this provision, beginning in 2014, business owners with at least 50 full-time or full-time equivalent employees who do not offer health coverage to their full-time employees may be subject to a shared responsibility payment under the health care law (Olafson, 2013).

employment interests and pursuits: Identifying and selecting work opportunities based on personal assets, limitations, likes, and dislikes relative to work (adapted from Mosey, 1996).[AOTA Framework]

employment seeking and acquisition: Identifying job opportunities, completing and submitting appropriate application materials, preparing for interviews, participating in interviews and following up afterwards, discussing job benefits, and finalizing negotiations.[AOTA Framework]

empowerment: "Personal and social processes that transform visible and invisible relationships so that power is shared more equally" (CAOT, 1997a, 2002, p. 180).[CAOT] To enable; to gain mastery over one's affairs.

emulator: Device that imitates the action of another (e.g., a terminal emulator is a system that is not a terminal per se but is designed to operate like one).

enablement continuum (EC): The portrayal of a range of variations from ineffective to effective enablement, resulting from complex practice conditions and decisions that support or limit enablement (E. Townsend, G. Whiteford, & H. Polatajko, personal communication, July–December, 2006).[CAOT]

enablement foundations (EF): The interests, values, beliefs, ideas, concepts, critical perspectives, and concerns that inform and shape decision-making priorities in enabling occupation. [CAOT]

enablement reasoning: Integrates narrative, conditional, clinical (positivistic), and other forms of reasoning; a component of occupational therapy professional reasoning based on conceptual foundations (including values, beliefs, and concepts), framed by the practice context with different clients in different situations, and influencing the application of competence in key and related enablement skills, which are highly inter-related, dynamic, and evolving.[CAOT]

enabling/enablement: Focused on occupation, it is the core competency of occupational therapy—what occupational therapists actually do—and draws on an interwoven spectrum of key and related enablement skills, which are value-based, collaborative, attentive to power inequities and diversity, and charged with visions of possibility for individual and/or social change.[CAOT]

enabling occupation: Enabling people to "choose, organize, and perform those occupations they find useful and meaningful in their environment" (CAOT, 1997a, 2002, p. 180).[CAOT]

enactive representation: Motoric encoding of information about the world (e.g., child thinks "rattle" and shakes hand).

encephalitis: Disease characterized by inflammation of the parenchyma of the brain and its surrounding meninges, usually caused by a virus.

encephalopathy: Any disease that affects the tissues of the brain and its surrounding meninges.

encoding (cognitive): Processes or strategies used to initially store information in memory.

encopresis: A condition often confused with diarrhea, it is associated with constipation in which watery content bypasses the hard fecal masses and passes through the rectum.

encourager: Person in this role uses words of praise and accepts other ideas from the group.

enculturation: The acquisition of cultural knowledge that allows one to function as a member of a particular society.

end-diastolic volume: The amount of filling of the ventricles of the heart during diastole.

end feel: Sensation imparted to the hands of the clinician at the end point of range of motion; the point where movement of a joint stops when performing passive range of motion on an individual.

endocarditis: Inflammation of the endocardium, a disease generally associated with acute febrile or rheumatic diseases and marked by dyspnea, rapid heart action, and peculiar systolic murmurs.

endocardium: The thin endothelial membrane lining the cavities of the heart.

endocrine: Designating any gland producing one or more hormones, such as the thyroid and its hormone thyroxine.

endogenous: Growing from within. Developing or originating within the organism.

endometriosis: Abnormal proliferation of the uterine mucous membrane into the pelvic cavity.

endothelial: Pertaining to the epithelial cells that line the heart cavities, blood vessels, lymph vessels, and serous cavities of the body.

endotracheal: Within or through the trachea. Performed by passage through the lumen of the trachea (e.g., endotracheal tube).

end-systolic volume: The amount of blood remaining in each ventricle after each heartbeat.

endurance: Sustaining cardiac, pulmonary, and musculoskeletal exertion over time; ability to sustain effort over time.

endurance testing: Used to determine the capacity of an individual to sustain the energy output needed to fulfill a task.

endures: Persists and completes the task without obvious evidence of physical fatigue, pausing to rest, or stopping to "catch one's breath."AOTA Framework

energy: Sustained effort over the course of task performance. AOTA Framework

energy conservation techniques: Applying procedures that save energy; may include activity restriction, work simplification, time management, and organizing the environment to simplify tasks.

enfolded activity: Performing multiple activities in a given time frame.

engage/engagement: A historical cornerstone of occupational therapy and is the enablement skill to involve clients in doing, in participating, that is to say, in action beyond talk by involving others and oneself to become occupied (Answers.com). In the *Profile of Occupational Therapy Practice in Canada* (CAOT, in press), occupational therapists engage others through the core competency role as experts in enabling occupation.[CAOT]

engagement: The act of sharing activities.[OTPF 2008] Psychiatric rehabilitation program that focuses on stabilizing symptoms and/or developing a trusting relationship with the consumer.[C]

engagement in occupation: Performance of occupations as the result of choice, motivation, and meaning within a supportive context and environment.[OTPF 2014]

engaging skills: Interpersonal skills a practitioner uses when working with consumers.[C]

engineering controls: Strategy used in ergonomics to eliminate the hazard (problem) at the source.

enrichment services: Focus on maintaining and/or achieving a satisfactory quality of life.[C]

enteral: Administration of a pharmacologic agent directly into the gastrointestinal tract by oral, rectal, or nasogastric routes.

enteric: Pertaining to the intestines.

enterocele: Herniation of the intestine below the cervix associated with congenital weakness or obstetric trauma.

enthesopathy: Any inflammation of a joint.

entropion: Inversion of the edge of the eyelid.

entry level: Individual with less than 1 year of work experience.

enucleation: Removal of an organ or other mass from its supporting tissues.

enuresis: Inability to control urine, usually bedwetting.

environment: External physical and social conditions that surround the client and in which the client's daily life occupations occur.[OTPF 2014] External social and physical conditions or factors that have the potential to influence an individual.

environmental approaches: Interventions based on changing the environment (e.g., changing support systems, modifying job, home).

environmental assessment: Process of identifying, describing, and measuring factors external to the individual that can influence performance or the outcome of treatment. These can include space and associated objects, cultural influences, social relationships, and system available resources.

environmental barrier: Any type of obstacle that interferes with a person's ability to achieve optimal occupational performance.

environmental contingencies: Factors in the environment that influence the patient's performance during an evaluation.

environmental control unit (ECU): Device that allows those with limited physical ability to operate other electronic devices by remote control.

environmental elements: "Cultural, institutional, physical, and social forces that lie outside individuals, yet are embedded in individuals' actions" (CAOT, 1997a, 2002, p. 180).[CAOT]

environmental factors: The physical, social and attitudinal environment in which people live and conduct their lives.[ICF] "All aspects of the external or extrinsic world that form the context of an individual's life"; physical, social, and attitudinal (WHO, 2001, p. 193).[CAOT]

environmental fit: The process of matching an individual's capacities with opportunities for action in the physical, social, and cultural environments.

environmental press: Tendency of environments to encourage or require certain types of behavior.

environmental specificity: Focus on the real world context in which the person lives, learns, works, or socializes.[C]

environmental support: Any environmental element that facilitates an individual's ability to attain his or her optimum occupational performance.

enzyme: A protein functioning as a biochemical catalyst, necessary for most major body functions.

epicardium: The layer of the pericardium that is in contact with the heart.

epicritic sensation: Ability to localize and discern fine differences in touch, pain, and temperature.

epidemic: When a large number of people get a specific disease from a common source.

epidemiology: Science concerned with factors, causes, and remediation as related to the distribution of disease, injury, and other health-related events.

epidural: Anesthesia injected into the epidural space of the spine, which can produce a loss of sensation from the abdomen to the toes.

epigenesis: The development of an organism from an undifferentiated cell, consisting in the successive formation and development of organs and parts that do not preexist in the fertilized egg.

epilepsy: Group of disorders caused by temporary, sudden changes in the electrical activity of the brain that results in convulsive seizures or changes in the level of consciousness or motor activity.

epinephrine: A hormone secreted by the adrenal medulla in response to splanchnic stimulation and stored in the chromaffin granules that is released predominantly in response to hypoglycemia. It increases blood pressure, stimulates heart muscle, accelerates the heart rate, and increases cardiac output.

episode of care: All patient/client management activities provided, directed, or supervised by the physical therapist from initial contact through discharge.

episodic memory: Memory for personal episodes or events that have some temporal reference.

epispadias: Congenital opening of the urethra on the dorsum of the penis, or opening by separation of the labia minora and a fissure of the clitoris.

epistaxis: Nosebleed.

epistemology: Dimension of philosophy that is concerned with the questions of truth by investigating the origin, nature, methods, and limits of human knowledge.

Epstein-Barr virus (EBV): A virus that causes infectious mononucleosis. It is spread by respiratory tract secretions (eg, saliva, mucus).

equality: Requires that all individuals be perceived as having the same fundamental rights and opportunities.

equilibrium reaction: Reaction that occurs when the body adapts and posture is maintained, and when there is a change of the supporting surface; any of several reflexes that enables the body to recover balance. Begins to develop at approximately age 6 months.

equinovarus: Deformity of the foot in which the foot is pointing downward and inward. *Also known as* clubfoot.

equipment: Device that usually cannot be held in the hand and is electrical or mechanical (e.g., table, electrical saw, or stove); devices can be specifically designed to assist function or compensate for absent function or they can be labor-saving and convenience gadgets.

Erb's palsy: Injury to the brachial plexus involving the fifth and sixth cervical roots, usually occurring at birth, causing musculature weakness in the shoulder and upper arm. The arm is typically rotated internally, hanging limp in extension.

ergometer: Device that can measure work done.

ergometry: Measurement of work.

ergonomics: Field of study that examines and optimizes the interaction between the human worker and the nonhuman work environment.

ergonomic work site analysis: Analysis that categorizes jobs on the basis of the qualifications and physical demands they require to ensure that a person is capable of performing a given job safely.

Erhardt Developmental Prehension Assessment (EDPA): Provides a sequential description of fine motor skills, measures voluntary and involuntary arm-hand patterns from the prenatal period to 15 months, and measures pencil grasp/prewriting skills from ages 1 to 6 years.

eructation: Producing gas from the stomach, often with a characteristic sound; belching.

erythema: First-degree reddening of the skin due to a burn or injury.

***Escherichia coli* (*E. coli*):** A species of organisms constituting the greater part of the intestinal flora. In excess, causes urinary tract infections and epidemic diarrheal disease.

escrow accounts: Funds placed in trust with a third party by a borrower for a specific purpose and to be delivered to the borrower only on the fulfillment of certain conditions.Small Business Administration

essential fat: Stored body fat that is necessary for normal physiologic function and found in bone marrow, the nervous system, and all body organs.

essential functions: Fundamental, not marginal, job duties. In deciding whether a function is essential, the following questions are considered: Are employees in the position required to perform the function? Will removing that function fundamentally change the job?

essential health benefits: The Affordable Care Act ensures that health plans offered in the individual and small group markets, both inside and outside of the health insurance Marketplace, offer this comprehensive package of items and services. Essential health benefits must include services within at least 10 core categories, among them emergency services, maternity and newborn care, prescription drugs, and preventive and wellness services. For more information on these requirements, visit healthcare.gov.

essential hypertension: High blood pressure that is idiopathic, self-existing, having no obvious external cause. *Also known as* intrinsic hypertension.

establishment: A single-location business unit, which may be independent—called a single-establishment enterprise—or owned by a parent enterprise.Small Business Administration

estrogen: The female hormone that is responsible for maintenance of female sex characteristics and is formed in the ovary, placenta, testis, and adrenal cortex.

ethical dilemma: Conflict of moral choices with no satisfactory solution, which is often caused by attempting to balance two or more undesirable alternatives with no overriding principle to tell an individual what to do.

ethical investigator: Researcher who protects participants from physical and mental discomfort, harm, and danger.

ethical jurisdiction: Right or authority to interpret the system of values imposed by a group. In the profession of occupational therapy, the American Occupational Therapy Association, National Board for Certification in Occupational Therapy, and state regulatory boards have jurisdiction.

ethical relativism: View that each person's values should be considered equally valid.

ethical research practice: Refers to the investigator's obligations to respect the individual's freedom to decline to participate in research or to discontinue participation at any time.

ethics: System of moral principles or standards that govern personal and professional conduct.

ethnic: Member of, or pertaining to, groups of people with a common racial, national, linguistic, religious, or cultural history.

ethnicity: Component of culture that is derived from membership in a racial, religious, national, or linguistic group or subgroup, usually through birth.

ethnocentrism: Process of judging different cultures or ethnic groups only on the basis of one's own culture or experiences.

ethnogerontology: Study of ethnicity in an aging context.

ethnographic approach: A strategy for data collection using observation, interview, and other qualitative methods.

ethnography: The study and detailed description of human groups using direct observation and interview.

ethologic theory: Branch of developmental theory that emphasizes innate, instinctual qualities of behavior that predispose individuals to behave in certain patterns.

ethology: The systematic study of the formation of the core characteristics of being human. The study of animal and human behavior. Central to the ethologist's approach is the principle that animal behavior (like physical characteristics) is subject to evolution through natural selection, through the development of the individual, and, in humans, in cultural history.

etiology (ETIOL): Dealing with the causes of disease.

etiquette: Particular behaviors that are observed by a certain society as being acceptable.

euthanasia: The deliberate ending of life of a person suffering from an incurable disease; has been broadened to include the withholding of extraordinary measures to sustain life, allowing a person to die.

evaluation: "Process of obtaining and interpreting data necessary for intervention. This includes planning for and documenting the evaluation process and results" (AOTA, 2010, p. S107).[OTPF 2014]

eversion: Turning outward.

evidence: A ground for a belief that which tends to prove or disprove any conclusion (Brown, 1993). In health care, evidence is conceived in a scientific context and can be defined as "an observation, fact or organized body of information offered to support or justify inferences or beliefs in the demonstration of some proposition or matter at issue" (Upshur, 2001, p. 7). Evidence consists of many things besides research, including things such as clinical and other reasoning. Occupational therapists collect and use evidence generated from clients, the literature, and their peers and from reflecting on their personal experiences (Dubouloz, Egan, Vallerand, & von Zweck, 1999).[CAOT]

evidence-based practice: Includes experiential, qualitative, and quantitative evidence. "The occupational therapist provides knowledge of client, environment and occupational factors relevant to enabling occupation. Ideally, this evidence is derived from a critical review of the research literature, expert consensus and professional experience" (CAOT, ACOTUP, ACOTRO, & PAC, 1999, p. 267). Practice founded on research that supports its effectiveness.[CAOT]

evisceration: Removal of the contents of a cavity.

evolution: Gradual process of development or change.

Ewing's sarcoma: Malignant bone tumor that often attacks the shaft of the long bones.

exacerbation: Increase in the severity of a disease or any of its symptoms.

examination: The process of obtaining a history, performing relevant systems reviews, and selecting and administering specific tests and measures.

excess disability: Disability that occurs above and beyond that which should occur given the person's actual limitations.

exchange relationship: Social concept that views interaction as exchanges of value (e.g., the grandfather who teaches his grandson how to fish is exchanging knowledge and experience for the company and affection that the grandson may bring to the interaction).

excitation: An act of irritation or stimulation.

excretion: Process through which metabolites of drugs (and active drug itself) are eliminated from the body through urine and feces, evaporation from skin, exhalation from lungs, and secretion into saliva.

excursion: A range of movement regularly repeated in performance of a function.

executive function: Higher level, multistep, cognitive functions or abilities requiring skill/precision.

exercise therapy: Manages musculoskeletal disorders by restoring strength to weakened muscles, restoring mobility or increased range of motion, correcting postural faults, preventing joint deformity, and improving joint stability.

exertional angina: Paroxysmal thoracic pain due most often to anoxia of the myocardium precipitated by physical exertion. *Synonym*: angina.

exhaustion: Depletion of energy with a consequent inability to respond to stimuli.

existential humanism: Philosophical movement emphasizing individual existence, freedom, and choice.

existentialism: A philosophical movement that rejects the metaphysical and centers on an individual person as a being in the world. It has as a major tenet that every person is unique and cannot be explained in reductionist physiological terms. It aims toward a comprehensive concept of human existence and uses phenomenological methods to grasp the "essence" of a person's consciousness, feelings, moods, experiences, and relationships.

exocrine: Secreting outwardly (the opposite of endocrine).

exophthalmos: Abnormal protrusion of the eyeball, which results in a marked stare.

expectorate: To expel mucus or phlegm from the lungs; to spit.

expert in enabling occupation: Occupational therapy practitioners use evidence-based processes that focus on occupation—including self-care, productive pursuits, and leisure—as a medium for action. Practitioners take client perspectives and diversity into account. Expert in enabling occupation is the central role, expertise and competence of an occupational therapy practitioner. Clients may include individuals, families, groups, communities, organizations or populations (CAOT, in press).[CAOT]

expertise: The possession of a large body of knowledge and procedural skill that allows the solution of most domain problems effectively and efficiently.

explanatory model: Model held by an individual about an illness episode containing knowledge, thoughts, and feelings about the etiology, timing, and mode of onset of an illness; the pathophysical process; the natural history and severity of the illness; the ethnoanatomy and ethnophysiology; and the appropriate treatments and their rationale.

exploratory laparotomy: Incision into the abdominal cavity used in order to view the condition of abdominal organs.

expresses: Displays affect/attitude.[AOTA Framework]

expressive aphasia: Loss of the ability to produce language, either spoken or written. *Also known as* Broca's aphasia.

extended care facility (ECF): Facility that is an extension of hospital care; derived from Medicare legislation.

extended school year programs: Programs run during the summer months or weekends for children.

extension (EXT): Straightening a body part.

external adjustment: Changes in other professionals' knowledge, skills, or attitudes that result from a learning situation.

external environment: Contexts such as climate, community, and economics.

external stimulation: Factors in the area where the activity is being performed that may enhance or impede performance.

external validity: The degree to which an experimental finding is predictable to the population at large.

exteroceptive: Receptors activated by stimuli outside of the body.

extinction: Behavioral approach to discouraging a particular behavior by ignoring it and reinforcing other more acceptable behaviors.

extrafusal muscle: Striated muscle tissue found outside the muscle spindle.

extrapyramidal: Outside of the pyramidal tracts.

extrapyramidal signs: Motor symptoms that mimic Parkinson's disease, dyskinesia, and other lesions in the extrapyramidal tract.

extrinsic motivation: Stimulation to achieve or perform that initiates from the environment.

exudate: Material, such as fluid, cells, or cellular debris, that has escaped from blood vessels and has been deposited in tissues or on tissue surfaces, usually as a result of inflammation. An exudate, in contrast to a transudate, is characterized by a high content of protein, cells, or solid materials derived from cells.

Facebook: A popular, free social networking website that allows registered users to create profiles, upload photos and videos, send messages to other users, and keep in touch with friends and family.

face validity: Dimension of a test by which it appears to test what it purports.

facilitation techniques: Manual methods used to encourage movement and sensory awareness.

facilitator: A person who helps people in an online group or forum to manage their conversations and have productive discussions. Often known to set rules, draw out topics for discussion, keep people on topic, and monitor discussions to ensure appropriate online behavior.

fact: Truth or reality.

fact-centered: An approach to teaching cultural competence focused on learning about the beliefs and behaviors of specific ethnic groups.

factitious disorder: A person simulates a mental or physical illness with the sole objective of assuming the patient role; for many, hospitalization is the primary objective.

factor analysis: Statistical test that examines the relationships of many variables and their contribution to the total set of variables.

failure to thrive: "A condition in which infants and children not only fail to gain weight but may actually lose it. It is seen more often in institutionalized and retarded children. The causes include chronic conditions, starvation, emotional deprivation, and social disruption" (Thomas & Craven, 1997, p. 703).

Jacobs, K., & Simon, L. (Eds.). *Quick Reference Dictionary for Occupational Therapy, Sixth Edition* (pp. 108-118).
© 2015 SLACK Incorporated.

Fair Housing Amendment Act (1988): U.S. federal law meant to prohibit discriminatory housing for those with disabilities.

family centered: The child functions within the family as a unit.

family therapy: Intervention that focuses on the context of the entire family system.

fascia: A thin layer of connective tissue covering, supporting, or connecting the muscles or inner organs of the body.

fasciculation: A small local contraction of muscles, visible through the skin, representing a spontaneous discharge of a number of fibers innervated by a single motor nerve filament.

fascitis: Inflammation of a fascia.

fat emboli: Embolus formed by an ester of glycerol with fatty acids that causes a clot in the circulatory system and can result in vessel obstruction.

fatigue: State of exhaustion or loss of strength and endurance; decreased ability to maintain a contraction at a given force.

favism: Familial Mediterranean fever. Hereditary biochemical lesion of the erythrocytes and consequent enzyme deficiency.

fecundity: The fertility of an organism. Normally all organisms, assuming they reach reproductive age, are sufficiently fecund to replace themselves several times over. Darwin noted this, together with the fact that population numbers nevertheless tended to remain fairly constant. These observations led him to formulate his theory of evolution by natural selection.

Federal Register: Publication where proposed federal U.S. rules and regulations, as well as requests for proposals for grants, are published.

feedback: Knowledge of the results of an individual's performance to the extent that the individual's behavior is changed or reinforced in a desirable direction.

feedback control: Refers to the postural control mechanism of automatic responses that occurs when there is a displacement of one's center of gravity that is not under voluntary control. Automatic postural responses.

feedforward control: Refers to the postural control mechanism of automatic responses that occurs during an intentional displacement of the center of gravity, as during voluntary movement.

feeding: "The process of setting up, arranging, and bringing food [or fluid] from the plate or cup to the mouth; sometimes called self-feeding" (AOTA, 2007b).[OTPF 2008]

fee-for-service: Payment method by which a health care provider is reimbursed for each encounter or service rendered.

fee schedule: List of accepted charges or established allowances for specified medical or dental procedures.

Felbatol: Drug administered for seizures. Side effects include anorexia, vomiting, nausea, and headache. *Generic name*: felbamate.

feminism: A doctrine and movement advocating the granting of the same social, political, and economic rights to women as the ones granted to men.

fenoprofen calcium: Anti-inflammatory drug for treating rheumatoid arthritis and osteoarthritis. Side effects include anemia, headache, dizziness, drowsiness, and renal problems. *Trade name*: Nalfon.

festinating gait: Patient walks on his or her toes as pushed. Starts slowly, increases, and may continue until the patient grasps an object in order to stop. Seen in patients with Parkinson's disease.

festination: A symptom characterized by small, quick forward steps.

fetal alcohol syndrome (FAS): Low birth weight, developmental delays, and physical defects in infants caused by mothers consuming alcohol during pregnancy.

fetal growth retardation: Condition of babies who are especially small for their gestational age at birth.

fetus: Describes the baby from the 8th week after conception until birth.

fibrillation: Small, local involuntary muscle contraction.

fibrin: A whitish, insoluble protein formed from fibrinogen by the action of thrombin, as in the clotting of blood. Fibrin forms the essential portion of a blood clot.

fibroblast: Chief cell of connective tissue responsible for forming the fibrous tissues of the body, such as tendons and ligaments.

fibrosis: Formation of fibrous tissue, fibroid degeneration.

fidelity: Duty to be faithful to the client and the client's best interest; includes the mandate to keep all client information confidential.

fieldwork: A crucial part of occupational therapy education. Fieldwork experiences provide role modeling and opportunities to perform professional responsibilities under supervision. Fieldwork takes place in a variety of settings and emerging areas of practice. Two types of fieldwork experiences are included within the occupational therapy curriculum: Level I and Level II fieldwork.

fieldwork coordinator: A fieldwork site's representative who assigns student placements and oversees the student's experience at the facility.

fieldwork educator: A fieldwork site's staff member who is assigned to supervise the student.

fieldwork site: A hospital, clinic, rehabilitation facility, outpatient program, school, private practice, day program, etc., where a student is placed for a Level I or Level II experience.

figure ground: Differentiating between foreground and background forms and objects[UTIII]; person's ability to distinguish shapes and objects from the background in which they exist.

financial management: Using fiscal resources, including alternate methods of financial transaction and planning and using finances with long- and short-term goals.[AOTA Framework]

financial reports: Reports commonly required from applicant's request for financial assistance, e.g.—balance sheet: a report of the status of a firm's assets, liabilities and owner's equity at a given time; income statement: a report of revenue and expense which shows the results of business operations or net income for a specified period of time; cash flow: a report which analyzes the actual or projected source and disposition of cash during a past or future accounting period.[Small Business Administration]

fine coordination/dexterity: Using small muscle groups for controlled movements, particularly in object manipulation.

fine motor coordination: Motor behaviors involving manipulative, discreet finger movements and eye/hand coordination.

fine motor pattern of development: Mastery of smaller muscles (i.e., fingers); takes place after gross motor development.

finger goniometer: Instrument used to measure the range of movement of the finger joints.

firm end feel: A muscular or ligamentous stretch with no give remaining.

fiscal management: Method of controlling the economics of problems at hand. It is concerned with discovering, developing, defining, and evaluating the financial goals of a department.

fissure: Deep groove.

fistula: Abnormal tube-like duct or passage from a normal cavity or tube to a free surface or another cavity.

Fit Chart: Illustrates the relationship of the components of occupational performance and engagement (H. Polatajko & J. Craik, personal communication, July–December, 2006).[CAOT]

fixator: Muscle that contracts to brace one bone, to which a mover attaches.

flaccid: Inability to move an extremity due to loss of motor control.

flaccidity: State of low tone in the muscle that produces weak and floppy limbs.

flashback: The return of images after the effects of hallucinogens have worn off; hallucinations may occur for extended periods.

flattened effect: Incongruous absence of appropriate emotional response.

flexibility: Range of motion at a joint or in a sequence of joints.

flexion (FLEX): Act of bending a body part.

flight of ideas: Rapid continuous speech with rapid, unclear shifts from subject to subject.

flooding: Behavioral technique in which the individual is inundated with an unpleasant stimulus on the theory that this will overwhelm and exhaust any anxiety response.

flow: A state of consciousness when people are so involved in an activity that nothing else seems to matter; of optimal experience, transcendence, and enjoyment when individuals are challenged but engaged within the scope of their abilities.

flow chart: A graphical representation for the definition, analysis, or solution of a problem in which symbols are used to represent operations, data, flow, equipment, etc.Small Business Administration

flows: Uses smooth and fluid arm and hand movements when interacting with task objects.AOTA Framework

fluid goniometer: Goniometer that has a circular chamber filled with fluid that has a 360-degree scale. It is used to measure the change in the angle of a joint.

fluid intelligence: Ability to use new information.

fluidotherapy: A dry heat agent that transfers energy by forced convection, providing heat. Warm air is circulated through a container holding fine cellulose particles. The solid particles become suspended when air is forced through them, thus the properties of fluidotherapy are similar to those of liquids. The viscosity of the air-fluidized system is low, permitting exercise with relative ease. Patients/clients with rheumatoid arthritis, osteoarthritis, silastic joint replacements, wounds, sprains and strains, and amputations benefit from this exercise/heat modality. It has been used to promote relaxation, increase blood flow to an area, and decrease pain.

focal epilepsy: Jerking or stiffening of many muscles on the same side of the body that crosses over to the opposite side and then continues. The person does not fully lose consciousness, but consciousness is altered.

focus: The predetermined set of interests one brings to interactions.

focuses: Directs conversation and behavior to ongoing social action.AOTA Framework

folkways: Social customs to which people generally conform; traditional patterns of life common to a people.

follicle-stimulating hormone (FSH): One of the gonadotropic hormones of the anterior pituitary, which stimulates the growth and maturation of graafian follicles in the ovary and stimulates spermatogenesis in the male.

follower: Person in this role passively accepts ideas of others and consents to the movement of the group.

foot-drop splint: Splint used to prevent the development of plantar flexion contractures.

force: Product of mass and acceleration; a kinematic measurement that encompasses the amount of matter, velocity, and its rate of change of velocity; also strength, energy, and power.

force couple: Body being acted upon by two equal and parallel forces from opposite directions; the points of application of these forces must be on opposite sides of the object and be operating at some distance apart from one another.

force plate: An embedded plate in the floor used to measure the force that a person exerts when walking.

forceps: Locked tong-like obstetrical instruments used to aid in the delivery of the fetal presenting part.

foreclosure: The act by the mortgagee or trustee upon default for the payment of interest or principal of a mortgage of enforcing payment of the debt by selling the underlying security.Small Business Administration

foreign language translator: An individual who speaks two languages and can translate from one to the other and back.

forensic: Pertaining to the law.

form constancy: Recognizing forms and objects as the same in various environments, positions, and sizes.

formal educational participation: Including the categories of academic (e.g., math, reading, working on a degree), nonacademic (e.g., recess, lunchroom, hallway), extracurricular (e.g., sports, band, cheerleading, dances), and vocational (prevocational and vocational) participation.AOTA Framework

forums: Similar to bulletin boards, these websites are used for discussion among members.

founder effect: The genetic consequences of founding a new population with few individuals. The founder population will most likely differ genetically from its parent population because it will contain only a fraction of the total genetic variation. Any recessive gene will increase in frequency.

fracture (Fx): Pertaining to broken bone(s).

fragile X syndrome: Sex-linked disorder that results when the bottom tip of the long arm of the X chromosome is pinched off.

Affected individuals can have delayed development of speech and language, intellectual disability, anxiety, hyperactive behavior, and fidgeting or impulsive actions. Some may show features of autism spectrum disorders that manifest in problems with communication and social interaction. Most males and some females with fragile X have characteristic physical features that include a long and narrow face, large ears, prominent jaw and forehead, unusually flexible fingers, and flat feet.

frame of reference (FOR): The viewpoint, context, or set of assumptions within which a person's perception and thinking seem always to occur, and which constrains selectively the course and outcome of action (Atherton, 2002). Occupational therapy frames of reference are sets of interrelated theories, constructs, and concepts that determine how specific occupational challenges will be perceived, understood, and approached (Mosey, 1986), and that guide occupational therapists' decision making through the practice process.[CAOT] Organization of interrelated, theoretical concepts used in practice.

franchising: A continuing relationship in which the franchisor provides a licensed privilege to the franchisee to do business and offers assistance in organizing, training, merchandising, marketing and managing in return for a consideration. Franchising is a form of business by which the owner (franchisor) of a product, service, or method obtains distribution through affiliated dealers (franchisees). The product, method, or service being marketed is usually identified by the franchisor's brand name, and the holder of the privilege (franchisee) is often given exclusive access to a defined geographical area.[Small Business Administration]

Frank-Starling mechanism: The intrinsic ability of the heart to adapt to changing volumes of inflowing blood.

freedom: Allows the individual to exercise choice and to demonstrate independence, initiative, and self-direction.

free radicals: Short-lived chemicals that cause changes in cells that are thought to result in aging.

frequency counts: Process of counting specific behaviors that occur during an identified time period.

frequency distribution curve: Raw scores (z scores) are plotted on the abscissa (x-axis) and the frequency of occurrence is plotted on the ordinate (y-axis).

Fresnel prism: Prism applied to a person's glasses that shifts images toward the center of the visual field.

frontal plane: Divides the body into front and back sections; motion occurs around the anterior-posterior axis.

frostbite: To injure the tissues of the body by exposure to intense cold.

fugue: Dissociative disorder in which an individual, while in an amnesic state, travels away from home and assumes a new identity.

fulcrum: The intermediate point of force application of a three- or four-point bending construct; entity on which a lever moves.

full-circle goniometer: Instrument that measures the motion of a joint in both directions; measures 0 to 180 degrees each direction.

full-thickness skin loss: Third-degree burn or wound in which skin is completely destroyed and underlying structures (e.g., muscles, vessels) can be visualized.

function (FUNC): "The skill to perform activities in a normal or accepted way (Reed & Sanderson, 1983) and/or adequately for the required tasks of a specific role or setting" (Christiansen & Baum, 1997; CAOT, 1997a, 2002, p. 181).[CAOT] Performance; action.

functional adaptation: The ability for another cortical pathway in a nontraumatized area to carry the same information as the original pathway that was derailed.

functional assessment: Observation of motor performance and behavior to determine whether a person can adequately perform the required tasks of a particular role or setting.

Functional Capacity Evaluation (FCE): Evaluation that determines the person's abilities and limitations.

functional communication: Using equipment or systems to send and receive information, such as writing equipment, telephones, typewriters, computers, communication boards, call lights, emergency systems, Braille writers, telecommunication devices for the deaf, and augmentative communication systems.[UTIII] Ability to participate in casual everyday conversation, and includes the ability to understand implied meaning and to enjoy humor.

functional electrical stimulation (FES): Stimulation of nerves from surface electrodes in order to activate specific muscle groups for facilitating function.

Functional Independence Measure (FIM): Instrument used to measure the extent of disability based on the responses to 18 items covering areas of self-care, sphincter control, mobility, locomotion, communication, and social cognition.

functional life scale: Measures the effects of a person's impairments on his or her ability to participate in daily activities at home rather than in a rehabilitation setting. It uses 44 items, each rated on a five-point scale.

functional limitation: Restriction of the ability to perform a physical action, activity, or task in an efficient, typically expected, or competent manner.

functional mobility: Moving from one position or place to another (during performance of everyday activities), such as in-bed mobility, wheelchair mobility, and transfers (wheelchair, bed, car, tub, toilet, tub/shower, chair, floor). Performing functional ambulation and transporting objects.[AOTA Framework]

functional muscle testing: Performance-based muscle assessment in particular positions simulating functional tasks and activities and usually under specific test conditions.

functional position: Hand configuration predominantly used in hand splinting in the past decades for hands that required immobilization. It involves 20 to 30 degrees wrist extension, 45 degrees metacarpal joint flexion, 30 degrees proximal interphalangeal joint flexion, and 20 degrees distal interphalangeal joint flexion, with the thumb abducted.

functional reach: A simple clinical measure of functional balance that quantifies one's forward reach capacity prior to loss of balance. Measures one's ability to move center of gravity to the margins of the base of support.

functional reserve: Refers to the excess or redundant function that is present in virtually all physiologic systems.

functioning: Focus on the performance of everyday activities.[C]

furuncle: A painful nodule formed in the skin by circumscribed inflammation of the corium and subcutaneous tissue, enclosing a central slough or "core." It is caused by bacteria, which enter through the hair follicles or sudoriparous glands.

G

gag reflex: Involuntary contraction of the pharynx and elevation of the soft palate is elicited in most normal individuals by touching the pharyngeal wall or back of the tongue.

gait: The manner or style of locomotion (walking), including rhythm, cadence, and speed.

galactosemia: Recessive, inherited metabolic disorder that prevents an individual from converting galactose to glucose, which results in serious physical and mental challenges.

Galileo, Galilei (1564–1642): Italian mathematician, physicist, and astronomer whose work anticipated and revolutionized the experimental methods of scientific inquiry. His support of Copernicus' work on the solar system led to 8 years of house arrest by the Inquisition.

galvanic skin response (GSR): Change in the electrical resistance of the skin as a response to different stimuli.

Galveston Orientation and Amnesia Test (GOAT): Ten-question test that measures amnesia and disorientation in persons with closed-head injury.

ganglion: A mass of nerve cells serving as a center from which impulses are transmitted. A cystic tumor on a tendon sheath.

gangrene: Decay of tissue in a part of the body when the blood supply is obstructed by disease or injury.

gastric intubation: Forced feeding, usually through a nasogastric tube.

gastric lavage: Washing out the stomach with repeated flushings of water.

gate control theory: The pain modulation theory developed by Melzak and Wall who proposed that presynaptic inhibition in

Jacobs, K., & Simon, L. (Eds.). *Quick Reference Dictionary for Occupational Therapy, Sixth Edition* (pp. 119-126).
© 2015 SLACK Incorporated.

the dorsal gray matter of the spinal cord results in blocking of pain impulses from the periphery.

gatekeeper: A primary care physician who is responsible for coordinating all services.

gathers: Collects together needed or misplaced tools and materials, including (a) collecting located supplies into the workspace and (b) collecting and replacing materials that have spilled, fallen, or been misplaced.[AOTA Framework]

gazes: Uses eyes to communicate and interact with others.[AOTA Framework]

gender expression: The manner in which a person represents or expresses their gender identity to others (Substance Abuse and Mental Health Services Administration, 2014).

gender identity: A person's internal sense of being male, female, or something else. Since gender identity is internal, one's gender identity is not necessarily visible to others (Substance Abuse and Mental Health Services Administration, 2014). Realization of a child that males and females are different due to physical characteristics. *Synonym*: core gender identity.

gender stability: Realization that gender will stay the same throughout a lifetime.

gene: A unit of heredity composed of DNA. In classical genetics, a gene is visualized as a discrete particle, forming part of a chromosome, that determines a particular characteristic.

gene flow: The exchange of genes among populations either directly by migration or by diffusion of genes over many generations.

General Adaptation Syndrome (GAS): Used by Hans Selye to describe the body's generalized defensive response to prolonged stress or noxious stimuli in the environment. This syndrome consists of an alarm reaction, a resistance stage, and an exhaustion stage.

generalization: Applying previously learned concepts and behaviors to a variety of new situations[UTIII]; skills and performance in applying specific concepts to a variety of related solutions.

generalized anxiety disorder: Persistent diffused sense of anxiety that is not triggered by any specific object, activity, or situation.

general systems theory: Conceptualizes the individual as an open system that evolves and undergoes different forms of growth, development, and change through an ongoing interaction with the external environment.

generational inequity: Social policy concerned with the condition in which an aging segment of society is unfair to younger members because older adults pile up advantages by receiving large allocations of resources such as Social Security and Medicare.

genes: Biologic unit that contains the hereditary blueprints for the development of an individual from one generation to the next.

genetic adaptation: Changes in biological characteristics to facilitate survival in a particular location, thought to be an evolutionary response to environmental circumstances.

genetic drift: The random change of gene frequencies over time, which happens in all populations but can take place rapidly in small populations.

geniculostriate system: Visual system pathways that transmit information for identifying the nature of the objects in the environment.

genital prolapse: The falling out or slipping out of place of an internal organ, such as the uterus, rectum, vagina, or bladder.

genome: The complete set of genetic information in every living organism. The human genome consists of 3 billion matching pairs of nucleotides.

genotype: The genetic constitution of an organism or group.

geriatric day care: Ambulatory health care facility for older adults.

Geriatric Functional Rating Scale: Assessment used to assist in making independent living decisions.

geriatrics: Area of study concerned with medical care in old age.

germinal period: Stage or interval of time from conception to implantation of the blastocyte to the uterus, approximately 8 to 10 days.

gerontological tripartite: Approach to the study of aging that collectively combines three phenomena of the aging process: the biological capacity for survival, the psychological capacity for adaptation, and the sociological capacity for the fulfillment of social roles.

gerontology (GER): Area of study concerned with care, health issues, and special problems of growing old.

Gesell Preschool Test: Norm-referenced test for children 2½ to 6 years that assesses personal, social, communication, gross motor, and fine motor skills.

gestation: Total period of time the baby is carried in the uterus, approximately 40 weeks in humans.

gestures: Uses movements of the body to indicate, demonstrate, or add emphasis.^{AOTA Framework}

getting older younger: Refers to children who are using clothes, make-up, etc., that are typically used at an older age. *Synonym*: down-aging.

Glasgow Coma Scale: Scale for assessing level of consciousness in trauma; specific numerical values are used.

glaucoma: Causes loss of vision when fluid pressure in the eye damages the optic nerve.

globin: The protein constituent of hemoglobin; also any member of a group of proteins similar to the typical globin.

glomerulus: A tuft or cluster; used in anatomical nomenclature as a general term to designate such a structure, as one composed of blood vessels or nerve fibers.

glottis: The vocal apparatus of the larynx, consisting of the true vocal cords and the opening between them (rima glottidis).

glucagon: A hyperglycemic-glycogenolytic factor thought to be secreted by the pancreas in response to hypoglycemia or stimulation by the growth hormone of the anterior pituitary gland.

glucocorticoid: Hormone from the adrenal cortex that raises blood sugar and reduces inflammation.

glucose: A thick, syrupy, sweet liquid generally made by incomplete hydrolysis of starch.

glucosuria: Presence of glucose in the urine.

gluten: A tenacious elastic protein substance found in foods processed from wheat and related grain species, including barley and rye.

gluten intolerance: Refers to people who experience unpleasant symptoms following gluten ingestion but do not have celiac disease. Has been replaced in some fields with the term *non-celiac gluten sensitivity*.

glycogenesis: The formation or synthesis of glycogen.

glycogenolysis: The splitting up of glycogen in the body tissue.

glycoprotein: A substance produced metabolically that creates osmotic force.

goal: Measurable and meaningful, occupation-based, long-term or short-term aim directly related to the client's ability and need to engage in desired occupations (AOTA, 2013a, p. S35).[OTPF 2014]

goal state: Predetermined situation in which a problem's solution is directed toward the goal.

Golgi tendon organ (GTO): Sensory receptors in the tendons of muscles that monitor muscle tension.

goniometer: Instrument for measuring movement at a joint.

goniometry: Measurement of the angle of the joint or a series of joints.

Google Scholar: A search engine that specifically looks for scholarly articles across the Internet. A useful tool to begin researching articles and to assemble reference lists.

gout: Painful metabolic disease that is a form of acute arthritis; characterized by inflammation of the joints, especially of those in the foot or knee.

graded activity: Activity that has been modified in one or more ways in order to provide the appropriate therapeutic demand or challenge for a person.

Graded Exercise Test: Physical performance of measured, incremental workloads with measurement of physiologic response. Used to assess physiologic response to exercise stress for the determination of cardiac and respiratory status.

grading: Viewing an activity on a continuum from simple to complex, typically grading an activity more challenging as a person has gained skill.

grandfather clause: Ruling or law that allows occupational therapy assistants not formally trained to earn credentials once formal training began for all occupational therapy assistants.

grandiosity: An exaggerated sense of one's importance, power, or status.

grand mal: Type of seizure in which there is a sudden loss of consciousness immediately followed by a generalized convulsion.

granulation tissue: The formation of a mass of tiny red granules of newly formed capillaries, as on the surface of a wound that is healing.

granulocyte: Any cell containing granules, especially a granular leukocyte. A heterogeneous class of leukocytes characterized by a multilobed nucleus and intracellular granules. Granulocytes include neutrophils, eosinophils, basophils, and mast cells.

granulocytosis: Increase in circulating granulocyte number.

graphesthesia: Ability to identify letters or designs on the basis of tactile input to the skin.

graphomotor: Pertains to movement involved in writing.

gratification: Ability to receive pleasure, either immediate (immediately upon engaging in an activity) or delayed (after completion of the activity).

gravitational insecurity: Overresponse to gravity/movement.

gravity: Constant force that affects almost every motor act characterized by heaviness or weight.

gray matter: Area of the central nervous system that contains the cell bodies.

greater trochanter: The bony prominence that gives attachment to the hip abductor muscles.

grip force: Pressure exerted on a held object or in lifting an object.

grips: Pinches or grasps task objects with no "grip slips."[AOTA Framework]

grooming: Obtaining and using supplies; removing body hair (use of razors, tweezers, lotions, etc.); applying and removing cosmetics; washing, drying, combing, styling, and brushing hair; caring for nails (hands and feet), skin, ears, and eyes; applying deodorant.[UTIII]

gross coordination: Using large muscle groups for controlled, goal-directed movements.[UTIII]

gross domestic product (GDP): Represents the market value of the total output of the goods and services produced by a nation's economy.

gross motor pattern of development: Mastery of larger muscles (proximal musculature); takes place before fine motor development.

grounded theory: A qualitative method of research that uses systematic inductive guidelines for collecting and analyzing data.

group: Collective of individuals (e.g., family members, workers, students, community members).[OTPF 2014] Plurality of individuals (three or more) who are in contact with one another, who take each other into account, and who are aware of some common goal.

group content: What a group is doing and saying at a particular point in time.

group development: Stages a group goes through as members progress from initiation to termination.

group dynamics: Forces that influence the interrelationships of members and ultimately affect group outcome.

group interaction skill: Ability to participate in a variety of primary groups.

group intervention: Skilled knowledge and use of leadership techniques in various settings to facilitate learning and acquisition by clients across the lifespan of skills for participation, including basic social interaction skills, tools for self-regulation, goal setting, and positive choice making, through the dynamics of group and social interaction. Groups may be used as a method of service delivery.[OTPF 2014]

group leader: Role of observer, group designer, role model, and climate setter.

group phases: Phases of group development in terms of leader, group member, and activity roles.

group polarization: The effect that causes a group to adopt a more extreme attitude after a group discussion than it had before the discussion.

group process: Interpersonal relationship among participants in a group.

group roles: Patterns of behavior shared by group members and necessary for the group to function and meet its goals; often categorized as expressive and instrumental.

group spokesperson: A religious authority, tribal elder, or public figure associated with a recognized organization who represents a member of an ethnic or social group, usually by making pronouncements on the ethical dimensions of an issue.

group therapy: Any intervention directed toward groups of individuals rather than an individual alone.

growth potential: Belief in each person's inherent capacity to grow.[C]

guided search: Person is cued to help identify relevant information needed for problem solving.

Guides to the Evaluation of Permanent Impairment (4th ed.): Commonly used tool for rating permanent impairments; written by the American Medical Association. Converts medical information into numerical values, such as 95% to 100% impairment (Hansen & Atchison, 2000).

Guillain-Barré syndrome (GBS): Increased sensitivity response in the peripheral nervous system. Inflammation of the spinal nerve roots, peripheral nerves, and occasionally the cranial nerves. It also results in rapid paralysis of the limbs, accompanied by sensory loss and muscle atrophy.

gustatory: Interpreting tastes.[UTIII]

Guttman scale: Specific type of behavioral measurement scale that, when scored, results in an inclusive hierarchy of performance. Items on such a scale are ordered to ensure that if one performs a given item satisfactorily, then one must also have the ability to perform all previous items at a designated criterion level of performance.

gyral atrophy: Decreases in the gray or white matter, or both, of the brain.

H

habilitation: Health care services designed to assist people in acquiring, improving, minimizing the deterioration of, compensating for an impairment of, or maintaining (partially or fully) skills, function, or performance for participation in occupation and daily life activities (AOTA policy staff, personal communication, December 17, 2013).[OTPF 2014] Process of giving a person the resources to promote improvement in activities of daily living, including specialized treatment and training, thereby encouraging maximum independence.

habits: "Acquired tendencies to respond and perform in certain consistent ways in familiar environments or situations; specific, automatic behaviors performed repeatedly, relatively automatically, and with little variation" (Boyt Schell et al., 2014a, p. 1234). Habits can be useful, dominating, or impoverished and can either support or interfere with performance in areas of occupation (Dunn, 2000b).[OTPF 2014]

habit spasm: Tic that lasts for a long period of time.

habit training: Developed by Slagle to provide routine and occupation to severely ill patients.

habituate: Process of accommodating to a stimulus through repeated diminishing exposure.

habituation subsystem: Conceptual subsystem in the Model of Human Occupation that houses the ability to organize skills into roles and routines.

half-circle goniometer: Instrument that is used to measure movement of the wrist joint. It only allows measurement in one direction.

Jacobs, K., & Simon, L. (Eds.). *Quick Reference Dictionary for Occupational Therapy, Sixth Edition* (pp. 127-139).
© 2015 SLACK Incorporated.

half-lapboard: An example of an adaptive device that provides support to a patient's or client's hemiplegic arm.

half-life: Measure of the amount of time required for 50% of a drug to be eliminated from the body.

hallucinate: Sense (e.g., sight, hearing, smell, taste, or touch) of something that does not exist externally.

halo effect: Error based on the fact that if a person is believed to possess one positive trait, he or she may possess others as well.

haloperidol: Tranquilizer used to relieve anxiety and tension in the treatment of schizophrenia and other psychiatric disorders. Common side effects are muscle incoordination and restlessness. *Trade name*: Haldol.

Halsted-Reitan Neuropsychological Battery: Battery that tests perceptual, intellectual, and motor skills and performance.

handicap: Disadvantage, resulting from an impairment or disability, that limits or prevents the fulfillment of a role that is normal (depending on age, sex, and social and cultural factors) for that individual.

handicapping situation: A barrier to the performance of an activity (a nonaccessible building, an attitude discrimination, a policy that denies access).

handles: Supports, stabilizes, and holds tools and materials in an appropriate manner that protects them from damage, falling, or dropping.AOTA Framework

hand-over-hand: Treatment technique where the occupational therapy assistant moves to assist the correct movement.

haptic technology: A tactile feedback technology that takes advantage of the sense of touch by applying forces, vibrations, or motions to the user.

hardiness: Personal characteristics that function to resist succumbing to the negative effects of dealing with stressful life events.

harmony with nature: A value orientation found in some cultures that suggests that humans must live in harmony with natural phenomena.

Hawaii Early Learning Profile (HELP): Criteria-referenced test for children age 0 to 36 months that assesses personal, social, communication, cognition, self-help, gross motor, fine motor, and visual-motor integration.

Hawthorne effect: Research error due to response differences paid to the participant by the researcher.

Hayflick's limit: Biologic limit to the number of times a cell is able to reproduce.

hazard: State that could potentially harm a person or do damage to property.

head injury (HI): Caused by direct impact to the head, most commonly from traffic accidents, falls, industrial accidents, wounds, or direct blows.

health: "State of complete physical, mental, and social well-being, and not merely the absence of disease or infirmity" (WHO, 2006, p. 1).[OTPF 2014] Health is more than the absence of disease (WHO, 1986); from an occupational perspective, health includes having choice, abilities, and opportunities for engaging in meaningful patterns of occupation for looking after self, enjoying life, and contributing to the social and economic fabric of a community over the lifespan to promote health, well-being, and justice through occupation (adapted from CAOT, 1997a, 2002).[CAOT]

Health Belief Model (HBM): This model is based on the concept that a person's health-related behavior depends on the person's perception of four critical areas: the severity of a potential illness or injury, the person's susceptibility to that illness, the benefits of taking preventative action, and the barriers to taking action.

healthcam: Camera that takes pictures of movement and is calibrated to measure the distance moved.

health education: A combination of educational, organizational, economic, and environmental supports for behavior conducive to health.

health informatics: Use of information technologies for health care data collection, storage, and analysis to enhance health care decisions and improve quality and efficiency of health care services (AOTA, 2014a).

health literacy: An individual's ability to read, understand, and use health care information to make decisions and follow instructions for treatment.

health maintenance: Developing and maintaining routines for illness prevention and wellness promotion, such as physical fitness, nutrition, and decreasing health risk behaviors.

health maintenance organization (HMO): Prepaid organized health care delivery system.

Health Maintenance Organization Act of 1973: U.S. federal law that provided for the planning and development of health maintenance organizations; encourages less ambulatory care.

health management and maintenance: Developing, managing, and maintaining routines for health and wellness promotion, such as physical fitness, nutrition, decreasing health risk behaviors, and medication routines.AOTA Framework

health policy: Set of initiatives taken by government to direct resources toward promoting, improving, and maintaining the health of its citizens.

health promotion: "Process of enabling people to increase control over, and to improve, their health. To reach a state of complete physical, mental, and social well-being, an individual or group must be able to identify and realize aspirations, to satisfy needs, and to change or cope with the environment" (WHO, 1986). OTPF 2014

health status: A condition in which one successfully and satisfactorily performs occupations (adapted from McColl, Law, & Stewart, 2002).AOTA Framework

hearing: The act of perceiving sound.

heart disease: Any of the diseases of the heart.

heart failure (HF): The inability of the heart to pump enough blood to maintain an adequate flow to and from the body tissues.

heart-lung machine: Performs functions of the heart and lungs during open heart surgery so these organs may be operated on.

heat therapy: Application of heat on a body part used to relieve the symptoms of musculoskeletal disorders.

heavy work: Exerting up to 50 to 100 pounds of force occasionally, 25 to 50 pounds of force frequently, or 10 to 20 pounds of force constantly to move objects.

heeds: Uses goal-directed task actions that are focused toward the completion of the specified task (i.e., the outcome originally agreed on or specified by another) without behavior that is driven or guided by environmental cues (i.e., "environmentally cued" behavior).^{AOTA Framework}

hegemony: Domination or leadership, especially the predominant influence of one state over another.

helplessness: Psychological state characterized by a sense of powerlessness or the belief that one is not capable of meeting an environmental demand competently.

hemangioma: Benign tumor composed of newly formed blood vessels clustered together.

hematocrit (Hct): The volume percentage of erythrocytes in whole blood.

hematoma: Localized collection of blood in an organ or within a tissue.

hemianesthesia: Total loss of sensation to either the left or right side of the body.

hemianopsia: Blindness in one half of the field of vision in one or both eyes.

hemiparesis: Weakness of the left or right side of the body.

hemiplegia (hemi): Condition in which half of the body is paralyzed.

hemoglobin (Hgb): The oxygen-carrying pigment of the erythrocytes, formed by the developing erythrocyte in bone marrow.

hemolysis: The liberation of hemoglobin. The separation of the hemoglobin from the corpuscles and its appearance in the fluid in which the corpuscles are suspended.

hemolytic: Pertaining to, characterized by, or producing hemolysis.

hemophilia: Lack of clotting factors that results in a hemorrhage.

hemoptysis: Expectoration of blood due to hemorrhage in the respiratory system.

hemorrhage: The escape of large quantities of blood from a blood vessel; heavy bleeding.

hemothorax: A collection of blood in the pleural cavity.

hepatitis: Inflammation of the liver.

here-and-now experience: Immediate experience in the group is examined as a projection of the person's past and provides members with an opportunity to test new and more adaptive interpersonal skills.

hereditary: The genetic transmission of a particular quality or trait from parent to offspring.

hernia: The protrusion of all or part of an organ through a tear in the wall of the surrounding structure, such as the protrusion of part of the intestine through the abdominal muscles.

herniated vertebral disc: Weakness in the annulus allowing the nucleus pulposus to protrude; presses against nerve root and spinal cord.

heroin: Highly addictive narcotic from the opium family.

heterograft: Grafted skin taken from an animal, usually a pig. *Also known as* xenograft.

heterotopic ossification: Abnormal calcifications at shoulder, elbow, hip, or knee joint, resulting in redness, swelling, limitations in range of motion, and pain.

HET Model (Human-Environment-Technology Model): Conceptual framework designed to convey the relationship between human performance deficits and the use of technologies to address these deficits.

heuristic: Clinical reasoning strategies, or shortcuts, that simplify complex cognitive tasks.

hidrosis: Formation and excretion of sweat.

hierarchy: A ranking system having a series of levels running from lowest to highest.

high longevity: Long life.

high power distance (HPD): Describes a culture or organization where inequality is accepted.

high technology: Systems and devices with more complex components (which may have alternative features) and individualized adjustments (which are not routinely used or commonly available to the public).

hilus: A depression or pit at the part of an organ where the vessels and nerves enter.

hip fracture: Break in the femur in the neck region, trochanter, or upper shaft. Five types exist based on fracture location: subcapital, transcervical, basilar, intertrochanteric, or subtrochanteric. Four classifications exist based on degree of bone segment displacement: incomplete, complete with no displacement, partially displaced, or completely displaced.

hippocampus: A nuclear complex forming the medial margin of the cortical mantle of the cerebral hemisphere forming part of the limbic system.

hippotherapy (HPOT): Treatment that uses the multidimensional movement of the horse to help patients/clients achieve functional outcomes.

hirsutism: Excessive growth of hair in unusual places, especially in women.

histogram: Bar graph.

history (Hx): Type of interview (structured, semi-structured, or unstructured) during which information about specific areas of functional performance is elicited. Historical information can be gathered directly from the person or indirectly through the reports of others who are familiar with his or her past performance.

history of ideas: Discipline that studies the history and development of ideas and theories in terms of their origins and influences.

history-taking interview: An interview used to elicit information about the patient's medical, family, marriage, sexual, and occupational histories.

histrionic personality disorder: A personality disorder characterized by attention seeking, excitability, emotional instability, and self-dramatization (Levine, Walsh, & Schwartz, 1996).

holism: A "view of persons as whole beings, integrated in mind, body, and spirit" (CAOT, 1997a, 2002, p. 181).[CAOT] Philosophical theory that wholes are greater than the sum of their parts. In health care, treating of the whole person rather than the symptoms of a disease. First used in modern times by J.C. Smuts in 1928.

holistic: A concept in which understanding is gained by examination of all parts working as a whole.

holophrase: Infants' one-word utterances.

home establishment and management: Obtaining and maintaining personal and household possessions and environment (e.g., home, yard, garden, appliances, vehicles), including maintaining and repairing personal possessions (clothing and household items) and knowing how to seek help or whom to contact.[AOTA Framework]

home health program: Health or rehabilitation services provided in a client's home.

homeostasis: Physiological system used to maintain internal processes despite changes in the environment.

hominid: Of the primate family including humans and their fossil ancestors (Latin: Homo, homin = man).

***Homo*:** The genus of primates that includes modern humans (modern *Homo sapiens* sometimes known as *Homo sapien sapiens*, the only living representative) and various extinct species, of which four or five are usually recognized although the number is uncertain.

- ***H. habilis*:** the earliest species (small and large forms, probably two species)

- ***H. erectus*:** descended from *H. habilis*

- ***H. sapiens*:** descended from *H. erectus*

- Neanderthal man (***H. neanderthalensis***)

***Homo erectus*:** A direct ancestor of modern man who appeared about 1.5 million years ago and lived to 300,000 years ago. Fossils of *H. erectus*, which are sometimes called Pithecanthropus (ape man), are similar to present-day man except that there was a prominent ridge above the eyes and no forehead or chin. They had crude stone tools and used fire.

homogamy: Notion that similar interests and values are important in forming strong, lasting personal relationships.

homogeneity of variance: Assumption that the variability within each of the sample groups should be fairly similar.

Homo habilis: The oldest of the species. Fossils of *H. habilis* were found in the Olduvai Gorge in Tanzania. Estimated to have lived 2.3 to 1.5 million years ago. Gracile or delicate-boned toolmaker.

homologous: Corresponding in structure, position, and origin. Derived from an animal of the same species but of different genotype.

homonymous hemianopsia: Loss of the same side of the field of vision in both eyes usually due to optic tract damage.

homoscedasticity: Standard deviations of the Y scores along the regression line is fairly equal.

homosexuality: Sexual attraction to another of the same sex.

homunculus: Commonly used illustration representing anatomical structures and functions of the primary motor and/or sensory areas of the brain.

hope: "Perceived ability to produce pathways to achieve desired goals and to motivate oneself to use those pathways" (Rand & Cheavens, 2009, p. 323).[OTPF 2014]

horizontal or job extension: Used as an administrative control in ergonomics, the job content is increased by giving the worker a greater number of tasks to perform all within the same level of responsibility.

horizontal plane: Runs transversely across, dividing the body into upper and lower parts. *Synonym*: transverse plane.

Hormic School of Psychology: An early psychological school of thought centered on vital or purposeful energy and related to Jung's view of the importance of an individual's search for meaning in life.

hormones: Chemical substances produced in the body that have a specific effect on the activity of a certain organ; applied to substances secreted by endocrine glands and transported in the blood stream to the target organ on which their effect is produced.

Hospice Assessment of Occupational Function (HAOF): Designed to integrate hospice philosophy and practice, occupational therapy history and philosophy, occupational science, and occupational behavior. The person is viewed through all characters of his or her personality, including culture, religion, and primary caregiver situations.

hospice programs: Care for terminally ill clients and emotional support for them and their families.

hot-cold belief system: Folk medical system in which certain substances in the environment and the individual are classified as hot or cold and have specific illness-causing or curative properties related to that classification.

household maintenance: Maintaining home, yard, garden, appliances, vehicles, and household items.[UTIII]

human: An organism that maintains and balances itself in the world of reality and actuality by being in active life and active use.

human chorionic gonadotropin (HCG): A growth hormone that influences the gonads.

human development: Ongoing changes in the structure, thought, or behavior of a person that occur as a function of both biologic and environmental influences.

human factors engineering: Profession that investigates and optimizes function of interactions between humans and machines.

human immunodeficiency virus (HIV): Virus that causes AIDS, which is contracted through exposure to contaminated blood or bodily fluid (e.g., semen or vaginal secretions).

humanism: A nonreligious philosophy based on belief in potential of human nature rather than in religious or transcendental values.

human subject: Living individual about whom an investigator conducting research obtains data through intervention or interaction with the individual or identifiable private information.

humerus: Long bone of the upper arm.

humoral immunity: Immune function via soluble factors found in blood and other body fluids.

Huntington's chorea: Degenerative disease of the basal ganglia in the brain. It is characterized by abnormalities in postural reactions, trunk rotation, distribution of tone, and extraneous movements.

hyaluronic acid: Substance that lubricates cells under compressive forces.

hydrocele: Accumulation of serous fluid in a sac-like cavity, especially in the testes.

hydrocephalus: Enlargement of the head due to an increase in cerebrospinal fluid within the brain, which may lead to necrosis of brain tissue by compromising its blood supply. **overt:** Head enlarges if onset is before age 2 years. **occult:** Head size remains normal.

hydrocephaly: Condition characterized by abnormal accumulation of cerebrospinal fluid within the ventricles of the brain, which leads to enlargement of the head.

hydrostatic weighing: Underwater weighing to determine body volume; body volume is used to determine body density from which body composition can be calculated.

hydrotherapy: Intervention using water.

hyperactivity: Excessive level of activity.

hyperbaric oxygen: Oxygen under greater pressure than normal atmospheric pressure.

hyperbilirubinemia: An excess of bilirubin in the blood.

hypercalcemia: Excessive amount of calcium in the blood.

hypercapnia: Excessive amount of carbon dioxide in the blood.

hypercard: Software program available for the computer that aids in the programming of user-friendly mouse or pushbutton-oriented applications.

hypercholesterolemia: An excess of cholesterol in the blood.

hyperglycemia: Abnormally increased content of sugar in the blood.

hyperkalemia: Excessive amount of potassium in the blood.

hyperlipidemia: Abnormally high concentration of lipids in the blood.

hypermetria: Distortion of target-directed voluntary movement. The limb moves beyond its target.

hypermobility: Condition of excessive motion in joints.

hypernatremia: Excessive amount of sodium in the blood.

hyperplasia: Increased number of cells.

hyperpnea: Abnormal increase in the depth and rate of the respiratory movements.

hyperreflexia: Hyperactive or repeating (clonic) reflexes. These usually indicate an interruption of corticospinal and other descending pathways that influence the reflex arc, usually due to a lesion above the level of the spinal reflex pathways.

hypersomnia: Sleeping for excessive lengths of time.

hypertension (Htn): High arterial blood pressure, ranging from 140 to 200 mm Hg systolic and 90 to 110 mm Hg diastolic. Any abnormally high blood pressure or a disease of which this is the chief sign.

hyperthesias: Abnormally increased sensitivity to stimulation.

hypertonus: Muscular state wherein muscle tension is greater than desired; spasticity; hypertonus increases resistance to passive stretch.

hypertrophic scarring: Excessive markings left by the healing process in the skin or an internal organ.

hypertrophy: Increased cell size leading to increased tissue size.

hyperuricemia: Excess of uric acid in the blood.

hyperventilation: Increased expiration and inspiration.

hypnagogic hallucinations: Vivid, dream-like experiences that occur while dozing or falling asleep.

hypnotic: Drugs that produce sleep.

hypochondriasis: In the absence of medical evidence, a sustained conviction that one is ill or about to become ill; abnormal concern about one's health.

hypokinetic disease: Complications arising from inactivity. *Synonym*: disuse syndrome.

hypometria: Distortion of target-directed voluntary movement in which the limb falls short of reaching its target.

hyponatremia: Decreased amount of sodium in the blood.

hypoplasia: Defective or incomplete development (e.g., osteogenesis imperfecta).

hyporeflexia: An absent or diminished response to tapping. It usually indicates a disease that involves one or more of the components of the two-neuron reflex arc.

hypospadias: Abnormal congenital opening of the male urethra on the undersurface of the penis.

hypotension: Abnormally low blood pressure.

hypothesis: Conclusion drawn before all the facts are known; working assumption that serves as a basis for further investigation; a plausible explanation or best guess about a situation.

hypothetical-deductive reasoning: Form of problem solving in which several possible ideas are tested in order of probability to reach a solution.

hypotonicity: Decrease in the muscle tone and stretch reflex of a muscle resulting in decreased resistance to passive stretch and hyporesponsiveness to sensory stimulation.

hypotonus: Muscular state wherein muscle tension is lower than desired; flaccidity; hypotonus decreases resistance to passive stretch.

hypovolemia: Abnormally decreased volume of circulating fluid (plasma) in the body.

hypoxia: Deficiency of oxygen in the blood. *See* anoxia.

hysterectomy: Surgical removal of the uterus.

hysterical conversion: Somatoform disorder characterized by the loss of functioning of some part of the body not due to any physical disorder but apparently due to psychological conflicts.

iatrogenic illnesses or injuries: Illnesses and injuries caused by the process of health care.

ICD code: International Classification of Diseases code used for billing and reimbursement purposes.

ICF: International Classification of Functioning, Disability and Health developed by the World Health Organization.

icing: "Ice is applied in small, overlapping circles for 5 to 10 minutes until skin flushing and numbness occur" (Trombly, 1995, p. 662).

iconic representation: Memory of the stimuli in terms of pictorial images or graphics that stand for a concept without defining it fully.

id: In psychoanalytic theory, the unconscious part of the psyche, which is the source of primitive, instinctual drives and strives for self-preservation and pleasure. The primary process element of personality.

ideation: An internal process in which the nervous system gathers information from stimuli in the environment or recruits information from memory stores to formulate an idea about what to do.

ideational apraxia: Inability to formulate a plan to complete request commanded (i.e., attempt to strike a cigarette instead of a match).

identity: "A composite definition of the self and includes an interpersonal aspect. . .an aspect of possibility or potential (who we might become), and a values aspect (that suggests importance and provides a stable basis for choices and decisions). . . . Identity can be viewed as the superordinate view of ourselves that includes both self-esteem and self-concept but also importantly reflects and is influenced by the larger social world in which we find ourselves" (Christiansen, 1999, pp. 548-549). [OTPF 2008] Gradually emerging and continually changing sense of self; used in Erik Erikson's theory of development.

identity diffusion: Eriksonian psychosocial crisis in which integration of childhood skills, goals, and roles does not occur.

ideomotor apraxia: Interference with the transmission of the appropriate impulses from the brain to the motor center; results in the inability to translate an idea into motion (e.g., a person who knows what he or she wants to do but cannot do it).

idiopathic: Designating a disease whose cause is unknown or uncertain.

illness: Experience of devalued changes in being and in social function. It primarily encompasses personal, interpersonal, and cultural reactions to sickness.

illusion: A misinterpretation of a real experience, such as a mirage in which it appears that water is on a road that is known to be dry.

imaginative play: Activities that include make-believe games.

imbalance: Lack of balance, as in proportion, force, and functioning.

immediate recall: Ability to recall information within 1 minute of it being received.

immediate return economies: Hand-to-mouth subsistence existence.

immunoglobulin (Ig): Glycoprotein found in blood and other body fluids that may exert antibody activity. All antibodies are Ig molecules, but not all Ig exhibits antibody activity.

immunosuppression: Decrease in responsiveness of the immune system with an imbalance of the antigen-antibody relationship.

impaired auditory processing: Difficulty utilizing auditory information efficiently and effectively.

impairments: Problems in body function or structure such as a significant deviation or loss.[ICF]

impingement: To trap and compress.

implementation: The "process of activating a plan, versus intervention which implies doing to or for people" (CAOT, 1997a, 2002, p. 181).[CAOT]

impotence: Weakness, especially inability of the male to achieve or maintain erection.

impulsive: To act without planning or reflection.

inattention: Lack of attention span or concentration.

incidence rate (IR): Number of new cases per 100 workers years (which is equivalent to 200,000 work hours).

$$IR = \frac{\text{number of new cases during a time period} \times 200{,}000 \text{ hours}}{\text{total hours worked by all employees for that time period}}$$

inclusion area: Midpoint area of the normal curve.

inclusion stage: In group development, the stage where the individual is concerned with being accepted.

incoherence: Inability to express oneself in a way that others can understand; ideas are not presented in a related order.

incompetence: Failing to meet requirements; incapable; unskillful. Lacking strength and sufficient flexibility to transmit pressure, thus breaking or flowing under stress.

incontinence: Inability to control excretory functions.

indemnity: Standard fee-for-service insurance policies provided by employers, organizations, or individuals. Usually the most expensive type, this insurance covers service from any provider.

indemnity insurance: Type of insurance based on payments only when an illness or accident has occurred.

independence: "Self-directed state of being characterized by an individual's ability to participate in necessary and preferred occupations in a satisfying manner irrespective of the amount or kind of external assistance desired or required" (AOTA, 2002a, p. 660).^OTPF 2014

independent living movement: A political movement to promote a view of disability as a socially constructed phenomenon. Independent living represents a new attitude, a new set of organizing principles, and a new approach to service delivery aimed to ensure people with disabilities access to housing, health care, transportation, employment, education, and mobility. These aims are achieved through self-help and peer support, research and service development, and referral and advocacy.

independent practice association (IPA): Partnership, corporation, association, or other legal entity that has entered into an arrangement for provision of its services with persons who are licensed to practice medicine.

independent variable: Antecedent variable.

index individual: A person of interest in any social group; in studies of social support, the person who receives the support.

indirect patient care activities: Scheduling, setting up, supervision, documentation, meetings, education, etc.

indirect services: Those activities, strategies, and interventions provided to agencies and others to assist them in providing direct care services.

individual change: Stretching beyond former ways of thinking and doing, given time and openness to give voice to experiences of changing identity and to integrate new assumptions and perspectives, on a continuum and is interconnected with enabling social change.[CAOT]

individual habilitation plan (IHP): A written multidisciplinary plan of care for a developmentally disabled adult that identifies needs, strategies for meeting these needs, and the individuals involved in providing the program. This may be a part of a referral to physical therapy.

individualism: A social theory that emphasizes the importance of the individual.

individuality: Social relationship structure defined by degree of autonomy of the individual.

individualization: Focus on the unique differences of each person.[C]

individualized education plan (IEP): Interdisciplinary plan required for special education students in the United States under the provisions of Public Law 94-142. Allows parents or guardians to examine all school records and to participate with professionals in making educational placement decisions and in developing written diagnostic-prescriptive plans for school-aged children.

individualized family service plan (IFSP): Multidisciplinary, family-centered treatment plan documenting how the infant's or toddler's developmental and family needs will be addressed.

individual shared responsibility: This provision of the law applies to the self-employed and requires that each individual, beginning in January 2014, have basic health insurance coverage (known as minimum essential coverage) for each month, qualify for an exemption, or make a payment when filing a federal income tax return starting in 2015. Individuals will not have to make a payment under these rules if coverage is unaffordable, you spend less than 3 consecutive months without coverage, or you qualify for an exemption for several other reasons, including hardship and religious beliefs (Olafson, 2013).

Individuals with Disabilities Education Act (IDEA) (1990): U.S. federal legislation that provides resources to school-aged children with disabilities.

individual transition plan (ITP): Plan of activity and instruction based on a student's individual needs that will promote transition from school to post-school activities; ITP must be documented in the student's individualized education plan by age 14 years.

inductive fallacy: Overgeneralizing on the basis of too few observations.

inductive reasoning: Generation and testing of a hypothesis on the basis of evidence to indicate its validity.

industry: According to Erik Erikson and his theory of development, this is when children in elementary school focus on applying themselves in doing certain activities that are reflective of being successful in the adult world.

inelastic traction: Splinting method in which a series of splints that apply a minimal amount of tension or force are used and refitted every 2 or 3 days. This method has demonstrated effectiveness in increasing passive motion of joints that are stiffened. Inelastic traction is especially effective for chronically stiffened joints.

infancy: Time of development of a child from a few weeks after birth until the second year of life.

infantile myoclonic: Sudden, brief, involuntary muscle contractions producing head drops and flexion of extremities.

infarct: An area of coagulation necrosis in a tissue due to local anemia resulting from obstruction of circulation to the area.

infection: The state of being infected especially by the presence in the body of bacteria, protozoans, viruses, or other parasites.

inference: Possible result or conclusion that could be deduced from evaluation data.

inferential (predictive) statistics: Utilizing the measurements from the sample to anticipate characteristics of the population.

inferential therapy: Form of electrotherapy that applies a large variety of low-level frequencies to deep structures in the body. It is useful in treating swelling.

inferior (inf): From anatomical position, located away from the head.

inflammatory: Pertaining to or characterized by inflammation.

informal social network: People who provide support but are not connected with any formal social service agency.

informant interview: Interview in which a therapist gathers information about the client or environment from significant others.

informational support: A type of social support that informs, thereby reducing anxiety over uncertainty.

informed consent: Requirement that the person must be given adequate information about the benefits and risks of planned treatments or research before he or she agrees to the procedures.

inhalant: Compound or medication that is suitable for inhaling.

inhibition: Arrest or restraint of a process.

initiates: Starts or begins the next action or step without hesitation. AOTA Framework

innate goodness: View presented by Swiss-born French philosopher Jean-Jacques Rosseau, who stressed that children are inherently good.

innovation: Culture change through development of new technologies or ideas.

inotropic: Affecting the force or energy of muscular contractions. Either weakening or increasing the force of muscular contraction.

inpatient: Services delivered to the patient/client during hospitalization.

inquires: (a) Seeks needed verbal or written information by asking questions or reading directions or labels or (b) asks no unnecessary information questions (e.g., questions related to where materials are located or how a familiar task is performed).^{AOTA} Framework

inquiry-centered approach: A method of asking questions and gathering information to learn about culture in a specific situation.

insertion: Distal attachment of a muscle that exhibits most of the movement during muscular contraction.

inservice education: In-house seminars or special training sessions, either inside or outside the facility.

insiders: Members of a cultural group.

insight: Self-understanding.

in situ: Localized site, confined to one place (e.g., cancer that has not invaded neighboring tissues).

insomnia: Abnormal or prolonged inability to sleep.

instability: Description of a joint that has lost its structural integrity and is overtly hypermobile.

Instagram: An online photo-sharing and social networking service that enables its users to take pictures, apply digital filters to them, and post them online.

instant messaging (IMing): Sending short instantaneous messages to other users anywhere in the world who have Internet or phone data access. Many conversations are now conducted via instant messages.

instinctual drives: Aspect of the psychodynamic theory in which Freud believes that there are two primary instinctual impulses that demand gratification: sex and aggression.

institution: Any public or private entity or agency.

institutional ethnography: Examination of the social organization of institutions.

institutionalization: Effects of dehumanizing and depersonalizing characteristics of the environment that result in apathy, a significant decrease in motivation and activity, and increased passivity of an individual. Also refers to confinement.

instrumental activities of daily living (IADLs): Activities that support daily life within the home and community and that often require more complex interactions than those used in ADLs.^{OTPF 2014} Essential self-maintenance activities that are used to measure independent living capability that are not considered as basic daily living activities or self-care tasks.

insufficiency: Deficiency or inadequacy. The failure or inability of an organ or tissue to perform its normal function.

insurance denial: When a third party has denied payment for a service; organizations may appeal denials if they believe the criteria have not been equitably applied.

intake interview: Interview in which the therapist identifies the client's needs and his or her suitability for treatment.

integration: Unifying or bringing together; in children, the developmental ability to link successive actions instead of viewing each action as a separate, unrelated event; usually acquired by 2 years of age.

integumentary: Pertaining to or composed of skin.

intellectual disability: A disability characterized by significant limitations both in intellectual functioning and in adaptive behavior, which covers many everyday social and practical skills. People with intellectual disabilities may have limitations in skills such as communicating, taking care of him- or herself (activities of daily living), and social skills. Children with intellectual disabilities (sometimes called cognitive disabilities or mental retardation) may take longer to learn to speak, walk, and take care of their personal needs such as dressing or eating.

intelligence: Potential or ability to acquire, retain, and use experience and knowledge to reason and problem solve.

intelligence quotient (IQ): A measure of intelligence that takes into account both mental and chronological age.

intention tremor: Rhythmical, oscillatory movement initiated with an arm or hand.

interactional moment: A point in time in the interaction between two or more individuals.

interactive reasoning: One of three clinical reasoning styles used by occupational therapists. The process involves individualizing treatment for the specific needs of the client.

intercultural: Across or among multiple cultures.

interdecile range: Scores including the central 80% of a distribution.

interdependence: "Reliance that people have on one another as a natural consequence of group living" (Christiansen & Townsend, 2010, p. 419). "Interdependence engenders a spirit of social inclusion, mutual aid, and a moral commitment and responsibility to recognize and support difference" (Christiansen & Townsend, 2010, p. 187).[OTPF 2014] A concept that recognizes the mutual dependencies of individuals within social groups.

interdisciplinary: Relating to, or involving, two or more disciplines that are usually considered distinct, as in occupational and physical therapy.

interdisciplinary treatment plan: A plan of care, includes goals and interventions of all disciplines working with a patient.

interests: "What one finds enjoyable or satisfying to do" (Kielhofner, 2008, p. 42).[OTPF 2014]

interface: Program or device that links the way two or more pieces of equipment or person/machine units work together.

intermediate care facilities (ICF): Designed to give personal care, simple medical care, and intermittent nursing care.

intermediate-level practice: Competent entry-level skills practitioner with 1 to 3 years of experience.

intermittent positive-pressure breathing: Mechanical device that uses air pressure to inflate and deflate the lungs for breathing.

internal adjustment: Changes in individual beliefs or behavior that result from a learning situation.

internal environment: Aspects such as motivation, wellness, and emotional state.

internality: General term given for the extent to which people feel that their actions can influence their environment.

internal postural control: Ability of the body to support and control its own movement without reliance on supporting structures in the environment.

internal validity: The cause and effect relationship can be identified by the results of an experiment.

International Classification of Diseases (ICD): Disease classification system developed by the World Health Organization.

International Classification of Functioning, Disability and Health Framework (ICF): Recognizes disability as a universal human experience, placing all health conditions on an equal footing and allowing the focus to shift from cause to impact.

interneuron: Nerve cell that links motor and sensory nerves.

internodal: The space between two nodes; the segment of a nerve fiber connecting two nodes (often called internodal bundles or pathways).

interoceptive: Receptors activated by stimuli from within visceral tissues and blood tissues.

interpersonal: Occurring between oneself and others.

interpersonal skills: Using verbal and nonverbal communication to interact in a variety of settings.[UTIII]

interprofessional: Involving multiple health professions.

interprofessional education (IPE): Involves educators and learners from two or more health professions and their foundational disciplines who jointly create and foster a collaborative learning environment. The goal of these efforts is to develop knowledge, skills, and attitudes that result in interprofessional team behaviors and competence (Buring et al., 2009).

interval data: Measurements that are assigned values so the order and intervals between numbers are recognized.

intervention: "Process and skilled actions taken by occupational therapy practitioners in collaboration with the client to facilitate engagement in occupation related to health and participation. The intervention process includes the plan, implementation, and review" (AOTA, 2010, p. S107).[OTPF 2014]

intervention approaches: Specific strategies selected to direct the process of interventions on the basis of the client's desired outcomes, evaluation data, and evidence.[OTPF 2014]

intervention implementation: Ongoing actions taken to influence and support improved client performance. Interventions are directed at identified outcomes. Client's response is monitored and documented.[AOTA Framework]

intervention plan: A plan that will guide actions taken and that is developed in collaboration with the client. It is based on selected theories, frames of reference and evidence. Outcomes to be targeted are confirmed.[AOTA Framework]

intervention review: A review of the implementation plan and process as well as its progress toward targeted outcomes.[AOTA Framework]

intervertebral discs: Pads of fibrous elastic cartilage found between the vertebrae. They cushion the vertebrae and absorb shock.

intracranial: Occurring within the cranium.

intracultural variability: Difference among individuals within a group identified as representing a specific culture.

intradisciplinary: Treatment within a discipline.

intrafusal muscle: Striated muscle tissue found within the muscle spindle.

intrapersonal: Occurring within oneself.

intrinsic motivation: Concept in human development that proposes that people develop in response to an inherent need for exploration and activity.

intubation: The insertion of a tube; especially the introduction of a tube into the larynx through the glottis, performed for the introduction of an external source of oxygen.

intussusception: Telescoping of the bowel within itself.

invalid occupations: Coined by Tracy as activities for the disabled.

inventory: Assessment composed of a list of items to which the person gives responses.

inversion: Turning inward or inside out.

involuntary movement: Movement that is not done of one's own free will; not done by choice. Unintentional, accidental, not consciously controlled movement.

involution: A rolling or turning inward over a rim such as a toenail growing back into the soft tissue of the toe. Also a term used to describe the return of the uterus to the nonpregnant size and position following delivery of a baby.

involvement: Focus on the active participation of consumer.[C]

iodine: Element important for the development and functioning of the thyroid gland.

iontophoresis: A electrotherapeutic modality that creates ion transfer. It is the introduction of topically applied, physiologically active ions into the epidermis and mucous membranes of the body by the use of continuous direct current. The electrical principle of iontophoresis is that an electrically charged electrode will repel a similarly charged ion. This modality is used to "drive in" local anesthetics, anti-inflammatory agents, and edema reduction agents and is used to treat a variety of skin conditions. It has been found to be helpful in the treatment of calcium deposits, softening scars and adhesions, fungus infections, musculoskeletal inflammation conditions, edema reduction, muscle relaxant and vasodilatation, hyperhydrosis, bursitis, neuritis, and slow-healing wounds and ulcers.

ipsilateral: Situated on or affecting the same side.

ischemia: Reduced oxygen supply to a body organ or part.

ischemic heart disease: Lack of blood supply to the heart.

Islets of Langerhans: Irregular structures in the pancreas composed of cells smaller than the ordinary secreting cells. These masses (islands) of cells produce an internal secretion (insulin), which is connected with the metabolism of carbohydrates, and their degeneration is one of the causes of diabetes.

isoenzyme: One of the multiple forms in which a protein catalyst may exist in a single species, the various forms differing chemically, physically, and/or immunologically.

isokinetic strength: Force generated by a muscle contracting through a range of motion at a constant speed.

isolation: To separate from other people during an infectious disease or because of a fear of interrelating.

isometric contraction: Contraction of a muscle during which shortening or lengthening is prevented.

isometric strength: Force generated by a contraction in which there is no joint movement and minimal change in muscle length.

isotonic contraction: Contraction of a muscle during which the force of resistance remains constant throughout the range of motion.

isotonic strength: Force of contraction in which a muscle moves a constant load through a range of motion.

isthmus: Narrow structure connecting two larger parts.

itinerant: Traveling from place to place.

Jacobs Prevocational Skills Assessment (JPSA): Fifteen-task battery designed to provide a profile of skills and behaviors of adolescents with learning disabilities using a work sample system. Tasks include filing, money concept, work attitude, and environment mobility.

Jamar grasp dynamometer: Instrument used to measure the strength of a person's grip.

jamming: A proprioceptive technique in which intermittent joint approximation is used to facilitate co-contraction around a joint by eliciting postural responses.

jaundice: A condition in which the eyeballs, skin, and urine become abnormally yellowish as a result of increased amounts of bile pigments in the blood. Usually secondary to conditions such as hepatitis or liver failure.

jaw jerk: Closure of the mouth caused by striking the lower jaw while it hangs passively open; this reflex is rare.

JCAHO (Joint Commission on Accreditation of Healthcare Organizations): A private quality-measurement organization.

Jebsen-Taylor Hand Function Test: Dexterity test made up of seven subtests that measure different aspects of hand function often used in activities of daily living. Subtests include writing, card turning, picking up objects, simulated feeding, and stacking checkers.

Jewett brace: A hyperextension trunk brace that provides a single three-point force system via a sternal pad, suprapubic pad, and a thoracolumbar pad that restricts forward flexion in the thoracolumbar area.

Jacobs, K., & Simon, L. (Eds.). *Quick Reference Dictionary for Occupational Therapy, Sixth Edition* (pp. 153-155).
© 2015 SLACK Incorporated.

job acquisition: Identifying and selecting work opportunities and completing the application and interview processes.[UTIII]

job capacity evaluation: Assessment of the match between the person's capabilities and critical demands of a specific job.

job description: Provides a written statement of a particular position in order to identify, define, and describe its parameters.

job performance: Including work habits, such as attendance, punctuality, appropriate relationships with coworkers and supervisors, completion of assigned work, and compliance with the norms of the work setting (adapted from Mosey, 1996, p. 342).[AOTA Framework]

job satisfaction: Positive feelings arising from work-related tasks.

job specification: Based on a job description and used primarily in the hiring process, it states the minimum requirements needed for a position (e.g., level of education, length of experience, and skills).

joint capsule: Any sac or membrane enclosing the junction of the bones.

joint mobility: Functional joint play and flexibility allowing for freedom of joint movement.

joint mobilization: Passive movements performed on the patient that assist with increasing range of motion.

joint protection: Application of procedures to minimize joint stress.

joint range of motion (JROM): Freedom of motion in joints. A goniometer is used to measure joint mobility on a 180-degree scale.

joint receptor: Anatomically localized in joint capsules and ligaments, they include the Golgi-type endings, Golgi-Mazzoni corpuscles, Ruffini's corpuscle, and free nerve endings. In general, they detect joint movement in the gravitational field causing the discharge of receptors in the somatic, visual, and vestibular afferent systems to maintain posture and balance.

joints: Places in the body where bones articulate. The classifications are: synarthrosis (nonmoving joints), amphiarthrosis (slightly moving joints), and diarthrosis (freely moving joints).

Journal of Occupational Therapy Students (JOTS): Published by the American Occupational Therapy Association, a journal containing articles written by occupational therapy students.

judgment: The ability to use data or information to make a decision.

jump sign: A test that screens for binocular vision, which is when both eyes cannot focus on a single point or target. The patient/client focuses on an object and the therapist then covers one eye; if the uncovered eye "jumps" to refocus on the object, this is a positive jump sign.

junctional rhythm: Rapid heart rate with a characteristically inverted P wave often preceding, following, or falling within the QRS complex on an EKG. Causes are usually digitalis toxicity, acute inferior myocardial infarction, or heart failure.

justice: Notion that all cases should be treated alike and fairly in accord with general standards of right and wrong.

just right challenge: Refers to the right match between the challenge of the activity and the person's skills to perform it.

juvenile: Pertaining to youth or childhood diseases, such as juvenile diabetes or juvenile arthritis.

juvenile rheumatoid arthritis (JRA): A form of arthritis that affects children.

Kabat, Knott, and Voss Proprioceptive Neuromuscular Facilitation (PNF): This approach is based on the premise that stronger parts of the body are utilized to stimulate and strengthen the weaker parts.

kalemia: The presence of potassium in the blood.

Kegel exercises: Pelvic floor strengthening exercises developed by Dr. Arnold Kegel.

Keirsey-Bates test: Seventy-question temperament assessment tool. It breaks up personalities into 16 different combinations.

keratin: A scleroprotein that is the principal constituent of epidermis, hair, nails, and the organic matrix of the enamel of the teeth.

keratitis: Inflammation of the cornea.

keratosis: Any horny growth, such as a wart or callosity.

ketone: Any compound containing a carbonyl group.

ketosis: A condition characterized by an abnormally elevated concentration of ketone (acetone) bodies in the body tissues and fluids causing an acidosis. Also referred to as ketoacidosis.

keyboard emulating interface: Hardware device connected to the computer or a software program installed on the computer that allows input from an alternate device to be accepted as a standard keyboard input.

key informant approach: A needs assessment technique that asks information of individuals ("key informants") who are selected for their assumed familiarity with the needs of the community as a whole or with the target population for a potential program.

keyword method: Mnemonic system that uses a part of the word to be learned to make an association that triggers the recall of the desired meaning or information.

Jacobs, K., & Simon, L. (Eds.). *Quick Reference Dictionary for Occupational Therapy, Sixth Edition* (pp. 156-158). © 2015 SLACK Incorporated.

kinematic direction: Title of Splint Classification System category that defines which way the primary or major segments of joints are moved.

kinematics: Area of kinesiology that is not concerned with cause but rather with measuring, describing, and recording motions.

kinesics: The study of body movements, gestures, and postures as a means of communication. *Synonym*: body language.

kinesiology: Study and science of motion.

kinesthesia: Identifying the excursion and direction of joint movement[UTIII]; person's sense of position, weight, and movement in space. The receptors for kinesthesia are located in the muscles, tendons, and joints.

kinesthetic: Sense derived from end organs located in muscles, tendons, and joints and stimulated by movement; also called proprioception.

kinetics: Area of kinesiology that is concerned with cause, as well as the forces that produce, modify, or stop a motion.

kin selection: Natural selection of genes that tends to cause the individuals bearing them to be altruistic to close relatives. These relatives have a higher probability of bearing identical copies of those same genes than do other members of the population. Thus, kin selection for a gene that tends to cause an animal to share food with a close relative will result in the gene being spread through the population because it (unconsciously) benefits itself. The more closely two animals are related, the higher the probability that they share some identical genes and therefore the more closely their interests coincide. Parental care is a special case of kin selection.

kits: Pre-prepared materials for a craft project.

Klinefelter's syndrome: Characterized by the presence of an extra X chromosome in males, causing failure to develop secondary sex characteristics, enlarged breasts, poor musculature development, and infertility.

Klippel-Feil syndrome: Condition in which one or more vertebrae are fused together in the neck area, causing shortening of the cervical spine.

knowledge: Refers to the ability to seek and use task-related knowledge.[AOTA Framework]

knowledge translation: The exchange, synthesis, and ethically sound application of knowledge (CIHR, 2002), disseminated through empirical research, peers, and continuing education (Craik, 2003).[CAOT]

Kohlman Evaluation of Living Skills (KELS): Standardized test combining interview and task performance; used to evaluate an individual's ability to function safely and independently in the community.

Kohn's pores: Openings in the interalveolar septa of the lungs.

Korsakoff's psychosis: Memory disorder characterized by loss of long-term memory, confabulation, and confusion. Cause is often a vitamin B deficiency from chronic alcoholism.

Krebs cycle: Tricarboxylic acid cycle that results in the energy production of adenosine triphosphate.

Kurzweil reading machine: Computerized device that converts print into speech. The user places printed material over a scanner that "reads" the material aloud by means of an electronic voice.

Kussmaul's respiration: Air hunger (as seen in persons with chronic obstructive pulmonary disease).

kyphoscoliosis: Backward and lateral curvature of the spinal column, such as that seen in vertebral osteochondrosis (Scheuermann's disease).

kyphosis: Abnormal anteroposterior curving of the spine; hunchback or roundback.

labeling theory: Sociological theory that questions the medical model of psychiatric diagnosis and treatment.

labile: Changeable.

labyrinthine righting reflexes: Begins at birth and continues through life. The head orients to a vertical position with the mouth horizontal when the body is tipped or tilted. Tested with the eyes blindfolded.

laissez-faire style: Low involvement.

laminectomy: Surgical excision of the posterior arch of the vertebra.

Landau reflex: Seen with infants at 3 months to 2 years. Lifting under the thorax in a prone position. First the head and then the back and legs will extend. If the head is pushed into flexion, the extensor tone will disappear.

laryngospasm: Spasmodic closure of the larynx.

latent period: Time during which a disease is in existence but does not manifest itself.

latent stage (latency): Fourth of Freud's stages of psychosexual development, characterized by the development of the superego (conscience) and by loss of interest in sexual gratification; typically occurs from the ages of 6 to 11 years in Western cultural groups.

lateral (Lat): From anatomical position, located further from the midline of the body.

lateral corticospinal tract (LCST): Contralateral descending motor tract. Upper motor neurons influencing lower motor neurons either directly or indirectly.

laterality: Using a preferred unilateral body part for activities requiring a high level of skill.[UTIII]

Jacobs, K., & Simon, L. (Eds.). *Quick Reference Dictionary for Occupational Therapy, Sixth Edition* (pp. 159-167).
© 2015 SLACK Incorporated.

lateralization: Tendency for certain processes to be more highly developed on one side of the brain than the other.

lateral spinothalamic tract: Pathway that provides precise sensation of pain and temperature.

lateral trunk flexion: Ability to move the trunk from side to side without moving the legs, which is essential for maintaining balance.

latissimus dorsi: Large muscle pair originating on the lower spine and ilium, which inserts on the proximal end of the humerus. Its fibers run superiorly and laterally. This muscle pair is responsible for extension and adduction of the humerus.

launching: Process in which youths move into adulthood and leave their family of origin.

learned helplessness: Process in which the person attributes his or her lack of performance to external factors rather than lack of effort.

learned nonuse: A process that occurs after an injury such as a cerebrovascular accident. Immediately following the injury, motor function is extremely impaired due to diaschisis (cortical shock). Attempts to use the affected limb at this time fail, and the client learns that the limb is useless. Compensation with the unaffected limb begins and produces successful results (a reward behavior), and further attempts at using the involved limb continue to be unsuccessful (a punished behavior). This pattern of reinforcement results in a strong learned response of not trying to use the affected limb. Thus, the client does not realize that a return of function of the affected limb may have gradually occurred.

learning: Acquiring new concepts and behaviors.[UTIII] Enduring ability of an individual to comprehend and/or competently respond to changes in information from the environment and/or from within the self. As one learns about the environment, alterations occur in the definition of the self and possible behaviors; as one learns about the self, alterations occur in the definition of the environment and possible behaviors.

learning disability (LD): Learning problem that is not due to environmental causes, mental retardation, or emotional disturbances, often associated with problems in listening, thinking, reading, writing, spelling, and mathematics.

learning environment: All the conditions (internal and external), circumstances, and influences surrounding and affecting the learning of the patient/client.

learning stations: Activities or special equipment are placed around the room for an individual to use and be evaluated on for therapeutic feedback or educational achievement.

learning theory: Theoretical base behind the behavioral frame of reference in which behavior is best learned when environmental influences are introduced.

least restrictive environment: Most normal learning environment where a person with a disability can have his or her educational needs met.

legal hold: A court-ordered restraint often associated with a belief that an individual is a danger to self or others.

legislative review: Review of a bill by the legislature when they perceive that an agency has misinterpreted the intent or has excessively revised existing regulations.

leisure: "Nonobligatory activity that is intrinsically motivated and engaged in during discretionary time, that is, time not committed to obligatory occupations such as work, self-care, or sleep" (Parham & Fazio, 1997, p. 250).[OTPF 2014]

leisure activities: Tasks for pleasure.

leisure exploration: Identifying interests, skills, opportunities, and appropriate leisure activities.[AOTA Framework]

leisure participation: Planning and participating in appropriate leisure activities; maintaining a balance of leisure activities with other areas of occupation; and obtaining, using, and maintaining equipment and supplies as appropriate.[AOTA Framework]

length of stay (LOS): The duration of hospitalization, usually expressed in days.

lesion: Injury to the central or peripheral nervous system that may prevent the expression of some functions and/or may allow the inappropriate, uncoordinated, uncontrolled expression of other functions.

lethargy: Sluggishness or inactivity.

leukocyte: White cell; colorless blood corpuscles that function to protect the body against microorganisms causing disease.

leukocytosis: Increase in circulating lymphocyte number.

leukopenia: Decreased white blood cell count.

levator ani syndrome: Spasm of the muscles surrounding the anus causing severe rectal pain.

level: Sloped no more than 1:50 or 2%.

level of arousal: Demonstrating alertness and responsiveness to environmental stimuli.[UTIII]

Levels of Cognitive Function Scale (LCFS): Eight stages of cognitive function and recovery following a traumatic brain injury developed at Rancho Los Amigos Hospital in 1972.

levels of processing: Durability of the memory trace is a function of the level to which the information was encoded.

lever system: System consisting of a rigid bar (lever), an axis (fulcrum), a force, and a resistance to that force. The distance between the axis and the point of application of force is known as the force arm; the distance between the axis and the point of application of resistance is known as the resistance arm. First-class lever system—axis lies between the two forces. In the human body, the triceps brachii muscle is an example of a first-class lever. Second-class lever system—resistance is between the effort force and the axis. In the human body, a person rising up on his or her toes while standing (gastrocnemius and soleus muscles) is an example of a second-class lever. Third-class lever system—effort is located between the axis and the resistance. In the human body, the biceps brachii muscle and most of the musculoskeletal levers are examples of third-class levers.

Librium: Anti-anxiety drug in the benzodiazepine class. *Generic name*: chlordiazepoxide.

licensure: Process established by a governmental agency to determine professional qualification.

life as narrative: A perspective that holds that life is experienced primarily as an unfolding and then as a remembered story.

life cycle: Place in important life phases, such as career cycle, parenting cycle, and educational process.[UTIII]

life expectancy: Number of years in the lifespan of an individual in a particular cultural group.

life review: Process in which one looks back at one's life experiences, evaluating, interpreting, and reinterpreting them.

life roles: Daily life experiences that occupy one's time, including roles of student, homemaker, worker (active or retired), sibling, parent, mate, child, and peer.

lifespan perspective: Makes seven basic contentions about development: it is lifelong, multidimensional, multidirectional, plastic, historically embedded, multidisciplinary, and contextual.

life stages: "Consecutive time spans in the individual's life that provide an overarching structure for understanding development. Integral to each life stage are biological, psychosocial, cognitive, and occupational tasks that must be carried out by the individual to meet his developmental needs" (Trombly, 1995).

lifestyle: Pattern of daily occupations over time that are stable and predictable, through which an individual expresses his or her self-identity.

lifestyle redesign: Assisting clients in examining how occupations contribute to healthy or unhealthy states and customizing change. Helping clients to acquire and implement self-directed habits and daily routines.

life tasks: Daily activities.

lifts: Raises or hoists task objects, including lifting an object from one place to another, but without ambulating or moving from one place to another.[AOTA Framework]

ligament: Inelastic fibrous thickening of an articular capsule that joins one bone to its articular mate, allowing movement at the joint.

light work: Exerting up to 20 pounds of force occasionally, or up to 10 pounds of force frequently, or a negligible amount of force constantly to move objects.

Likert scale: Point system that is used to rank a particular level of skill, function, or attitude.

limb apraxia: A disorder of skilled and purposeful movement of the arms and legs that occurs with neurological damage or disorders affecting the praxis system. People with limb apraxia often have functional deficits that impede everyday task performance and increase dependence on caregivers (Weiner, 2012).

limbic system: Primitive system thought to be associated with emotional and visceral functions in the body.

limitation: Act of being restrained or confined.

limiting charge: Statutory limit on the amount a nonparticipating health care provider can charge for services to Medicare patients.

limits of stability: The boundary or range that is the furthest distance in any direction a person can lean away from vertical (midline) without changing the original base of support (e.g., stepping, reaching, etc.) or falling.

lineality: Social relationship structure defined by biological and cultural relationship over time.

linear processing: Learning or solving a problem using a step-by-step process in which each step is dependent on what goes on before.

line of pull: Attachments of a muscle, direction of its fibers, and the location of its tendons at each joint at which the muscle crosses.

lingula: A small tongue-like structure. In the cerebellum, the part of the vermis of the cerebellum, on the ventral surface, where the superior medullary velum attaches (lingula cerebelli). In the lung, a projection from the lower portion of the upper lobe of the left lung, just beneath the cardiac notch, between the cardiac impression and the inferior margin (lingula of left lobe). In the lower jaw, the sharp medial boundary of the mandibular foramen, to which is attached the sphenomandibular ligament (lingula mandibulae). Lastly, the lingula sphenoidalis, a ridge of bone on the lateral margin of the carotid sulcus, projecting backward between the body and great wing of the sphenoid bone.

LinkedIn: A business-oriented social networking site that enables users to connect with colleagues, look for jobs, develop professional networks, and get answers to industry questions.

links: Underlined/bold text or images that, when clicked, jump you from one webpage or item of content to another. Also used to describe lists of recommended websites, often used as part of blog interfaces.

lithium carbonate: Drug treatment that can be effective for those with manic disorders but shows limited results for depression. Side effects are nausea, tremor, weakness, thirst, and excessive urination. *Trade name*: Eskalith.

lithotomy position: Position in which the client lies on his or her back with thighs flexed upon the abdomen and the lower legs on the thighs, which are abducted.

lobectomy: Excision of a lobe, as of the lung, thyroid, brain, or liver.

localization: Culture always situated in personally meaningful, interactive locations.

localized inflammation: Swelling, redness, and increased temperature that is isolated to the injured or infected part of the body.

locus of control: Psychological term referring to one's orientation to the world of events. Persons with an internal locus of control believe they can influence the outcome of events. Conversely, those with an external locus of control believe that the outcome of events is largely a matter of fate or chance (i.e., that they cannot have influence over the outcome of events).

Loewenstein Occupational Therapy Cognitive Assessment (LOTCA): Cognitive battery of tests for both primary assessment and ongoing evaluation in the treatment of individuals with brain injury.

logical classification: Ability to sort objects by their defining properties at the age of 5 or 6 years.

lol: A common Internet slang abbreviation that stands for "laugh out loud," "laughing out loud," or "lots of laughs."

long cane: Mobility device used by individuals with visual impairments who sweep it in a wide arc in front of them.

long distance exchange: The exchange of objects as currency a long distance from where the objects are found or made. Seashells found hundreds of miles inland are a particularly good example.

longevity: Long life or life expectancy.

long-handled reacher: Reacher with a long handle that can aid in dressing or retrieving objects that are out of arm's reach.

longitudinal arch: Composed of the motions of metacarpal, proximal interphalangeal, and distal interphalangeal joints of the digital ray. Splints involving these joints are said to involve the longitudinal arch.

longitudinal research: Subjects are measured over the course of their lives to gather data on potential trends in growth and development.

long-term care (LTC): Array of services needed by individuals who have lost some capacity for independence because of a chronic illness or condition.

long-term memory: Permanent memory storage for long-term information.

long-term support system: Ensuring that individuals have access to the services that are needed to support independent living.

loose associations: Thoughts shift with little or no apparent logic.

lordosis: Abnormal forward curvature of the lumbar spine; swayback.

low power distance (LPD): Cultures or organizations in which the majority of the members feel that any inequality in the society should be minimized.

low technology: Electronic or nonelectronic products or systems that have assumed a more commonplace role and accessibility in society.

low-temperature thermoplastics: Materials that are presently most often used for splinting. These materials soften and become more pliable with heat. After these materials are cooled, they remain in the shapes to which they were conformed.

low vision: Faulty vision that cannot be corrected by eyeglasses or contact lenses.

lower motor neuron (LMN): Sensory neuron found in the anterior horn cell, nerve root, or peripheral nervous system.

lumbar rotation: Rotating the client's pelvis away from the painful side; technique to treat spinal pain.

lumbar stabilization: Exercises whose objective is to strengthen the deep spine muscles as a foundation for good trunk stability.

lumpectomy: Excision of a small primary breast tumor leaving the rest of the breast intact.

Luria Nebraska Neuropsychological Battery (LNNB): General neuropsychological assessment of brain injury based on the work of Luria.

luteinizing hormone (LH): A gonadotropic hormone of the anterior pituitary that acts with the follicle-stimulating hormone to cause ovulation of mature follicles and secretion of estrogen by thecal and granulosa cells. It is also concerned with corpus luteum formation and, in the male, stimulates the development and functional activity of interstitial cells.

lymphadenopathy: Disease of the lymph nodes characterized by malaise and general enlargement of the nodes.

lymphatic system: The system containing or conveying lymph.

lymphedema: Swelling of an extremity caused by obstruction of the lymphatic vessels.

lymphoblast: T lymphocytes that have been altered during a viral attack to release a variety of chemicals, which encourage greater defensive activity by the immune system.

lymphocyte: A particular type of white blood cell that is involved in the immune response and produced by lymphoid tissue.

lymphoidectomy: Excision of lymphoid tissue.

lymphoma: Any of the various forms of cancers of the lymphoid tissue.

macular degeneration: Common eye condition in which the macula is affected by edema, pigment is dispersed, and the macular area of the retina degenerates. It is the leading cause of visual impairment in persons older than 50 years.

magnetic resonance imaging (MRI): The use of nuclear magnetic resonance to image brain areas.

main effects: The action of two or more independent variables each working separately.

mainstreamed: Concept in education that a child with a disability be put into a "typical" classroom for a portion or all of the school day.

maintain: An intervention approach designed to provide the supports that will allow clients to preserve the performance capabilities they have regained, that continue to meet their occupational needs, or both. The assumption is that, without continued maintenance intervention, performance would decrease, occupational needs would not be met, or both, thereby affecting health and quality of life.OTPF 2008

major depressive disorder: Mood disorder characterized by features such as downcast mood, loss of interest in activities, insomnia, and feelings of fatigue and worthlessness that cause impairment in daily functioning.

major medical insurance: Type of insurance designed to offset the heavy medical expenses resulting from a prolonged illness or injury.

make test: Form of muscle testing in which the therapist provides resistance against a muscle while it is moving through its range.

malaise: A vague feeling of bodily discomfort or uneasiness, as experienced early in an illness.

malingering: Pretending to be ill or suffering usually to escape work, receive compensation, or for sympathy.

malposition: Faulty or abnormal position.

malpractice: Performing tasks and/or duties in such a way that causes harm to the patient and/or others.

managed care: Integrated delivery systems. Cost containment approach that enables the payer to influence the delivery of health services prospectively (i.e., before services are provided).

management: The act, art, or manner of managing, handling, controlling, or directing.

management by objectives: Managerial system that improves the productivity of an organization by setting goals of progress that can be periodically measured, and using timetables and time limits to adhere to productivity goals.

management style: The beliefs and value system of the manager; the personality of the manager.

mandated reporter: Person who in the practice of his or her profession comes in contact with children and must make a report or see that a report is made when he or she has reason to believe that a child has been abused.

maneuvers: Moves one's body in relation to others.[AOTA Framework]

mania: Excessive activity, flight of thought, and grandiosity.

manipulates: Uses dexterous grasp-and-release patterns, isolated finger movements, and coordinated in-hand manipulation patterns when interacting with task objects.[AOTA Framework]

manipulation: A therapeutic movement, usually of small amplitude, accomplished at the end of the available range of motion but within the anatomical range at a speed over which the client has no control.

manipulative therapy: Passive movement technique that can be classified into either joint manipulation or mobilization. Manipulation is a sudden small thrust that is not under the patient's control, whereas mobilization is a passive movement technique where the patient can control the movement.

Mann-Whitney U Test: Test on rank-ordered data of the hypothesis of difference between two independent random samples. The independent t-test is its ordinal likeness.

manual muscle testing (MMT): Assesses the strength of a muscle through manual evaluation. Rating is done by moving the involved part through its full range of motion against gravity and then against gravity with resistance.

marked crossing: Crosswalk or other identified path intended for pedestrian use in crossing a vehicular way.

marketing: Managerial process by which individuals and groups obtain what they want by creating and exchanging products, services, or ideas with others.

markup: Difference between invoice cost and selling price. It may be expressed either as a percentage of the selling price or the cost price and is supposed to cover all the costs of doing business plus a profit. Whether markup is based on the selling price or the cost price, the base is always equal to 100 percent. Small Business Administration

Marxist structuralism: A philosophy of science or method of inquiry, which has affinities with Realism. It investigates "systems" in terms of totality, self-regulation, and transformation.

mass: Amount of space an object takes up without regard to gravity; a kinematic measurement.

massage: Manipulation of soft tissue of the body through stroking, rubbing, kneading, or tapping to increase circulation, improve muscle tone, and relax a patient.

master care plan: Treatment plan that includes the list of client problems and identifies the treatment team's intervention strategies and responsibilities.

mastery: Achievement of skill to a criterion level of success.

mastication: Chewing; tearing and grinding food with the teeth while it becomes mixed with saliva.

material culture: Artifacts, industry, architecture, and other material aspects of a particular society.

maturation: Sequential unfolding of behavioral and physiological characteristics during development.

maturational theory: Developmental theory that views development as a function of innate factors that proceed according to a maturational and developmental timetable.

mature group: Members take on all necessary roles, including leadership. The purpose is to balance task accomplishment with need satisfaction of all group members. The therapist is an equal member of this group.

maximal oxygen consumption (max VO$_2$, maximal oxygen uptake, aerobic capacity): The greatest volume of oxygen used by the cells of the body per unit time.

maximal voluntary ventilation (MVV): The greatest volume of air that can be exhaled in 15 seconds.

maximum heart rate (age predicted): Highest possible heart rate usually achieved during maximal exercise. Maximum heart rate decreases with age and can be estimated as 220 – age.

maximum voluntary contraction (MVC): Greatest amount of tension a muscle can generate and hold only for a moment, as in muscle testing.

McCarron-Dial System (MDS): Assessment used to determine the prevocational, vocational, and residential functioning levels of individuals with disabilities and the general population.

meal preparation and clean-up: Planning, preparing, and serving well-balanced, nutritional meals and cleaning up food and utensils after meals.[AOTA Framework]

Meals on Wheels: Program designed to deliver hot meals to the elderly, individuals with physical disabilities, or those who lack the resources to provide for themselves with nutritionally adequate warm meals on a daily basis.

mean (x): Measure of central tendency that specifies the arithmetic average.

meaning: To make sense out of a situation using everything a person brings to it, including perception, attitudes, feelings, and social and cultural values.

meaningfulness: Amount of significance or value an individual associates with an experience after encountering it.

meaningful occupations: "Chosen, performed and engaged in to generate experiences of personal meaning and satisfaction by individuals, groups, or communities" (CAOT, 1997a, 2002, p. 181).[CAOT]

meaninglessness: Lack of belief in the value, usefulness, or importance of daily occupations or lives.

meatus: Passage or opening within the body.

mechanical advantage (MA): In kinesiology, the ratio of the amount of effort expended to the work performed. MA = length of force arm/length of resistance arm

mechanical efficiency: Amount of external work performed in relation to the amount of energy required to perform the work; equal to force arm/resistance arm.

mechanical modalities: A broad group of agents that use distraction, approximation, or compression to produce a therapeutic effect.

mechanical ventilation: The use of a respirator for external support of breathing and the use of an ambu bag for inflating the lungs mechanically.

mechanics: Study of physical forces.

mechanistic view (reductionism): Belief that a person is passive and that his or her behavior must be controlled or shaped by the society or environment in which he or she functions. Supports that the mind and body should be viewed as separate and that the human being, like a machine, can be taken apart and reassembled if its structure and function are sufficiently well understood.

medial: From an anatomical position, located closer to the midline of the body.

medial longitudinal fasciculus (MLF): Pathway in the brainstem that connects the vestibular system with the cranial nerves that serve eye muscles (III, IV, VI).

median (Mdn): The value or score that most closely represents the middle of a range of scores.

mediastinum: The mass of tissues and organs separating the two lungs located from between the sternum in front and the vertebral column behind and from the thoracic inlet above to the diaphragm below. It contains the heart and its large vessels, the trachea, esophagus, thymus, lymph nodes, and other structures and tissues.

Medicaid: U.S. federally funded, state-operated program of medical assistance to people with low incomes, regardless of age.

medical necessity: Required medically.

medical skinfold caliper: Instrument used to measure body fat.

Medicare: U.S. federally funded health insurance program for the elderly, certain people with disabilities, and most individuals with end-stage renal disease, funded by Title VIII of the Social Security Act.

Medicare Part A: Hospital insurance program of Medicare, which covers hospital inpatient care, care in skilled nursing facilities, and home health care.

Medicare Part B: Supplemental medical insurance program of Medicare, which covers hospital outpatient care, physician fees, home health care, comprehensive outpatient rehabilitation facility fees, and other professional services.

medication routine: Obtaining medication, opening and closing containers, following prescribed schedules, taking correct quantities, reporting problems and adverse effects, and administering correct quantities using prescribed methods.[UTIII]

medicine: Any drug or remedy.

medicine ball: Heavy exercise ball used to increase strength and coordination of a client.

medium work: Exerting up to 20 to 50 pounds of force occasionally, 10 to 25 pounds of force frequently, or greater than negligible up to 10 pounds of force constantly to move objects.

MEDLINE: National Library of Medicine computer database that covers approximately 600,000 references to biomedical journal articles published currently and in the 2 preceding years.

megabyte: A megabyte is equal to 1,000 kilobytes of 1,000,000 bytes of electronic information; measure of the capacity of memory, disk storage, etc.

meiosis: Sperm and ova are produced by the reduction division process. Each contains only half of the parent cell's original complement of chromosomes (23 in humans).

melatonin: Hormone produced by the pineal gland; secreted into blood stream.

member checking: A form of triangulation in which the "other" data source is the client him- or herself.

memory: Recalling information after brief or long periods of time[UTIII]; the mental process that involves registration and encoding, consolidation and storage, and recall and retrieval of information.

memory notebook: Used with clients who have sustained a brain injury resulting in memory loss.

memory processes: Strategies for dealing with information that are under the individual's control.

memory structure: Unvarying physical or structural components of memory.

menarche: First menstrual period of a female; usually occurs between age 9 and 17 years.

Mendelian genetics: The theory of heredity that forms the basis of classical genetics, proposed by Gregor Mendel (1822–1884) in 1866. Mendel suggested that individual characteristics were determined by inherited "factors."

Meniere's disease: Disorder of the labyrinth of the inner ear that leads to progressive loss of hearing, characterized by ringing in the ear, dizziness, nausea, and vomiting.

meningitis: Infection of the cerebrospinal fluid within the cranium and spinal cord; may produce damage to the cerebral cortex, which may affect motor function, sensation, and perception, as well as other areas of the central nervous system.

meningocele: Protrusion of the meninges through the spinal column or skull.

menopause: Transition in women marking the end of the reproductive cycle; accompanied by cessation of menstruation, increases in hormonal levels, and alteration of the reproductive organs.

menstruation: Periodic discharge of a bloody fluid from the uterus through the vagina occurring at more or less regular intervals from puberty to menopause.

mental health (MH): A psychological state of well-being, characterized by personal growth, sense of purpose, and positive relations with others.

mental retardation: *See* intellectual disability.

mental status exam: Diagnostic procedure used to evaluate intellectual, emotional, psychological, and personality function.

mentor: A senior professional who acts as a role model to foster professional orientation and growth in a new professional.

meprobamate: Anti-anxiety drug that reduces muscle tension. *Trade names*: Miltown, Equanil.

mesoderm: Middle layer of cells that develops from the inner cell mass of the blastocyst, eventually becoming the muscles, the bones, the circulatory system, and the inner layer of the skin.

meta-analysis: Type of research in which previous research studies are examined to determine outcome trends.

metabolic acidosis: Metabolic environment of acidity. A pathologic condition resulting from accumulation of acid or loss of base in the body, characterized by an increase in hydrogen ion concentration (decrease in pH).

metabolic alkalosis: A pathologic condition resulting from the accumulation of base or loss of acid in the body, and characterized by a decrease in hydrogen ion concentration (increase pH).

metabolic equivalent level (MET): Method used to measure endurance levels; represents the energy requirements needed to maintain metabolic functioning, as well as perform varying activities. It is an abbreviation for oxygen consumption during activities. The greater the exertion, the greater the METs required for an activity (e.g., an individual who is semi-reclined uses 3.5 mL of oxygen per minute per kilogram of body weight or 1 MET; thus MET is required just to maintain metabolic functioning).

metabolism: Process by which the body inactivates drugs. *Synonym*: biotransformation.

metacognition: The process of thinking about one's thoughts; this allows reflection and behavioral change.

meta-ethics: Branch of philosophy that examines similarities in ways decisions between right and wrong are made.

methylamphetamine: Drug with actions and side effects similar to amphetamine. It is used to treat narcolepsy, parkinsonism, and some depressed states and to reduce appetite.

methylmethacrylate: A self-curing, acrylic resin adherent that is applied in paste form and becomes bone-like when hardened.

methylphenidate hydrochloride: Sympathomimetic drug that also stimulates the central nervous system. It is used to improve mental activity in convalescence and some depression states to overcome lethargy associated with drug treatment. Side effects include nervousness and insomnia. *Trade name*: Ritalin.

mHealth: The delivery of health-related information and services using mobile communication technology (e.g., Smartphone, electronic tablet, or other mobile devices) (AOTA, 2014a).

microbacteria: A genus of microorganism made up of gram-positive rods found in dairy products and characterized by relatively high resistance to heat.

microcephalus: Condition in which an atypically small skull results in brain damage and mental retardation.

microchip: Electronic device that consists of thousands of electronic circuits, such as transistors on a small sliver or chip of plastic. Such devices are the building blocks of computers. *Synonym*: integrated circuit.

microcomputer: Medium-sized computer that usually serves as a central computer for many individuals. Used primarily in academic and research settings.

micrographia: Abnormally small writing.

middle childhood: The years from 6 to 12.

migraine: Headache associated with periodic instability of the cranial arteries; may be accompanied by nausea.

Milani-Comparetti: Motor development screening test for infants and young children. Standardized screening tool for neurodevelopmental disorders.

milieu therapy: Treatment in which the environment is designed to provide specific levels of press and feedback.

Miller Assessment for Preschoolers (MAP): Developmental assessment that is based on the neurodevelopmental and sensory integration frames of reference but includes cognitive elements. It is regarded as being highly reliable in measuring performance components of children aged 3 to 6 years in the areas of cognition, communication, mobility, visual perceptual skills, and social integration.

mind-body relationship: The effect of the mind (and mental disorders) on the body and the effect of the body (and physical disorders) on the mind.

minimal brain damage (MBD): Superficial damage to the brain that cannot be detected using objective instruments. Such damage is usually assessed from deviations in behavior.

minimal risk: The probability and magnitude that harm and discomfort anticipated in the research are not greater in and of themselves than those ordinarily encountered in daily life or during the performance of routine physical or psychological examinations or tests.

minimal supervision: Contact provided on a need basis and may be less than monthly.

Mini-Mental State Exam (MMSE): Brief psychological test designed to differentiate between dementia, psychosis, and affective disorders.

Minimum Data Set (MDS): Comprehensive screening tool reflecting quality of life concerns, includes activities of daily living, self-performance, disease diagnosis, and activity pursuits (requirement for nursing homes using third-party payers).

ministration: Feeling closeness with co-workers.

Minnesota Rate of Manipulation Test (MRMT): Measures hand dexterity through five tasks using wooden disks: placing, turning, displacing, one-hand turning and placing, and two-hand turning and placing.

minority group: Group differing, especially in race, religion, or ethnic background, from the majority of a population.

minute ventilation: The volume of air inspired and exhaled in 1 minute. The highest minute ventilation achieved during exercise is also called the maximum breathing capacity.

mission statement: The statement of purpose of an agency or organization.

mitogen: A substance that stimulates cell division (mitosis) in lymphocytes.

mitosis: Cell duplication and division that generates all of an individual's cells except for the sperm and ova.

mnemonics: Memory-enhancing learning techniques that link a new concept to an established one.

mobile arm support (MAS): Frictionless arm support that is mounted to a wheelchair, table, or belt around the waist and uses gravity in an inclined plane to assist movement of the arms when shoulder and elbow muscles are weak.

mobility: Relates to moving the entire body or a body part in space as necessary when interacting with task objects.^{AOTA Framework}

mobility sphere: Territory within which individuals regularly travel in their daily activity patterns. Its dimensions depend on distances that the person can travel by ambulation or available modes of transportation, as well as on the accessibility features of the environment.

mobilization: A passive therapeutic movement at the end of the available range of motion at variable amplitudes and speed.

modality: A broad group of agents that may include thermal, acoustic, radiant, mechanical, or electrical energy to produce physiologic changes in tissues for therapeutic purposes.

mode (Mo): Value or score in a distribution that occurs most frequently.

model: An approach, framework, or structure that organizes knowledge to guide reasonable decision making.

modeling: Process by which a behavior is learned through observation and imitation of others.

Model of Human Occupation (MOHO): Gary Kielhofner's and Janice Burke's general systems theory-based view of the human being as an open system and the fact that a person's occupational behavior is the output of that system.

modem: Device that enables communication between two computers via the telephone line signals.

modernization theory: Theory that looks at how a society is organized as a basis for how older adults are treated.

modulates: Uses volume and inflection in speech.^{AOTA Framework}

modulation: A variation in levels of excitation and inhibition over sensory and motor neural pools.

molding: The shaping of the fetal head by the overlapping fetal skull bones to adjust to the size and shape of the birth canal.

molecular pharmacology: Study of interaction of drugs and subcellular entities.

money management: Budgeting, paying bills, and using bank systems.[UTIII]

monitoring: Determining a client's status on a periodic or ongoing basis.

monoamine oxidase (MAO) inhibitor: Drug used to treat depression by blocking the action of monoamine oxidase. It allows serotonin and norepinephrine to gather at receptor sites in the synapses of the nerve cells in the brain. It is believed to alleviate symptoms of depression.

monocular: Pertaining to one eye.

monocyte: A circulating phagocytic leukocyte, which can differentiate into a macrophage upon migration into tissue.

mood: Pervasive and sustained emotion that, when extreme, can color one's whole view of life; generally refers to either elation or depression.

moral treatment: The first systematic treatment, which commenced in the last decade of the 18th century, providing responsible care for an appreciable number of people with mental illness. "Moral" was used in this early context as the equivalent of "emotional" or "psychological" (from the same root as morale) and has to do with custom, conduct, way of life, and inner meaning.

morbidity: Illness or abnormal condition.

mores: Very strong norms; often laws.

Moro's reflex: Normal neurological response in early infancy that involves stiffened extension of arms and legs and the flexion and abduction of extremities, often with crying.

morphine: Highly addictive narcotic from the opium family. Food and Drug Administration–controlled substance; used as a sedative and painkiller.

mortality: Being subject to death.

motivation: Individual drives toward the mastery of certain goals and skills; may be intrinsic or involve inducements and incentives.

motivational theory: Theory in which motivation is described as an arousal to action, initiating molding and sustaining specific action patterns. Certain reinforcers may be used to increase or decrease motivation. Internal rewards appear to be better motivators than extrinsic ones.

motor: Actions or behaviors a client uses to move and physically interact with tasks, objects, contexts, and environments (adapted from Fisher, 2006). Includes planning, sequencing, and executing novel movements. *Also see* praxis.[OTPF 2008]

motor coordination: Functions that are traditionally defined as motoric. This includes gross motor, fine motor, and motor planning functions.

motor deficit: Lack or deficiency of normal motor function that may be the result of pathology or other disorder. Weakness, paralysis, abnormal movement patterns, abnormal timing, coordination, clumsiness, involuntary movements, or abnormal postures may be manifestations of impaired motor function (motor control and motor learning).

motor development: Growth and change in the ability to do physical activities, such as walking, running, or riding a bike.

Motor-Free Visual Perception Test (MVPT): Norm-referenced test for children 4 to 8 years that assesses visual perception.

motor lag: A prolonged latent period between the reception of a stimulus and the initiation of the motor response.

motor learning: How one learns the highly complex skills that are used every day; requires time and practice.

motor neuron: Nerve cell that sends signals from the brain to the muscles throughout the body.

motor planning: Ability to organize and execute movement patterns to accomplish a purposeful activity.

motor skills: "Occupational performance skills observed as the person interacts with and moves task objects and self around the task environment" (e.g., activity of daily living [ADL] motor skills, school motor skills; Boyt Schell et al., 2014a, p. 1237). [OTPF 2014]

motor strip: Precentral sulci—controls movement of all muscles.

motor unit: One alpha motor neuron, its axon, and all muscle fibers attached to that axon.

mouse: Device that moves on a horizontal plane and controls the cursor on a computer monitor.

mouthstick: Assistive device; tool that has a mouthpiece with a pen, pencil, eraser, or paintbrush attached to it. It can also be used to push the buttons of a computer keyboard.

Movement Assessment of Infants: Observation test for children 0 to 12 months that assesses gross motor and reflexes.

moves: Pushes, pulls, or drags task objects along a supporting surface.^{AOTA Framework}

moxibustion: Therapeutic burning as a form of cure for ailments such as malaria, hepatitis, and abdominal problems used by an array of cultures.

multicultural: Including or reflective of many cultures.

multicultural counseling: Process in which a therapist from one ethnic or racial background interacts with a person of a different background in order to assist in the psychological and interpersonal development and adjustment to the dominant culture.

multiculturalism: Awareness and knowledge about human diversity in ways that are translated into more respectful human interactions and effective interconnections.

multidimensional maps: Pictures of the self and environment that are created within the central nervous system after receipt and analysis of multisensory input.

multidisciplinary: Several disciplines treat the person.

multidisciplinary team: Health care workers who are members of different disciplines, each one providing specific services to the patient/client.

multigenerational model: Model of family therapy that focuses on reciprocal role relationships over a period of time and thus takes a longitudinal approach.

multi-infarct dementia: Form of organic brain disease characterized by the rapid deterioration of intellectual functioning, caused by vascular disease.

multilingual: Speaking many languages fluently.

Multiphasic Environmental Assessment Procedure (MEAP): Collection of checklists and questionnaires designed to evaluate the quality of living in a given sheltered care facility. The assessment focuses on the structural components of the facility, the social atmosphere, programs offered, and the attributes of the resident and staff.

multiple myeloma: Primary malignant tumor of the plasma cells usually arising in bone marrow.

multiple personality: Dissociative disorder in which more than one distinct personality exists in the same individual, and each personality is relatively integrated and stable.

multiple regression: Making predictions of one variable (using the multiple R) based on measures of two or more others.

multiple sclerosis (MS): Disease characterized by the progressive destruction of the myelin sheaths of neurons in the central nervous system.

multiple sleep latency test: Test that measures the degree of daytime sleepiness and rapid eye movement sleep of an individual.

multiple subjectivities: A viewpoint that individuals may perceive a single event or experience in diverse ways.

multiskilled practitioner: Person from one profession who has established competence in specific skills usually associated with another profession.

muscle endurance: Sustained muscular contraction, measured as repetitions of submaximal contraction (isotonic) or submaximal holding time (isometric).

muscle spindles: Sensory receptors in the tendons of muscles that monitor tension of muscles.

muscle strength: Nonspecific term relating to muscle contraction, often referring to the force generated by a single maximal isometric contraction.

muscle testing: Method of evaluating the contractile unit, including the muscle, tendons, and associated tissues, of a moving part of the body by neurologic or resistance testing.

muscle tone: Demonstrating a degree of tension or resistance in a muscle at rest and in response to stretching[UTIII]; amount of tension or contractibility among the motor units of a muscle; often defined as the resistance of a muscle to stretching or elongation.

muscle weakness: Lack of the full tension-producing capability of a muscle needed to maintain posture and create movement.

muscular atrophies: Diseases of unknown etiology that are caused by the breakdown of cells in the anterior horn of the spinal cord.

muscular dystrophy (MD): Degenerative inherited neuromuscular disorder characterized by progressive muscle weakness and atrophy.

muscular system: Framework of voluntarily controlled skeletal muscles in the body.

musculoskeletal: System in the human body that is associated with the muscles and the bones to which they attach.

mutability: The muscle fiber's ability to change in response to a new demand.

mutation: Error in gene replication that results in a change in the molecular structure of genetic material.

mutism: The inability to speak.

mutual cultural accommodation: The process by which individuals make modest adaptations in their behavior based on new knowledge from a previous contact with another culture.

mutual support group: Type of group in which members organize to solve their own problems, usually led by the group members themselves who share a common goal and use their own strengths to gain control over their lives.

myalgia: Pain in a muscle or muscles.

myasthenia gravis (MG): Chronic progressive autoimmune disorder of striated muscles that leads to weakness in the voluntary muscles, particularly those innervated by the bulbar nucleus.

myelin: A fat-like substance forming the principal component of the sheath of nerve fibers in the central nervous system.

myelination: The process of forming the "white" lipid covering of nerve cell axons; myelin increases the conduction velocity of the neuronal impulse and forms the white matter of the brain and spinal cord.

myelitis: Inflammation of the spinal cord with associated motor and sensory dysfunction.

myelography: Radiograph process used to view spinal lesions in the subarachnoid space after injection with dye or air.

myelopathy: A general term denoting functional disturbances and/or pathological changes in the brain.

Myers-Briggs Test: Based on Karl Jung's profile of psychological types, this test describes 16 trait combinations and their associated patterns of action.

myocardial infarction (MI): Caused by partial or complete occlusion of one or more of the coronary arteries. *Also known as* a heart attack.

myoclonus: Sudden quick spasms of a muscle or group of muscles.

myoelectric prostheses: Artificial limbs that are operated electronically using the client's remaining muscle function.

myofascial release (MFR): Techniques used to release fascial tissue restrictions secondary to tonal dysfunction.

myokymia: Continual, irregular twitching of a muscle often seen around the eye in the facial region.

myoma: Benign tumor consisting of muscle tissue.

myopathy: Abnormal muscle function.

myorrhaphy: Suture of a muscle.

myotasis: Stretching of muscle.

myringoplasty: Reconstruction of the eardrum.

myringotomy: Puncture of the eardrum with evacuation of fluids from the middle ear.

myxoma: A tumor composed of mucous tissue.

naproxen: Drug administered for arthritis and dysmenorrhea that may cause drowsiness, headache, dizziness, vomiting, and rash.

narcissism: Egocentricity; dominant interest in one's self.

narcissistic personality disorder: A personality disorder characterized by grandiosity, exaggerated sense of self-importance, arrogance, exploitation of others, a preoccupation with receiving attention, fragile self-esteem, and hypersensitivity to the perceptions of others (Levine, Walsh, & Schwartz, 1996).

narcolepsy: Chronic sleep disorder manifested by excessive and overwhelming daytime sleepiness.

narcotic: A drug that suppresses the central nervous system, producing sleep or stupor.

narrative: The interpretation of events through stories.

narrative documentation: System of documentation that uses summary paragraphs to describe evaluation data and treatment progress.

narrative reasoning: An aspect of clinical reasoning requiring understanding the "life stories" of clients.

National Board for Certification in Occupational Therapy, Inc. (NBCOT): Formerly known as the American Occupational Therapy Certification Board, Inc. (AOTCB), the NBCOT is an independent certification board responsible for the certification examinations taken by graduates of accredited occupational therapy and occupational therapy assistant programs. The board maintains the examinations, screens test questions, assesses the content of examinations, determines certification procedures, and issues documentation to those who successfully pass the examination. The NBCOT is also responsible

Jacobs, K., & Simon, L. (Eds.). *Quick Reference Dictionary for Occupational Therapy, Sixth Edition* (pp. 185-192).
© 2015 SLACK Incorporated.

for disciplinary measures against occupational therapists and occupational therapy assistants and for ensuring continuing competence of practitioners in fulfilling its mission to protect the public.

National Consumer Health Information and Health Promotion Act of 1976: U.S. federal legislation that attempted to set rational goals for health information and education.

national health insurance: Form of insurance sponsored by a national government intended to pay for health services used by its citizens.

National Health Planning and Resource Development Act of 1974: U.S. federal legislation that established regional health systems agencies to assume responsibility for health care planning for community needs and for cost containment.

National Society for the Promotion of Occupational Therapy (NSPOT): Founded on March 15, 1917, for the promotion of occupational therapy; forerunner of the American Occupational Therapy Association.

natriuresis: The excretion of sodium in the urine.

natural environments: All integrated community settings.

naturalistic observation: Technical term that refers to a qualitative research technique of observing an individual in his or her natural environment.

natural killer (NK) cell: A large granular lymphocyte capable of killing certain tumors and virally infected cells.

natural kinds: Method of grouping objects, usually animals, based on common external characteristics that are intrinsic to all members of that category.

nature/nurture controversy: Debate over the extent to which inborn, hereditary characteristics as compared to life experiences and environmental factors determine a person's identity and psychological make-up.

navigates: Modifies the movement pattern of the arm, body, or wheelchair to maneuver around obstacles that are encountered in the course of moving through space such that undesirable contact with obstacles (e.g., knocking over, bumping into) is avoided (includes maneuvering objects held in the hand around obstacles).^{AOTA Framework}

nebulizer: An atomizer; a device used for throwing a spray or mist.

neck extension splint: Holds the neck extended and prevents the fusion of the chin to the chest.

neck righting reflex: Involuntary response in newborns in which turning the head to one side while the infant is supine causes rotation of the shoulders and trunk in the same direction. The reflex enables the child to roll over from a supine to prone position.

necrosis: Death of tissue usually resulting in gangrene.

needs assessment: Systematic gathering of information about strengths, problems, resources, and barriers in a given population or community. Results of needs assessments are the basis of program planning.

negative reinforcement: Removing an adverse stimulus to increase the probability of a desired behavior.

negligence: Commission of an act that a prudent person would not have done or the omission of a duty that a prudent person would have fulfilled that results in injury or harm to another person. May be the basis for a malpractice suit.

neocerebellum: Those parts of the cerebellum that receive input via the corticopontocerebellar pathway.

neo-Darwinism: *See* synthetic Darwinism.

neologism: A new, meaningless word often spoken by fluent aphasic patients/clients.

neonate: Represents the first 4 weeks of an infant's life.

neophilia: Love for, great interest in what is new; novelty.

neoplasm: A new and abnormal formation of tissue, such as a tumor.

nephrotoxicity: The quality of being toxic or destructive to kidney cells.

nepotism: Favoritism shown to relatives, especially in conferring offices.

nerve conduction test: Measurement of electrical conductivity of motor and sensory nerves by application of an external electrical stimulus to the nerve and evaluation of parameters such as nerve conduction time, velocity, amplitude, and shape of the resulting response as recorded from another site on the nerve or from a muscle supplied by the nerve.

nervios: Nerves (Hispanic idiom).

nervous system: The network of neural tissues in the body composed of the central and peripheral divisions, which are responsible for the processing of impulses.

network: Communication link between computers, communication between a central computer and users, or any group of computers that are connected in order to send messages to each other.

networking: Process that links people and information in order to accomplish objectives; often informal.

net worth: Property owned (assets), minus debts and obligations owed (liabilities), is the owner's equity (net worth).Small Business Administration

neural Darwinism: Gerald Edelman's theory of the biological development of the brain within an individual's lifespan, rooted in Darwinian notions of natural selection. *See* neuronal group selection.

neuralgia: Attacks of pain along the entire course or branch of a peripheral sensory nerve.

neural plasticity: Innate healing ability of the brain via "re-routing" neural pathways in an effort to compensate for areas of tissue damage.

neurapraxia: Interruption of nerve conduction without loss of continuity of the axon.

neuritic plaques: Normative age-related change in the brain involving amyloid protein collecting on dying or dead neurons.

neuritis: Condition causing a dysfunction of cranial or spinal nerve; in sensory nerves, paresthesia is present.

neuroanatomy: Structures within the central, peripheral, and autonomic nervous systems.

neurobehavioral approach: Analysis of tactile, kinesthetic, visual, auditory, and olfactory sensations and their required motor, visual, and verbal responses for each activity. Neurological integration of the input from the senses and muscular responses is included.

neurodevelopment: The progressive growth and development of the nervous system.

Neurodevelopmental Treatment (NDT): Intervention approach developed to address abnormal tonicity in a muscle and elimination of unwanted muscle activity and retraining of normal, functional patterns of movement in individuals with acquired brain dysfunction due to stroke, etc.

neurofibromatosis: von Recklinghausen's disease. Growth of multiple tumors from the nerve sheath.

neurogenic pain: Pain in the limbs caused by neurologic lesions.

neurohypophysis: Posterior lobe of the pituitary gland.

neuroleptic: Drug or agent that modifies psychotic behavior; antipsychotic.

neurologic impairment: Any disability caused by damage to the central nervous system (brain, spinal cord, ganglia, and nerves).

neurologist: Specialist who diagnoses and treats diseases of the nervous system.

neurolysis: Destruction of nerve tissue or loosening of adhesions surrounding a nerve.

neuroma: Tumor or growth along the course of a nerve or at the end of a lacerated nerve, which is often very painful.

neuromuscular: Pertaining to the nerves and the muscles.

neuromuscular facilitation: Increasing the activity of the muscles through sensory stimuli.

neuromuscular inhibition: Decreasing the activity of the muscles through the specific application of sensory stimuli.

neuromuscular re-education: Specific treatment regimens carried out by occupational and physical therapists to improve motor strength and coordination in persons with brain or spinal cord injuries.

neuron: Nerve cell.

neuronal group selection: The central theory of Edelman's neural Darwinism. It has three major tenets: a dynamic selection process that sets up the neuroanatomical characteristics of individuals during development; patterns of responses selected from this anatomy during experience; and physiology and psychology that give rise to behavior through re-entry, a process of signaling between brain maps. *See* re-entrant signaling.

neuropharmacology: Study of the effects of drugs on the brain.

neuroplasty: Surgical repair of nerves.

neuropsychological: A specialty area of cognitive research that explores the neurological basis of behavior.

neurosis: Mental disorder in which reality testing is not seriously disturbed; diagnostic category used prior to DSM-III.

neurotic: Analytic concept that reflects psychodynamic conflicts that cause difficulty for an individual to remain in contact with reality.

neurotmesis: Damage to the axon or complete transection of a nerve. Regeneration is less successful than in axonotmesis.

neurotransmitters: Chemical substances that convey new impulses at the synapses (gaps between nerve cells).

new public health: Global Public Health initiatives of recent years based on the Declaration of Alma Ata and the Ottawa Charter for Health Promotion. Emphasis is on primary health care, illness prevention, and health promotion.

nitroglycerin: Taken for pain in the heart due to angina pectoris. Reduces the amount of blood returning to the heart, lessening the workload by dilating peripheral blood vessels.

nominal (or categorical) data: Numbers are utilized to name mutually exclusive categories.

nominal scales: Measurement scales that contain information that is categorical and mutually exclusive (i.e., it can only be contained in one category).

nonhuman environment: Everything that is not human.

nonjudgmental acceptance: Therapist or group therapist lets the client know that his or her ideas and thoughts will be valued and not rejected.

nonmaleficence: Obligation to avoid doing harm to another individual or creating a circumstance in which harm could occur.

nonmaterial culture: Nontangible aspects of a society such as language, knowledge, skills, beliefs, and values.

nonmoral values: Operational beliefs utilized with the sole purpose of meeting personal preferences.

nonparametrics: Statistical tests that do not predict the population parameter, μ, or normality of the underlying population distribution.

nonrapid eye movement (NREM): Sleep state in which brain waves become slower and less regular.

nonverbal communication: Information exchange that does not require oral or written forms of language (e.g., gestures, positioning of the body).

normal curve: When scores and frequency of occurrence are plotted on the x- and y-axes, respectively, this frequency distribution curve ensues.

normality: Range of behavior considered acceptable by a social group or culture.

normative behavior: Behavior consistent with the beliefs, values, and expectations of a cultural group.

normative ethics: Examination of daily debates between group members about what is right and what is wrong.

norm-referenced test: Any instrument that uses the typical scores of members of a comparison group as a standard for determining individual performance.

norms: Standards of comparison derived from measuring an attribute across many individuals to determine typical score ranges.

nosocomial: Diseases originating in hospitals.

notes: Notations made by the therapist in the patient's/client's chart that are made each time treatment/service/evaluation is provided.

notes and accounts receivable: A secured or unsecured receivable evidenced by a note or open account arising from activities involving liquidation and disposal of loan collateral.Small Business Administration

notices/responds: Responds appropriately to (a) nonverbal environmental/perceptual cues (i.e., movement, sound, smell, heat, moisture, texture, shape, consistency) that provide feedback with respect to task progression and (b) the spatial arrangement of objects to one another (e.g., aligning objects during stacking). Notices and, when indicated, makes an effective and efficient response.AOTA Framework

noticing: Act of knowing; awareness of critical issues.

novitiate: Beginning stages or apprenticeship within a professional career.

noxious: Harmful to health; injurious (e.g., noxious gas, noxious stimuli).

NSAID: Nonsteroidal anti-inflammatory drug, such as ibuprofen or aspirin.

nuchal rigidity: Reflex spasm of the neck extensor muscles resulting in resistance to cervical flexion.

null hypothesis: The belief that results are solely a result of chance.

nyctalopia: Inability to see well in faint light or at night.

nystagmus: Rhythmic, constant, and rapid involuntary movement of the eyeball.

ObamaCare: See Appendix 33.

objective measure: Method of assessment that is not influenced by the emotions or personal opinion of the assessor.

object relations: In psychoanalytic theory, the investment of psychic energy in objects and events in the world; sometimes seen exclusively as the bond(s) between two persons.

obligatory reflexive response: Reflex that is consciously present in a motor pattern; this reflex may dominate all other movement components.

observation (OBS): Watching; a judgment or opinion.

observer bias: When the previous experiences of the individual influence his or her observations and interpretation of behaviors being assessed or evaluated.

obsession: Irresistible thought pattern, usually anxiety provoking, that intrudes on normal thought processes.

obsessive-compulsive disorder: Anxiety disorder characterized by recurrent uncontrollable thoughts, irresistible urges to engage repetitively in an act, or both such that they cause significant anxiety or interfere with daily functioning.

obtrusive observation: When the individual is aware of being observed by the therapist for the purpose of evaluation of cognitive, physical, and/or psychosocial performance.

Occident: Europe and America as distinct from the Orient (Latin: occidens; entis = setting, sunset, west).

occipitofrontal: A line from the root of the nose to the most prominent portion of the occipital bone of the fetus at term.

occipitomental: Diameter from the chin of the fetus to the most prominent portion of the occipital bone; the correct angle for the application of forceps during delivery.

occupation: Daily life activities in which people engage. Occupations occur in context and are influenced by the interplay among client factors, performance skills, and performance patterns. Occupations occur over time; have purpose, meaning, and perceived utility to the client; and can be observed by others (e.g., preparing a meal) or be known only to the person involved (e.g., learning through reading a textbook). Occupations can involve the execution of multiple activities for completion and can result in various outcomes. The *Framework* identifies a broad range of occupations categorized as activities of daily living, instrumental activities of daily living, rest and sleep, education, work, play, leisure, and social participation.[OTPF 2014]

occupational adaptation: A response to occupational challenges (Schkade & Schultz, 1992) with all clients, from individuals to populations, given that "individuals continuously adapt their occupations" (Meltzer, 2001, p. 17).[CAOT]

occupational adaptation (the process): A series of actions, internal to the individual, that unfold as the individual is faced with occupational challenge. The individual engages in this process with the intention to produce a response that will result in an experience of relative mastery over the challenge.

occupational adaptation (the state): State of competency toward which human beings aspire. The existence and strength of this state in an individual is a function of the extent to which occupational responses have been effective in producing relative mastery over occupational challenges and the extent to which such responses have been successfully generalized to a variety of occupational challenges.

occupational alienation: "The outcome when people experience daily life as meaningless or purposeless" (Stadnyk, Townsend, & Wilcock, in press).[CAOT] Sense of isolation, powerlessness, frustration, loss of control, estrangement from society or self as a result of engagement in occupation, which does not satisfy inner needs.

occupational analysis: *See* activity analysis.^OTPF 2014 Previously known as activity or task analysis; requires competency to analyze and adapt the parts, steps, processes or components of an occupation. Occupational analysis is a form of assessment focused on occupation, and the competency to use that information is to consider and implement various forms of adaptation or transformation.^CAOT

occupational apartheid: A willful exclusion of a group, "refers to the segregation of groups of people through the restriction or denial of access to dignified and meaningful participation in occupations of daily life on the basis of race, color, disability, national origin, age, gender sexual preference, religion, political beliefs, status in society or other characteristics. Occasioned by political forces, its systematic and pervasive social, cultural and economic consequences jeopardize health and wellbeing as experienced by individuals, communities and societies" (Kronenberg & Pollard, 2005, p. 67).^CAOT

occupational balance: A balance of engagement in occupation that leads to well-being. For example, the balance may be among physical, mental, and social occupations; between chosen and obligatory occupations; between strenuous and restful occupations; or between doing and being.

occupational balance/imbalance: "Is a temporal concept since it refers to allocation of time use for particular purposes and is based on the reasoning that human health and well-being require a variation in productive and leisure occupations" (Stadnyk et al., in press).^CAOT

occupational behavior: Set of responses that allow the individual to maintain role competence.

occupational behaviour: Aspect or class of human action that encompasses mental and physical doing.^CAOT

occupational capacity: The actual or potential ability to engage in occupations.^CAOT

occupational capacity evaluation: Assessment of the match between the person's capabilities and critical demands of a specific job.

occupational change: Occurs by adding, abandoning, or altering occupations through the use of adapting, restructuring, refraining and reconstructing strategies to (a) develop through occupational transitions across the life course, (b) monitoring occupational engagement, health and well-being, (c) restore occupational potential and performance, or (d) prevent occupational losses and deprivation, occupational alienation or other forms of occupational justice.[CAOT]

occupational citizenship: Optimal engagement as a fully integrated citizen in a just and inclusive society with entitlement for all people to participate, enabled by the opportunities and resources they require, in the occupations of everyday life that foster health and well-being.[CAOT]

occupational competence: Adequacy or sufficiency in an occupational skill, meeting all requirements of an environment; develops as a progression from novice to master in the performance of occupations; an iterative process repeated again and again with the addition of mastery in each new occupation.[CAOT]

occupational demands: *See* activity demands.[OTPF 2014]

occupational deprivation: "A state of prolonged preclusion from engagement in occupations of necessity and/or meaning due to factors which stand outside of the control of the individual" (Whiteford, 2000, p. 201); the influence of an external circumstance that prevents a person from acquiring, using, or enjoying occupation over an extended period of time (Whiteford, 1997; Wilcock, 1996, 2006).[CAOT] Deprivation of occupational choice and diversity because of circumstances beyond the control of individuals or communities.

occupational development: A systematic process of change in occupational behaviors across time resulting from the growth and maturation of the individual in interaction with the environment; the constellation of occupations an individual accumulates across the life span, her or his life course occupational repertoire; marked by the changes in the specific occupations that an individual can and does perform over the course of life; governed by the principles underlying the occupational trajectories and transitions that occur across the life course, and the

processes whereby these occur (Davis & Polatajko, 2006, p. 138).
CAOT Systematic progression of change which occurs across the
lifespan in response to an individual's role-based challenges.

occupational disruption: "May appear to be similar to occupational deprivation. . .but it refers to a temporary or transient disruption. . .and results from factors that are internal or individual,
such as illness" (Whiteford, 2004, p. 223).CAOT

occupational engagement: To involve oneself or become occupied, to participate in occupation (Houghton Mifflin Company,
2004). Involvement for being, becoming, and belonging, as well
as for performing or doing occupations (Wilcock, 2006).CAOT

occupational enrichment: The "deliberate manipulation of environments to facilitate and support engagement in a range of
occupations congruent with those that the individual might
normally perform" (Molineux & Whiteford, 1999, p. 127).CAOT

occupational factors: Include the self-maintenance, work, home,
leisure, and family roles and activities of the person.

occupational form: The objective set of physical and sociocultural
circumstances, external to the person, that guides, structures, or
suggests what is to be done by the person (the occupational performance). In occupational therapy, the therapist collaborates
with the person in synthesizing (designing) the occupational
form, so that a therapeutic occupational performance can result.

occupational grouping: A set of occupations grouped by a theme,
primarily named by the individual or society (e.g., such as self-
care, productivity, leisure) (Polatajko et al., 2004).CAOT

occupational history: A record of how one progresses from one
occupation to another, often due to a transitional event such as a
marriage or divorce (Meltzer, 2001).CAOT A process used to gain
understanding of the life conditions and circumstances that
have influenced the ways in which one has learned to approach
tasks (activities) and to fulfill roles (Bruce & Borg, 2001).

occupational identity: "Composite sense of who one is and wishes
to become as an occupational being generated from one's history of occupational participation" (Boyt Schell et al., 2014a,
p. 1238).OTPF 2014 "How an individual sees the self in terms of

various occupational roles, an image of the kind of life desired" (Kielhofner, Mallinson, Forsyth, & Lai, 2001, p. 261).[CAOT]

occupational imbalance: A lack of balance or disproportion of occupation resulting in decreased well-being.

occupational issues (OI): Challenges to occupational engagement or to inclusive and just participation in occupations, including yet not limited to occupational performance issues, occupational alienation issues, occupational balance issues, occupational development issues, occupational deprivation issues, occupational marginalization issues.[CAOT]

occupational justice: "A justice that recognizes occupational rights to inclusive participation in everyday occupations for all persons in society, regardless of age, ability, gender, social class, or other differences" (Nilsson & Townsend, 2010, p. 58). Access to and participation in the full range of meaningful and enriching occupations afforded to others, including opportunities for social inclusion and the resources to participate in occupations to satisfy personal, health, and societal needs (adapted from Townsend & Wilcock, 2004).[OTPF 2014]

occupational justice/injustice: "Whilst social justice addresses the social relations and social conditions of life, occupational justice addresses what people do in their relationships and conditions for living" (Wilcock & Townsend, 2000, p. 84). Motivating this exploration is a utopian vision of an occupationally just world governed to enable all individuals to flourish in diverse ways by doing what they decide they can do that is most meaningful and useful to themselves and to their families, communities, and nations (Wilcock & Townsend, 2008).[CAOT]

occupational life course: The occupational repertoire that accumulates across the life course; an occupational life course narrative is the history of occupational experiences and transitions over the life course (Davis & Polatajko, 2006).[CAOT]

occupational marginalization: When some social groups more than others are denied or restricted in making choices and decisions about their participation in everyday occupations, often resulting from invisible expectations, norms, and standards (Townsend & Wilcock, 2004).[CAOT]

occupational mastery: Competent occupational functioning (adapted from Schkade & Schultz, 1992).CAOT

occupational nurse: First training of nurses in the use of occupation in treatment.

occupational participation: Involvement in a life situation (WHO, 2001) through occupation.CAOT

occupational pattern: The "regular and predictable way of doing; occurs when human beings organize activities and occupations" (Bendixon et al., 2006, p. 4).CAOT

occupational performance: Act of doing and accomplishing a selected action (performance skill), activity, or occupation (Fisher, 2009; Fisher & Griswold, 2014; Kielhofner, 2008) that results from the dynamic transaction among the client, the context, and the activity. Improving or enabling skills and patterns in occupational performance leads to engagement in occupations or activities (adapted in part from Law et al., 1996, p. 16).OTPF 2014 The "result of a dynamic, interwoven relationship between persons, environment, and occupation over a person's lifespan; the ability to choose, organize, and satisfactorily perform meaningful occupations that are culturally defined and age appropriate for looking after oneself, enjoying life, and contributing to the social and economic fabric of a community" (CAOT, 1997a, 2002, p. 181).CAOT

occupational performance areas: Tasks related to self-care/self-maintenance, work/productive activities, and play/leisure.

occupational performance component: Any subsystem that contributes to the performance of self-care/self-maintenance, work/productive activities, and play/leisure (e.g., fine motor coordination).

occupational performance contexts: Situations or factors that influence an individual's engagement in desired and/or required performance areas (AOTA, 1994, p. 1047).

occupational performance goal (OPG): Directed toward choosing, organizing, or performing a meaningful occupation. An OPG is essential for the initiation of an occupational therapy process. An OPG becomes relevant for occupational therapy when attaining the goal becomes a challenge.CAOT

occupational performance issue (OPI): "An actual or potential issue (or problem)" (Fearing & Clark, 2000, p. 184) in the "ability to choose, organize, and satisfactorily perform meaningful occupations" (CAOT, 1997a, 2002, p. 30). An OPI becomes relevant for occupational therapy when solutions to choosing, organizing, or performing an occupation become a challenge.[CAOT]

occupational performance model (OPM): A "1991 portrayal of the interacting elements of individual performance components, areas of occupational performance, and the environment" (CAOT, 1997a, 2002, p. 182).[CAOT]

Occupational Performance Process Model (OPPM): A seven-stage process of practice for focusing on occupational performance using client-centered approaches with individual, organization, and other clients (CAOT, 1997a, 2002; Fearing, Law, & Clark, 1997).[CAOT]

occupational potential: What might be in the future beyond what is in the present; a combination of capacity, opportunity, resources, and social structure that enable engagement in occupations by individuals, families, groups, communities, organizations, and populations to reach beyond an existing occupational status to a predictable or unpredictable occupational status. [CAOT] Future capability to engage in occupation toward needs, goals, and dreams for health, material requirement, happiness, and well-being.

occupational profile: Summary of the client's occupational history and experiences, patterns of daily living, interests, values, and needs.[OTPF 2014]

occupational reasoning: The component of occupational therapy professional reasoning which integrates environmental, conditional reasoning about the context of practice and client lives, and biomedical clinical reasoning, both narrative and empirical, about the body, persons, and clinical practice.[CAOT]

occupational repertoire: "The set of occupations an individual has at a specific point in the life course" (Davis & Polatajko, 2006, p. 137).[CAOT]

occupational role: The rights, obligations, and expected behavior patterns associated with a particular set of activities or occupations, done on a regular basis, and associated with social cultural roles (adapted from Hillman & Chapparo, 1995, p. 88). CAOT

occupational satisfaction: The state of being satisfied or content with one's occupational performance or engagement. CAOT

occupational science: An interdisciplinary academic discipline in the social and behavioral sciences dedicated to the study of the form, the function, and the meaning of human occupations (Zemke & Clark, 1996). OTPF 2008 The rigorous study of humans as occupational beings (Wilcock, 2006). CAOT

occupational status: Collective term encompassing occupational performance components, occupational performance, and occupational role performance.

occupational technology: Means and tools by which material things are produced in a particular civilization which change ways of "doing."

occupational therapy (OT): Therapeutic use of everyday life activities (occupations) with individuals or groups for the purpose of enhancing or enabling participation in roles, habits, routines, and rituals in home, school, workplace, community, and other settings. Occupational therapy practitioners use their knowledge of the transactional relationship among the person, his or her engagement in valued occupations, and the context to design occupation-based intervention plans that facilitate change or growth in client factors (values, beliefs, and spirituality; body functions, body structures) and performance skills (motor, process, and social interaction) needed for successful participation. Occupational therapy practitioners are concerned with the end result of participation and thus enable engagement through adaptations and modifications to the environment or objects within the environment when needed. Occupational therapy services are provided for habilitation, rehabilitation, and promotion of health and wellness for clients with disability- and non-disability-related needs. These services include acquisition and preservation of occupational identity for those who have or are at risk for developing an illness, injury, disease, disorder, condition, impairment, disability, activity limitation, or participation restriction (adapted from AOTA, 2011).[OTPF 2014] The art and science of enabling engagement in everyday living through occupation; of enabling people to perform the occupations that foster health and well-being; and of enabling a just and inclusive society so that all people may participate to their potential in the daily occupations of life.[CAOT]

occupational therapy aide: According to the American Occupational Therapy Association's *Position Paper—Use of Occupational Therapy Aides in OT Practice*, individual assigned by an occupational therapy practitioner to perform delegated, selected, skilled tasks in specific situations under the direction and close supervision of an occupational therapy practitioner.

Occupational Therapy *Code of Ethics*: Refers to the document created by the American Occupational Therapy Association to provide clear parameters under which occupational therapy practitioners should practice their profession. It also promotes and maintains the highest standards of ethical behavior among occupational therapy personnel.

occupational therapy diagnosis: Descriptive problem statement that succinctly describes actual or potential occupational status dysfunctions that are amenable to intervention with occupational therapy procedures and modalities.

Occupational Therapy Functional Assessment Compilation Tool (OTFACT): Method of integrating and reporting the full range of functional performance by organizing occupational therapy assessment results, generating a functional profile of the client.

Occupational Therapy Global Day of Service (OTGDS): A unique opportunity for occupational therapy colleagues around the world to come together to provide a cohesive and organized global effort of community service and social participation (www.promotingot.org).

Occupational Therapy Intervention Process Model (OTIPM): A professional reasoning model that helps to ensure an occupation-centered perspective to guide reasoning and plan/implement occupation-based and occupation-focused services.

occupational therapy practitioner: Individual who is credentialed as an occupational therapist (OT) or an occupational therapy assistant (OTA).

occupational therapy support personnel: Persons who are supervised by occupational therapists and who have formal or on-the-job training in the basic theory and methods of occupational therapy.[CAOT]

occupational therapy treatment process: The generalization of the steps or stages that typically occur in professional interactions with clients.

Occupational Therapy Uniform Evaluation Checklist: Official document of the American Occupational Therapy Association that suggests guidelines for occupational therapy assessment by identifying areas of occupational performance.

occupational well-being: An experience in which people derive feelings of satisfaction and meaning from the ways in which they have orchestrated their occupational lives (Caron Santha & Doble, 2006; Doble, Caron Santha, Theben, Knott, & Lall-Phillips, 2006).[CAOT]

occupation-based intervention: A type of occupational therapy intervention—a client-centered intervention in which the occupational therapy practitioner and client collaboratively select and design activities that have specific relevance or meaning to the client and support the client's interests, needs, health, and participation in daily life.[OTPF 2008]

occupations: Groups of activities and tasks of everyday life, named, organized, and given value and meaning by individuals and a culture; occupation is everything people do to occupy themselves, including looking after themselves (self-care), enjoying life (leisure), and contributing to the social and economic fabric of their communities (productivity); the domain of concern and the therapeutic medium of occupational therapy (CAOT, 1997a, 2002); a set of activities that is performed with some consistency and regularity; that brings structure and is given value and meaning by individuals and a culture (adapted from Polatajko et al., 2004; and Zimmerman et al., 2006).[CAOT]

ocular dysmetria: The eyes are unable to fix gaze on an object or follow a moving object with accuracy.

oculomotor: Pertains to movements of the eyeballs.

old age: Arbitrary or societally defined period of life; specifically, over 65 years of age in the United States.

Older Americans Act: Enacted in 1965 as the major piece of legislation for provision of social and health-related services for older Americans; established federal, state, and local government network for advocacy and service delivery.

older person: Term used to refer to individuals in the later years of the life span. Arbitrarily set between 65 and 70 years in American society for the purpose of age-related entitlements.

oldest old: Persons older than 85 years of age.

old old: Persons older than 75 years of age.

olfactory: Interpreting odors[UTIII]; pertaining to the sense of smell.

olfactory defensiveness: Sensitivity to odors.

oligoclonal banding: A process by which cerebrospinal fluid immunoglobulin G is distributed, following electrophoresis, in discrete bands. Approximately 90% of patients/clients with multiple sclerosis show oligoclonal banding.

oligodendroglia: Myelin-producing cells in the central nervous system.

oliguria: Diminished amount of urine formation.

ombudsman: An official appointed to receive and investigate complaints made by individuals against public officials and institutions.

Omnibus Budget Reconciliation Act of 1987 (OBRA '87): U.S. federal legislation that recognizes quality of life as most important to nursing home residents.

Omnibus Reconciliation Act (1981): U.S. federal legislation designed to finance community-based services for people with developmental disabilities when that treatment is less expensive than an institution.

Omnibus Social Security Act (1983): U.S. federal legislation that established a prospective payment system based on a fixed price per diagnosis related group for inpatient services.

one-tail (directional) test: A test of the null hypothesis where only one tail of the distribution is utilized.

online: Computer linked to another computer or network.

onlooker play: Level of social play in which a child watches other children at play. The child may verbally interact but does not participate in the activity.

on-screen keyboard: Virtual keyboard provided on the computer monitor by specific software. An individual can then touch the on-screen keyboard with an alternate access device, such as an optical scanner or head pointer.

on-the-job evaluation: Assesses the physical demands, psychosocial factors, cognitive factors, analysis of essential functions, tools and machines used, description of the work environment, and hazards and stress factors in a competitive employment situation, as well as the person's ability to perform under such circumstances.

ontogeny: Course of development during an individual's lifetime: from egg to adult throughout the life span.

onychia: Inflammation of the nail bed.

onychogryphosis: Ingrown nail, either finger or toe.

onychosis: Any disease of the nails.

oocyte: A primitive cell in the ovary that becomes an ovum after meiosis.

open-chain movements: The distal end (insertion) of a kinematic chain moves (e.g., swing a baseball bat).

open-ended question: Question that may have multiple correct responses rather than a finite correct answer.

open enrollment period: Period of time in which new subscribers may elect to enroll in a health insurance plan.

open seclusion: Temporary placement in an isolated room with no windows or furniture, but the door is open.

open system: System of structures that function as a whole and maintains itself by means of input from the environment and organismic change occurring as needed.

operant conditioning: Form of conditioning in which reinforcement is contingent upon the occurrence of the desired response.

ophthalmologist: Medical doctor specializing in the eye.

ophthalmoplegia: Paralysis of ocular muscles.

opioid: Synthetic drugs that have pharmacological properties similar to opium or morphine.

opisthotonus: Position of extreme hyperextension of the vertebral column caused by a tetanic spasm of the extensor musculature.

opposition: The movement in which the thumb is brought across to meet the little finger.

Optacon: Camera that allows people who are blind to read by converting print to an image of letters, which are then produced onto the finger using vibrations.

optical character recognition: Technology used in scanning to convert the images of typed text into a computer code (i.e., translating the analog signal from the voltage of reflected light to a digital value readable by the computer).

optical pointers: Devices that sense light and feedback the stimulus to indicate where the device is pointing.

optokinetic nystagmus: Nystagmus induced by watching stripes on a drum revolving around one's face.

optometrist: Medical professional specializing in the correction of vision.

oral defensiveness: Avoidance of certain textures of food and irritation with activities using the mouth.

oral hygiene: Obtaining and using supplies; cleaning mouth; brushing and flossing teeth; or removing, cleaning, and reinserting dental orthotics and prosthetics.[UTIII]

oral-motor control: Coordinating oropharyngeal musculature for controlled movements.[UTIII]

order: The desired state of affairs, which is an absence of disease in medicine and competence in the performance of work, play, or self-care. Disorder is defined as disease in medicine and performance dysfunction in occupational therapy.

ordinal data: Rank-ordered data.

ordinal scales: Measurement scales that contain information that can be rank ordered.

ordinary interest: Simple interest based on a year of 360 days, contrasting with exact interest having a base year of 365 days.[Small Business Administration]

ordinate: In the coordinate system, the ordinate is the vertical axis (*also known as* the y-axis).

organic brain syndrome: Cluster of mental disorders characterized by impaired cerebral function resulting from damage to or changes in the brain.

organic communities: Societies in which natural functions, role perspectives, mutual interdependence, and intrinsic relationships are paramount.

organismic view: Concept that an individual is active in determining and controlling his or her own behavior and can change that behavior if it is desirous to do so.

organization: Entity composed of individuals with a common purpose or enterprise, such as a business, industry, or agency.[OTPF 2014]

organizational patterns: Hierarchic patterns of personnel ranking that indicate the underlying chain of command in an organization.

organizational skills: The ability to organize materials, space, and time in order to complete a task.

organizes: Logically positions or spatially arranges tools and materials in an orderly fashion (a) within a single workspace and (b) among multiple appropriate workspaces to facilitate ease of task performance.[AOTA Framework]

orgasm: The apex and culmination of sexual excitement.

orientation: Identifying person, place, time, and situation; initial stage of group development that includes a search for structure, goals, and dependency on the leader.

orients: Directs one's body in relation to others and/or occupational forms.[AOTA Framework]

origin: Proximal attachment of a muscle that remains relatively fixed during normal muscular contraction.

orthokinetic cuff: Device made from an elastic bandage applied to a weak muscle to provide tactile stimulation to the muscle via movement of the cuff–skin interface during muscle contraction.

orthopedic (Orth): Branch of medical science that deals with the prevention or correction of disorders involving locomotor structures of the body.

orthopedic impairment: Any disability caused by disorders to the musculoskeletal system.

orthopnea: Inability to breathe except in an upright position.

orthosis: Device added to a person's body to support, position, or immobilize a part; to correct deformities; to assist weak muscles and restore function; or to modify tone.

orthostatic hypotension: Lowered blood pressure when a person changes from a horizontal to an erect position.

orthotic: An external device utilized to apply forces to a body part to limit movement, increase the velocity or power of a movement, stop movement, or hold the body part in a particular position. Previously called braces.

oscilloscope: Instrument that displays a visual representation of an electrical wave such as a muscle contraction.

Osgood's Semantic Differential: Paper-and-pen rating scale to measure the meaning of activities.

osmosis: The passage of pure solvent from the lesser to the greater concentration when two solutions are separated by a membrane that selectively prevents the passage of solute molecules but is permeable to the solvent. An attempt to equalize concentrations on both sides of a membrane.

osteoarthritis (OA): Inflammation of the bones and joints (typically of older ages) due to years of body movement.

osteoblast: Any cell that develops into bone or secretes substances producing bony tissue.

osteochondrosis: A disease of one or more of the growth or ossifications centers in children that begins as a degeneration or necrosis followed by regeneration or recalcification.

osteoclast: Any of the large multinucleate cells in bone that absorb or break down bony tissue.

osteogenesis imperfecta: Autosomal dominant disorder that occurs once in 30,000 births. It is characterized by increased susceptibility to fractures. Normal intelligence and possible hearing loss are associated.

osteomyelitis: An infection usually caused by bacterial disease of the bone marrow and adjacent bone, in which chronic inflammation occurs due to infection reaching the bone through an opening in the skin as a result of trauma or surgery.

osteoplasty: Plastic surgery of the bones; bone grafting.

osteoporosis: Reduction in bone mass associated with loss of bone mineral and matrix occurring when bone resorption is greater than formation; found in sedentary, post-menopausal women or following steroidal therapy.

osteotomy: Operation to cut across a bone.

otitis media: Inflammation of the inner ear.

otolaryngology: The science of laryngology, rhinology, and otology.

otosclerosis: Hardening of the bony tissue of the ear resulting in conductive hearing loss.

ougenics movement: Set of policies from the early 1900s that viewed people with disabilities as "defectives" and "deviates."

outcome: End result of the occupational therapy process; what clients can achieve through occupational therapy intervention.[OTPF 2014]

outcome analysis: A systematic examination of patient/client outcomes in relation to selected patient/client variables (e.g., age, sex, diagnosis, interventions performed); outcomes analysis may be used in quality assessment, economic analysis of practice, and other processes.

outcome measure: Instrument designed to gather information on the efficacy of service programs; a means for determining whether goals or objectives have been met.

outcome orientation: Focus on evaluation of the person's success in terms of the impact on outcomes.[C]

outlays: Net disbursements (cash payments in excess of cash receipts) for administrative expenses and for loans and related costs and expenses (e.g., gross disbursements for loans and expenses minus loan repayments, interest and fee income collected, and reimbursements received for services performed for other agencies).[Small Business Administration]

out-of-pocket payment or costs: Costs borne solely by an individual without the benefit of insurance.

outpatient services: Ambulatory care provided in outpatient departments of health facilities.

output: Production or yield during a given time.

outreach services: Services that seek out and identify hard-to-reach individuals and assist them in gaining access to needed services.

outrigger: Projecting support attached to a splint from which finger loops are suspended.

outsiders: Those who are not members of a cultural group.

overflow: Clinical term for unwanted movement in a part of the body inappropriate to the action being performed.

overuse syndrome: Musculoskeletal disorder manifested from repetitive upper extremity movements occurring during activities. Symptoms include persistent pain in joints, muscles, tendons, or other soft tissues of the upper extremities. *Synonyms*: cumulative trauma disorder, repetitive strain disorder.

ovoid of motion: The curved path of motion through which a bone moves. It is always convex away from the joint at which motion occurs.

oximeter: A photoelectric device for determining the oxygen saturation of the blood.

oxygen consumption: The amount of oxygen used by the tissues of the body, usually measured in oxygen uptake in the lung; normally about 250 mL/minute, and it increases with increased metabolic rate.

oxygen saturation: The degree to which oxygen is present in a particular cell, tissue, organ, or system.

oxytocin: A hormone stored in the pituitary that causes contraction of the uterus.

pacemaker: Electrical device implanted to control the beating of the heart.

paces: Maintains a consistent and effective rate or tempo of performance throughout the steps of the entire task.^{AOTA Framework}

pachymeningitis: Acute inflammation of the dura mater.

Paget's disease: Disease characterized by a greatly accelerated remodeling process in which osteoclastic resorption is massive and osteoblastic bone formation is extensive. As a result, there is an irregular thickening and softening of the bones of the skull, pelvis, and extremities. It rarely occurs in people younger than 50 years.

pain character measurements: Any of the tools used to define the character of a patient's/client's pain.

pain estimates: A pain intensity measurement in which patient's/client's pain is rated on pain scale of 0 to 100.

pain intensity measurements: Any of the scales used to quantify pain intensity.

pain management: Use of treatment to control chronic pain, including the use of behavioral modification, relaxation training, physical modalities and agents, medication, and surgery.

pain modulation: Variation in the intensity and appreciation of pain secondary to central nervous system and autonomic nervous system effects on the nociceptors and along the pain pathways, as well as secondary to external factors such as distraction and suggestion.

pain pathway: The route along which nerve impulses arising from painful stimuli are transmitted from the nociceptor to the brain, including transmission within the brain itself.

Jacobs, K., & Simon, L. (Eds.). *Quick Reference Dictionary for Occupational Therapy, Sixth Edition* (pp. 211-242).
© 2015 SLACK Incorporated.

pain quality: A description of the nature, type, or character of pain (i.e., burning, dull, sharp, throbbing, or other).

pain response: Interpreting noxious stimuli.[UTIII]

paired t ratio: Statistical test between two sample means, where the sample selection is not independent.

Paleolithic: The earliest part of the Stone Age that began some 2.6 million years ago in Africa with the first recognizable stone tools, known as Oldowan, from Olduvai Gorge in Tanzania.

palliative care: Care rendered to temporarily reduce or moderate the intensity of an otherwise chronic medical condition.

palmar: Palm of the hand.

palmar arches: Natural curves in the palm created by the structure of joints, ligaments, and muscles.

palpate: To examine by touching and feeling.

palpation: Examination by touching and feeling.

palpitation: Rapid, violent, or throbbing pulsation in a body part.

palsy: The loss of movement or ability to control movement.

pancreatitis: Inflammation of the pancreas, with pain and tenderness of the abdomen, tympanites (gaseous pockets), and vomiting.

panic: Sudden acute fear or anxiety.

panic attack: State of extreme anxiety, usually including sweating, shortness of breath, chest pains, and fear. May come on unpredictably or as a result of a particular stimulus.

panic disorder: Anxiety disorder characterized by severe panic attacks, in which a person is overwhelmed with intense apprehension, dread, or terror; experiences an acute emergency reaction; thinks he or she might go crazy and die; and engages in fight-or-flight behavior.

papilledema: Edema and hyperemia of the optic disc.

paracrine: The method of extracellular hormonal communication.

paracyesis: Pregnancy that develops outside the uterus in the abdominal cavity.

paradigm: Refers to the organization of knowledge, as well as the changes in scientific thought over time; an organizing interaction. A pattern, example, or model.

paradox: A statement to the contrary of belief. A statement that is self-contradictory and, hence, false.

paraffin bath: A superficial thermal modality using paraffin wax and mineral oil.

parallel group participation: A group of people working on individual tasks with minimal requirements for interaction.

parallel interventions: Method of applying technology while at the same time providing therapy to maximize abilities for an individual for more powerful technology.

parallel play: Play in which children are doing the same activity at the same time and place, yet doing it separately.

parallel processing: Learning or solving a problem through a global approach integrating data into a whole experience.

parallel talk: A form of speech used during play therapy with children in which the clinician verbalizes actions, such as what is happening or what the child is doing, without requiring "answers" from the child. For example, "I'm building a tower. My tower is tall. You're building a tower, too. Your tower is tall, too." The clinician often repeats utterances of the child correctly and parallels the child's activities.

paralysis: Condition in which one loses voluntary motor control over a section of the body due to trauma or injury.

paranoia: Thought pattern that reflects a belief that others are persecuting or attempting to harm one, in the absence of a realistic basis for such fears.

paraphilias: Disorder characterized by intense, sexual arousing from fantasies, urges, or humiliation of oneself or others that is associated with distress or disability (Beers, Berkow, & Burs, 1999).

paraplegia (PARA): Paralysis of the spine affecting the lower portion of the trunk and legs.

parasomnia: Abnormal sleep behavior, including sleepwalking and bruxism (grinding the teeth).

parasympathetic nervous system: Autonomic nervous system that serves to relax the body's responses and is the opposite of the sympathetic nervous system.

parenchyma: Essential parts of an organ, which are concerned with its function rather than its framework.

parenteral: Administration by subcutaneous, intramuscular, or intravenous injection, thereby bypassing the gastrointestinal tract.

paresis: Weakness in voluntary muscle with slight paralysis.

paresthesia: Abnormal sensation, such as burning or prickling.

parietoalveolar: Pertaining to the cavities of the alveoli in the lungs.

Parkinson's disease: Degenerative disease, usually affecting the elderly population, that has three characteristic symptoms: tremor, rigidity, and bradykinesis.

paroxysm: Sudden, periodic attack or recurrence of symptoms of a disease.

participant observation: A process by which an ethnographer or fieldworker lives in a community and participates as much as possible in its routines while constantly observing.

participant-observer: Descriptor that can be applied when a therapist observes and evaluates an individual's performance while engaged in an activity with the person.

participation: "Involvement in a life situation" (WHO, 2001, p. 10). OTPF 2014

participation restriction: Problems an individual may experience in involvement in life situations.ICF

participatory style: Main assumption of this style is that people want to work and assume responsibility. Also, that if treated properly, people can be trusted and will put forth their best effort.

partnership: A legal relationship existing between two or more persons contractually associated as joint principals in a business.Small Business Administration

parturition: Act or process of giving birth to a child.

passive-aggressive personality disorder: Disorder that is characterized by resistance to social and occupational performance demands through procrastination, dawdling, stubbornness, inefficiency, and forgetfulness that appears to border on the intentional.

passive obedience: Research strategy wherein the researcher follows the participant's directions about what and how to do something.

passive range of motion (PROM): Amount of motion at a given joint when the joint is moved by the therapist.

passive stretch: Stretch applied with external force.

paternalism: Acting or making decisions on behalf of others without their consent.

pathology (PATH): The study of the characteristics, causes, and effects of disease, as observed in the structure and function of the body.

pathophysiology: An interruption or interference of normal physiological and developmental processes or structures.

patient management interview: Interview used by multiple professionals to identify the type of intervention or treatment needed.

patient-related consultation: When the health professional shares information with other professionals regarding individuals who are not presently receiving services.

patient's rights: The rights of patients to be informed about their conditions and prognoses and to make decisions concerning their treatment.

patterned responses: The programs either preprogrammed or created by the motor system to succeed at the presented task in the most efficient and integrated response possible at that moment in time.

patterns of help-seeking: Culturally distinct ways in which people go about finding help at particular times in an illness. It refers to both the range of options (often categorized as the biomedical, popular, and traditional health sectors) and the decision-making process.

pauciarticular: A form of juvenile rheumatoid arthritis that involves four joints or less and is generally asymmetrical.

Paxil: An orally administered antidepressant. *Generic name*: paroxetine hydrochloride.

Peabody Developmental Motor Scales (PDMS): Norm- and criteria-referenced test for children from birth to 7 years that assesses gross motor, praxis, fine motor, and visual-motor integration.

Peabody Picture Vocabulary: Untimed test that estimates the verbal intelligence of individuals ages 2½ to 18 years based on the measurement of hearing vocabulary. After the client hears a word, he or she chooses one of four pictures presented.

Pearson's *r*: Statistical technique that shows the degree of relationship between variables (also called the product-moment correlation).

pectus carinatum: Undue prominence of the sternum. *Synonyms*: chicken or pigeon chest or breast.

pectus excavatum: Undue depression of the sternum. *Synonyms*: funnel chest or breast.

pedagogy: Art and science of teaching children.

Pediatric Assessment of Self-Care Activities: Assessment that determines the child's degree of independence according to defined developmental sequences of feeding, toileting, hygiene, and dressing, including the use of fasteners.

peer culture: Stable set of activities or routines, artifacts, values, and concerns that a group of individuals produce or share.

peer review: Appraisal by professional coworkers of equal status of the way health practitioners conduct practice, education, or research.

peer support services: Focus on consumers helping one another with practical assistance, encouragement, advice, empowerment, and advocacy.[C]

pelvic floor: A sling arrangement of ligaments and muscles that supports the reproductive organs.

pelvimetry: A method of obtaining pelvic measurements by radiography.

pendular knee jerk: Upon elicitation of the deep tendon reflex of the knee, the lower leg oscillates briefly like a pendulum after the jerk, instead of returning immediately to resting position.

penicillin: Antibacterial drug used to treat infection.

percent body fat: Percent of body weight that is fat, includes storage fat (expendable), essential fat, and sex-specific fat reserve.

perception: Ability to organize and interpret incoming sensory information.

perceptual-motor: The interaction of the various channels of perception with motor activity, including visual, auditory, tactual, and kinesthetic channels.

perceptual motor skill: Ability to integrate perceptual (sensory) input with motor output in order to accomplish purposeful activities.

perceptual processing: Ability to integrate and understand perceptual (sensory) input in order to respond appropriately with motor output.

perceptual trace: Memory for past movement; the internal reference of correctness.

percussion (diagnostic): A procedure in which the clinician taps a body part manually or with an instrument to estimate its density.

percutaneous: Administration of a drug by inhalation, sublingual, or topical processes.

per diem rate: Fixed all-inclusive price for 1 day of hospital or nursing facility care, including all supplies and services provided to the patient during a day, excluding the professional fees of nonstaff physicians.

performance areas: Life tasks such as activities of daily living, work or productive activities, and play or leisure.

performance components: Sensorimotor, cognitive, integration, and psychosocial and psychological skills and abilities.

performance contexts: Temporal aspects of the physical, social, and cultural environment.

performance improvement: Planned, systematic, and organization-wide approach to designing, measuring, assessing, and improving organizational performance.

performance patterns: Habits, routines, roles, and rituals used in the process of engaging in occupations or activities; these patterns can support or hinder occupational performance.[OTPF 2014]

performance skills: Goal-directed actions that are observable as small units of engagement in daily life occupations. They are learned and developed over time and are situated in specific contexts and environments (Fisher & Griswold, 2014).[OTPF 2014]

performance subsystem: Subsystem in the Model of Human Occupation that includes neuromuscular skills, process skills, and communication/interaction skills.

perfusion: The act of pouring over or through, especially the passage of a fluid through the vessels of a specific organ or body part.

perinatal: Time period immediately before and after birth.

perineum: The area bounded by the pubis, coccyx, and thighs that is between the external genitalia and the anus.

period of concrete operations: Stage in the child's cognitive development where he or she is bound by immediate physical reality.

peripheral nerve injuries: Loss of precision pinch and grip due to crushing, severance, or inflammation/degeneration of the peripheral nerve fibers.

peripheral nervous system (PNS): Consists of all of the nerve cells outside the central nervous system, including motor and sensory nerves.

peripheral neuropathy: Any functional or organic disorder of the peripheral nervous system; degeneration of peripheral nerves supplying the extremities causing loss of sensation, muscle weakness, and atrophy.

peripheral pain: Pain arising from injury to a peripheral structure.

peristalsis: Movement by which a tube in the body (primarily the alimentary canal) sends contents within it to another part of the body. This is accomplished through alternative contractions and relaxations that resemble a wave- or worm-like movement.

peritonitis: Inflammation of the peritoneum; a condition marked by exudations in the peritoneum of serum, fibrin, cells, and pus. It is attended by abdominal pain and tenderness, constipation, vomiting, and moderate fever.

Perkins Brailler: Braille writing system with six keys, one for each of the six dots in a Braille cell, that leave an embossed print on paper.

perseveration: Inability to shift from thought to thought, persistence of an idea even when the subject changes.

person: Individual, including family member, caregiver, teacher, employee, or relevant other.^{OTPF 2014}

personal: "Features of the individual that are not part of a health condition or health status" (WHO, 2001, p. 17). Personal context includes age, gender, socioeconomic, and educational status. Can also include organizational levels (i.e., volunteers, employees) and population levels (i.e., members of a society).^{OTPF 2008}

personal care services: Services performed by health care workers to assist patients in meeting the requirements of daily living.

personal context: "Features of the individual that are not part of a health condition or health status" (WHO, 2001, p. 17). The personal context includes age, gender, socioeconomic and educational status and may also include membership in a group (i.e., volunteers, employees) or population (i.e., members of a society).^{OTPF 2014}

personal device care: Using, cleaning, and maintaining personal care items, such as hearing aids, contact lenses, glasses, orthotics, prosthetics, adaptive equipment, and contraceptive and sexual devices.^{AOTA Framework}

personal factors: The internal features of a person's life and living, including age, gender, educational background, coping styles, social background, profession, past and current experience, and other factors, which influence how disability is experienced by the person (WHO, 2001).

personal hygiene and grooming: Obtaining and using supplies; removing body hair (use of razors, tweezers, lotions, etc.); applying and removing cosmetics; washing, drying, combing, styling, brushing, and trimming hair; caring for nails (hands and feet); caring for skin, ears, eyes, and nose; applying deodorant; cleaning mouth; brushing and flossing teeth; or removing, cleaning, and reinserting dental orthotics and prosthetics.^{AOTA Framework}

personality: Individual's unique, relatively consistent, and enduring methods of behaving in relation to others and the environment.

personality disorder: Pervasive, inflexible, and stable personality traits that deviate from cultural norms and cause distress or functional impairment (Beers, Berkow, & Burs, 1999).

personality trait: Distinguishing feature that reflects one's characteristic way of thinking, feeling, and/or adapting.

personal protective equipment (PPE): Accessories provided on the worksite to protect workers from possible injuries and accommodate the physical requirements of workers and the job (e.g., gloves, eye wear, vibration and ear protection).

personal space: The area surrounding an individual that is perceived as private by the individual, who may regard movement into the space by another person as intrusive; although this varies in different cultures, it is usually 3 feet around the individual.

person-environment fit: Degree to which individuals have adapted to their unique environments.

person-environment interactions: Model proposing that behavior is a function of the person and his or her perceptions of the environment.

Person-Environment Occupational Performance Model: A model of occupational therapy practice that considers the individual, the situations, or the environments in which they find themselves and their engagement in daily occupations with the objective of providing multiple options for client-centered intervention.

person (intrinsic) factors: The neurobehavioral, cognitive, physical, and psychosocial strengths and deficits presented by the person.

person orientation: Focus on the individual first and foremost as a person with strengths and abilities, and not as a "case" exhibiting symptoms of disease.[C]

persons with disabilities: Individuals who experience substantial limitations in one or more major life activities, including but not limited to such functions as performing manual tasks, walking, seeing, hearing, speaking, breathing, learning, and working.

pervasive developmental disorder (PDD): The diagnostic category of PDD refers to a group of disorders characterized by delays in the development of socialization and communication skills. Parents may note symptoms as early as infancy, although the typical age of onset is before age 3 years. Symptoms may include problems with using and understanding language; difficulty relating to people, objects, and events; unusual play with toys and other objects; difficulty with changes in routine or familiar surroundings; and repetitive body movements or behavior patterns. Autism (a developmental brain disorder characterized by impaired social interaction and communication skills and a limited range of activities and interests) is the most characteristic and best studied PDD. Other types of PDD include Asperger's syndrome, childhood disintegrative disorder, and Rett's syndrome. Children with PDD vary widely in abilities, intelligence, and behaviors. Some children do not speak at all, others speak in limited phrases or conversations, and some have relatively normal language development. Repetitive play skills and limited social skills are generally evident. Unusual responses to sensory information, such as loud noises and lights, are also common (Office of Communications and Public Liaison, 2013).

pet therapy: *See* animal-assisted therapy (AAT).

petit mal: Type of seizure characterized by a momentary lapse of consciousness that starts and ends abruptly.

phacoemulsification: Method of treating cataracts by using ultrasonic waves to disintegrate the cataract, which is then aspirated.

phagocytosis: A process by which a leukocyte (monocyte, neutrophil) engulfs, ingests, and degrades a foreign particle or organism.

phalanges: Bones of the fingers and toes.

Phalen test: Test that confirms carpal tunnel syndrome.

phantom limb: Feeling of pressure or paresthesia as if it were coming from the amputated limb.

pharmacodynamics: The study of how drugs affect the body.

pharmacokinetics: The study of how the body handles drugs, including the way drugs are absorbed, distributed, and eliminated.

phenol block: An injection of phenol (hydroxybenzene) into individual nerves. Used as a topical anesthetic and produces a selective block of these nerves. Sometimes used to control severe spasticity in specific muscle groups.

phenotype: Observable characteristics of an organism that result from the interaction of the genotype with the organism's environment.

phenylketonuria (PKU): A hereditary disorder characterized by brain damage and mental retardation due to an inability to develop an essential enzyme, phenylalanine hydroxylase.

phenytoin: Anticonvulsant drug used to control major (grand mal) epileptic fits. Common side effects include dizziness, nausea, and skin rashes. *Trade name*: Dilantin.

philosophy: Logical study of nature and source of human knowledge or values; set of values and opinions of a group or individual.

philosophy of life: Personalized view of one's self and the world.

phlebotomy: Opening or piercing the vein.

phobia: Characterized by an extreme fear of a person, place, or thing when the situation is not hazardous.

phocomelia: The congenital absence or poor development of the proximal portion of the extremities. The hands and feet are thus attached to the trunk by an irregularly formed bone.

phonophoresis: The use of ultrasound waves to drive chemical molecules into the tissues for therapeutic purposes.

phototherapy: Intervention using the application of light.

phrenology: An approach to the study of neurology first proposed by Gall (1758–1828) in which it was proposed that the shape of the skull indicated the development and various mental functions of the underlying brain.

phylogeny: The evolutionary history of species.

physical: Nonhuman aspects of contexts. Includes the accessibility to and performance within environments having natural terrain, plants, animals, buildings, furniture, objects, tools, or devices.AOTA Framework

physical activities: Tasks using sensorimotor skills.

physical agent: A form of thermal, acoustic, or radiant energy that is applied to tissues in a systematic manner to achieve a therapeutic effect; a therapeutic modality used to treat physical impairments.

physical agent modalities (PAMs): Modalities such as hot packs, paraffin, electrical stimulation, and ultrasound used by qualified practitioners to prepare for or as an adjunct to purposeful activity.

physical demands: Physical requirements made on the worker by the specific job–worker situation as defined in the *Dictionary of Occupational Titles*. There are 20 demands: lifting, standing, walking, sitting, carrying, pushing, pulling, climbing, balancing, stooping, kneeling, crouching, crawling, reaching, handling, fingering, feeling, talking, hearing, and seeing.

physical environment: Natural and built nonhuman surroundings and the objects in them. The natural environment includes geographic terrain, plants, and animals, as well as the sensory qualities of the natural surroundings. The built environment includes buildings, furniture, tools, and devices.[OTPF 2014]

physical function: Fundamental component of health status describing the state of those sensory and motor skills necessary for mobility, work, and recreation.

physical therapy (PT): Health profession whose primary purpose is the promotion of optimal human health and function through the application of scientific principles to prevent, identify, assess, correct, or alleviate acute or prolonged movement dysfunction. See www.apta.org. From Section 6731 of New York State Education Law, the evaluation, treatment, or prevention of disability, injury, disease, or other condition of health using physical, chemical, and mechanical means including, but not limited to, heat, cold, light, air, water, sound, electricity, massage, mobilization, and therapeutic exercise with or without assistive devices, and the performance and interpretation of tests and measurements to assess pathophysiological, pathomechanical, and developmental deficits of human systems to determine treatment and assist in diagnosis and prognosis.

physician assistant: Health professionals licensed or, in the case of those employed by the federal government, credentialed to practice medicine with physician supervision.

***Physicians' Desk Reference* (PDR):** Provides a listing of medications, including the trade and generic names, the manufacturing company, the side effects and/or adverse reactions and appropriate interventions, and any incompatible medications.

physiological neophilia: Everything new is attractive in puberty.

physiologic flexion: The excessive amount of flexor tone that is normally present at birth because of the existing level of central nervous system maturation and fetal positioning in utero, or in adulthood, damage to the central nervous system.

physiology (PHYS): Area of study concerned with the functions of the structures of the body.

Piagentian: A set of concepts and constructs ascribed to Jean Piaget, a Swiss psychologist who studied child development.

pica: Compulsive eating of non-nutritious substances like dirt.

pinch meter: Type of dynamometer used to measure the strength of a client's pinch. It can be used to measure tip, lateral, and palmar pinching.

Pinterest: A pinboard-style photosharing website that allows users to create and manage theme-based image collections, such as events, interests, and hobbies. Users can browse the Internet or other pinboards for images, "re-pin" images to their own pinboards, and "like" photos.

piriformis syndrome: A condition characterized by overactivity of the piriformis muscle, causing external rotation of the leg and buttock pain.

pitocin: A synthetic oxytocic hormone administered through intravenous drip to induce or augment uterine contractions.

Pizzi Assessment of Productive Living (PAPL): Designed to assess all domains of function and occupational behaviors of people with AIDS or HIV. Takes into consideration their time and endurance limits.

PL 94-142 (1975): The Education for All Handicapped Children Act. U.S. federal law that mandated appropriate education in the least restrictive environment for all children ages 5 to 21 years with disabilities.

PL 99-457 (1986): Amended the Education for All Handicapped Children Act to create early intervention for infants and toddlers (birth to 2 years) and preschool programs (3 to 5 years) for children with disabilities.

PL 101-336 (1990): The Americans with Disabilities Act (ADA). U.S. federal law covering public accommodations, public services, transportation, employment, and telecommunication for individuals with disabilities.

PL 101-392 (1990): Carl D. Perkins Vocational and Applied Technology Education Act. U.S. federal law that mandated full vocational education for youths (until 22 years) with disabilities.

PL 101-476 (1990): Individuals with Disabilities Act (IDEA). U.S. federal law that reauthorized educational services for children (ages 3 to 21 years) with disabilities.

PL 102-119 (1991): Individuals with Disabilities Education Act (IDEA) Amendments. U.S. federal law that reauthorized early intervention for infants and toddlers with disabilities.

PL 102-569 (1992): Rehabilitation Act Amendments. U.S. federal law that mandated transition planning at high school graduation for students with disabilities.

PL 105-17 (1997): Individuals with Disabilities Education Act Amendments of 1997. U.S. federal law that restructured provisions of the act into four parts.

placebo effect: Improvement in a health condition as a result of provision of a substance or procedure believed to be inert (i.e., to have no observable chemical or physical effect).

placenta previa: Condition in which the placenta is implanted in the lower segment of the uterus, extending over the cervical opening. This often causes heavy bleeding during labor.

planes of motion: Imaginary lines that divide the body into right and left portions, front and back portions, and top and bottom portions.

plan of care: Statements that specify the anticipated long- and short-term goals and the desired outcomes, predicted level of optimal improvement, specific interventions to be used, duration, and frequency of the intervention required to reach the goals, outcomes, and criteria for discharge.

plaque: A lesion characterized by loss of myelin and hardening of tissue in diseases such as multiple sclerosis (peripherally) or Alzheimer's disease (in the brain).

plasma cell: Mature antibody secreting cell derived from the B cell.

plasmapheresis: A process by which blood is removed from the patient/client; plasma is discarded and replaced by normal plasma or human albumin. Reconstituted blood is then returned to the patient/client. This process is believed to rid the blood of antibodies or substances that are damaging.

plasticity: Ability of the central nervous system to adapt structurally or functionally in response to environmental demands.

platform crutches: Crutches designed to redirect stress from joints in the wrist and hand to the forearm under physical stress.

play: "Any spontaneous or organized activity that provides enjoyment, entertainment, amusement, or diversion" (Parham & Fazio, 1997, p. 252).[OTPF 2014]

play exploration: Identifying appropriate play activities, which can include exploration play, practice play, pretend play, games with rules, constructive play, and symbolic play (adapted from Bergen, 1988, pp. 64-65).[AOTA Framework]

play observation scale: Instrument developed by psychologist Kenneth Rubin to study children's behaviors when they are at play to identify children who may be at risk in terms of their social development.

play or leisure activities: Intrinsically motivating activities for amusement, relaxation, spontaneous enjoyment, or self-expression.[UTIII]

play participation: Participating in play; maintaining a balance of pay with other areas of occupation; and obtaining, using, and maintaining toys, equipment, and supplies appropriately.[AOTA Framework]

pleura: The serous membrane investing the lungs and lining the thoracic cavity, completely enclosing a potential space known as the pleural cavity. There are two pleurae, right and left, entirely distinct from each other.

pleurisy: Inflammation of the pleural membrane surrounding the lungs. *Synonym:* pleuritis.

pneumoencephalograph: Injection of air into the ventricles and subarachnoid spaces of the brain to assess their function.

pneumonectomy: The excision of lung tissue.

pneumopathology: Any disease involving the respiratory system.

pneumothorax: An accumulation of air or gas in the pleural cavity, which may occur spontaneously or as a result of trauma or a pathological process. Prevents the lung from expanding.

podiatrist: Licensed health care practitioners who treat clients with diseases or deformities of the feet.

point stimulation: The stimulation of sensitive areas of skin using electricity, pressure, laser, or ice for the purpose of relieving pain.

policy: A principle, law, or decision that guides actions (e.g., the sources and distribution of services and funds).

poliomyelitis: Viral infection of the motor cells in the spinal cord.

polyarticular: A form of juvenile rheumatoid arthritis that involves five joints or more.

polydrug abuse: Abuse of several psychoactive drugs (e.g., alcohol and cocaine).

polymorphism: Diversity occurring within biological populations.

polymyositis: Systemic connective tissue disease characterized by inflammatory and degenerative changes in the muscles. Leads to symmetric weakness and some degree of muscle atrophy; etiology unknown.

polyneuritis: Inflammation of many nerves at once.

polyp: Tumor with a stem (pedicle) that projects from a mucous membrane surface.

polyradiculopathy: Inflammation of multiple nerve roots.

polysomnogram: Instrument that continuously records an individual's sleep brain waves and a number of nerve and muscle functions while sleeping.

polysubstance dependence: Characterized by using at least three groups of substances (in the same 12-month period), but a single substance does not predominate.

Pomodoro technique: A time management method based on the idea that frequent breaks can help improve mental agility. Time is broken into 25-minute periods of focused work on one task, followed by a 5-minute break.

poor registration: When persons have difficulty registering stimuli due to high thresholds and act in accordance with those thresholds, they tend to have a dull or uninterested appearance. Their nervous systems fail to provide them with adequate activation to sustain focus on tasks or contextual cues.

population: Collective of groups of individuals living in a similar locale (e.g., city, state, country) or sharing the same or like characteristics or concerns.[OTPF 2014]

population at-risk: Group of people who share a characteristic that causes each member to be vulnerable to a particular event (e.g., non-immunized children exposed to the polio virus).

position in space: Determining the spatial relationship of figures and objects to self or other forms and objects[UTIII]; person's awareness of the place of his or her body in space.

position of deformity: Position of the hand in which the wrist is flexed, the metacarpals are in hyperextension, the interphalangeal joints are in flexion, and the thumb is adducted. Dorsal edema of the hand fosters this type of hand positioning.

positions: Positions body, arms, or wheelchair in relation to task objects and in a manner that promotes the use of efficient arm movements during task performance.[AOTA Framework]

positive reinforcement: Providing a desired reinforcer following an appropriate response.

positron emission tomography (PET): Dynamic brain imaging technique that produces a detailed image of the brain that can reflect changes in brain activity.

posterior: Toward the back of the body.

posterior cord syndrome: A rarely seen injury involving the dorsal columns with impairment of proprioception and kinesthesia.

posterolateral: In the rear and to one side.

post-formal thought: A theoretical construct used to describe the changes noted in adolescence and adulthood that flow on from more regular cognitive development models described by people such as Piaget.

Post-Occupancy Evaluation (POE): Generic, comprehensive, and systematic approach to assessing any physical environment that is currently in use.

post-polio syndrome: Collection of impairments occurring in persons who had poliomyelitis many years ago; related to chronic mechanical strain of weakened musculature and ligaments.

post-rotary nystagmus: Reflexive movement of the eyes that occurs after quick rotational movements have ceased; used as indicator of level of processing of vestibular information.

post-traumatic amnesia: The time elapsed between a brain injury and the point at which the functions concerned with memory are determined to have been restored.

post-traumatic stress disorder (PTSD): Characterized by intense negative feelings or terror in re-experiencing a traumatic or disastrous event in thoughts, nightmares, or dreams experienced over time. May also include physiological responses, such as excessive alertness, inability to concentrate or follow through on tasks, or difficulty sleeping.

postulates of change: How change occurs within a frame of reference.

postural alignment: Maintaining biomechanical integrity among body parts.[UTIII]

postural background movements: The subtle, spontaneous body adjustments that make overt movements of the hands easier (e.g., reaching for a distant object). These postural adjustments depend on good vestibular and proprioceptive integration.

postural control: Using righting and equilibrium adjustments to maintain balance during functional movements.[UTIII]

postural drainage: Positioning a person so that gravity aids in the drainage of secretions from the respiratory system.

postural insecurity: Fearfulness of movement or change in posture.

postural instability: Impaired balance and coordination.

postural tremor: A pathological tremor of 3 to 5 Hz that appears in a limb or the trunk when either is working against the pull of gravity.

posture: The attitude of the body. The position maintained by the body in standing or in sitting. The alignment and positioning of the body in relation to gravity, center of mass, and base of support. In the strictest sense, the position of the body or body part in relation to space and/or to other body parts. Functionally, the anticipation of, and response to, displacement of the body's center of mass.

power: Ability to impose one's will upon the behavior of other persons.

power distance index (PDI): Power distance defines the degree to which people accept hierarchical authority and how far they are willing to subordinate themselves.

powered wheelchair: Computerized wheelchair that allows a person to control speed and direction by pushing a button or using a joystick. It enables those without the use of their arms to move their wheelchairs without assistance.

power of attorney: Document authorizing one person to take legal actions on behalf of another who acts as an agent for the grantor.

practice settings: Various environments in which physical therapy is rendered, such as acute care, subacute care, rehabilitation settings, skilled nursing facilities, outpatient departments, assisted living environments, home care, fitness centers, and other community settings.

Prader-Willi syndrome: Characterized by severe obesity, mental retardation, small hands and feet, and small genitalia. In infancy, problems with poor tone, feeding, and body temperature control are common. More than 50% of children with Prader-Willi have a deletion of chromosome 15.

pragmatism: Practical way of solving problems. A philosophy of the late 19th and 20th centuries that interprets truth in terms of practical effects. "Meaning" can best be understood by examining its consequences on human activity.

praxis: Skilled purposeful movements (Heilman & Rothi, 1993). The ability to carry out sequential motor acts as part of an overall plan rather than individual acts (Liepmann, 1920). The ability to carry out learned motor activity, including following through on a verbal command, visual spatial construction, ocular and oral–motor skills, imitation of a person or an object, and sequencing actions (Ayres, 1985; Filley, 2001). Organization of temporal sequences of actions within the spatial context, which form meaningful occupations (Blanche & Parham, 2002). *Also see* motor.[OTPF 2008]

predictive validity: Positive correlation between test scores and future performance.

prednisone: Anti-inflammatory steroid used to treat arthritis and other severe inflammations.

pre-eclampsia: Illness of late pregnancy characterized by high blood pressure, swelling, and protein in the mother's urine. *Synonym*: toxemia.

preferred practice patterns: Boundaries within which physical therapists may select any number of clinical pathways, based on consideration of a wide variety of factors, such as individual patient/client needs; the profession's code of ethics and standards of practice; and patient/client age, culture, gender roles, race, sex, sexual orientation, and socioeconomic status. Preferred practice patterns for physical therapy are outlined and defined in the *Guide to Physical Therapist Practice* (2003) by the American Physical Therapy Association.

preferred provider organization (PPO): Acts as a broker between the purchaser of health care and the provider.

prefix: Word element of one or more syllables placed in front of a combining form in order to change its meaning.

pregnancy: Condition of carrying a fertilized ovum (zygote) in the uterus.

prehension: To use the hand to hold or manipulate objects.

prejudice: Unreasonable feelings, opinions, or attitudes directed against a race, religion, or national group.

preload: Conditions in the heart prior to beating (e.g., blood pressure, filling volume, etc.).

premature: Child born before the 37th week of gestation; can describe the birth or the infant.

premium: Amount paid to an insurer or third party for insurance coverage under an insurance policy.

premium tax credits: When enrolled in the Health Insurance Marketplace, consumers and self-employed individuals may be eligible for a new kind of tax credit that can be used to lower what you pay for your monthly health plan premiums. Starting in 2014, individuals who qualify can take the premium tax credit in the form of advance payments to lower their monthly health plan premiums, which can help make insurance more affordable.

premorbid personality: Psychosocial factor referring to personality characteristics that are present before the development of a disease and have either a positive or negative effect on the rehabilitative process.

premotor time (PMT): In a reaction time test, the time between the stimulus onset to the onset of electromyographic activity.

prenatal period: Time between conception and birth. The body does not change this much again during the entire lifespan as it does in these 38 weeks.

prepaid health plan: An insurance plan provided by health maintenance organizations and competitive medical plans. Preventive and wellness services are available in addition to care for illnesses.

preparatory methods and tasks: Methods and tasks that prepare the client for occupational performance, used either as part of a treatment session in preparation for or concurrently with occupations and activities or as a home-based engagement to support daily occupational performance. Often preparatory methods are interventions that are done to clients without their active participation and involve modalities, devices, or techniques.^OTPF 2014

prepared learning: Form of learning to which an individual is biologically predisposed.

presbyastasis: Age-related disequilibrium in the absence of known pathology.

presbycusis: Age-related hearing loss.

presbyopia: Impaired vision as a result of aging.

presenile: Pertaining to a condition in which a person manifests signs of aging in early or mid-life.

press: The behavioral influences exerted by an environment.

pressured speech: Loud and emphatic speech that is difficult to interrupt; often seen during a manic or other psychotic episode.

pressure point: Point over an artery where the pulse may be felt.

prevalence: The proportion of people who currently have a given condition, calculated as the number of existing cases of a disease divided by the total population at a given point in time.

prevention: Education or health promotion efforts designed to identify, reduce, or prevent the onset and reduce the incidence of unhealthy conditions, risk factors, diseases, or injuries (AOTA, 2013b).^OTPF 2014

prevention intervention: Occurs when therapists use their expertise to anticipate problems in the future and design interventions to keep negative outcomes from occurring.

preventive medicine: Care designed to deter disease and maintain optimal health.

prevocational skills: Antecedents to job skill development such as cooperative behavior, task focus, and motivation.

primacy effect: Tendency for an individual to remember the initial items of a list more accurately than those in the middle of the list.

primary aging: Term used to describe the characteristics of physical change, as a result of aging, that are part of the biological process and are inevitable to all humans.

primary appraisal: Part of the appraisal process in coping whereby the individual determines whether a stressful episode poses a situation of potential harm, threat, or challenge.

primary care: Ongoing monitoring of health status to prevent disease and sequelae of disease. First encounter in time or order of caregiving. Preventive interventions such as diet and exercise to prevent hypertension. The provision of integrated, accessible health care services by clinicians who are accountable for addressing the majority of personal health care needs, developing a sustained partnership with patients/clients, and practicing in the context of family and community.

primary care provider: Clinician who assumes ongoing responsibility for a client's overall health care needs.

primary circular reaction: Child's repetition of behavior in order to experience the pleasure the behavior produced the first time; the child is interested in the action itself.

primary health care: Basic level of health care that includes programs directed at health promotion, early diagnosis, and prevention of disease.

primary intracerebral hemorrhage: Syndrome in which bleeding occurs spontaneously in the brain.

primary lateral sclerosis (PLS): A disease of the upper motor neurons in the arms, legs, and face. Caused by nerve cell degeneration in the motor regions of the cerebral cortex and results in slow and effortful movements. The legs are often affected first; followed by the trunk, arms, and hands; and finally, the muscles that control speech, swallowing, and chewing. Symptoms include weakness, muscle stiffness and spasticity, clumsiness, slowing of movement, and problems with balance and speech.

primary prevention: Efforts that support or protect the health and well-being of the general population.

primary purpose: Title of Splint Classification System category that delineates whether the purpose of a particular splint is for immobilization or restriction of movement. Primary purpose immobilization splints cease motion, primary purpose mobilization splints enhance motion, and primary purpose restriction splints permit motion only within a partial range.

primary somesthetic area: Portion of the parietal lobe of the cerebrum that receives information about the general senses from receptors in the skin, joints, muscles, and body organs.

primatology: The study of primates.

prime mover: Muscle with the principal responsibility for a given action (e.g., the biceps brachii is the prime mover for flexing the arm at the elbow).

prime rate: Interest rate which is charged business borrowers having the highest credit ratings, for short-term borrowing.^{Small Business Administration}

primitive reflex (reaction): Any reflex normal in an infant or fetus. Its presence in an adult usually indicates serious neurologic disease (e.g., grasp reflex, Moro's reflex, and sucking reflex).

principle: A general truth or rule that emerges from the testing of assumptions and hypotheses; generally proven or tested.

principle of object permanence: Ability to realize that objects not within sight do exist; usually accomplished by children of 8 months of age.

principle of overload: Concept that repeated imposition of a stress above that normally experienced will produce physiologic adaptation.

privacy officer: A person designated by an organization that routinely handles protected health information to develop, implement, and oversee the organization's compliance with the U.S. Health Insurance Portability and Accountability Act privacy rules.

proactive interference (PI): Inability to recall recent experiences as a result of the memory of earlier experiences.

problem-based learning: Process of learning through solving everyday problems as they evolve in life.

problem-focused coping: Strategies that are directed at the source of stress itself rather than at feelings or emotions associated with the stress.

problem-oriented medical record (POMR): Patient-centered method of recording; includes database, list of patient's problems, interdisciplinary treatment plan, and progress notes.

problem-oriented process model: A conceptual model in which emphasis is on the process surrounding the problem definition.

problem solving: Recognizing a problem, defining a problem, identifying alternative plans, selecting a plan, organizing steps in a plan, implementing a plan, and evaluating the outcome[UTIII]; ability to manipulate knowledge and apply the information to new or unfamiliar situations.

problem space: The boundaries or limitations that define the problem definition and guide the area of concepts that need to be considered.

procedural memory: Knowledge for the necessary procedures to perform some activity; the so-called "knowing how."

procedural reasoning: One of three reasoning styles used by occupational therapists. It resembles the steps used in medical problem solving: cue acquisition, hypothesis generation, cue interpretation, and hypothesis evaluation.

procedures: The sequence of steps to be followed in performing an action; criteria for the way in which things are done.

process: Way in which occupational therapy practitioners operationalize their expertise to provide services to clients. The occupational therapy process includes evaluation, intervention, and targeted outcomes; occurs within the purview of the occupational therapy domain; and involves collaboration among the occupational therapist, occupational therapy assistant, and client.OTPF 2014

process-oriented approach to reasoning: A clinical problem is examined in terms of the problem-solving process or talk stages.

process skills: "Occupational performance skills [e.g., ADL process skills, school process skills] observed as a person (1) selects, interacts with, and uses task tools and materials; (2) carries out individual actions and steps; and (3) modifies performance when problems are encountered" (Boyt Schell et al., 2014a, p. 1239).OTPF 2014

prodromal: Preliminary phase of an illness that warns of upcoming major/primary symptoms.

productive activities: Work substitute tasks.

productivity: It is viewed as a controlling mechanism for top-level management. It is the ratio between the output and the resources expended to obtain the desired output.

product liability: Type of tort or civil liability that applies to product manufacturers and sellers.Small Business Administration

product line: Services that are labeled to ensure that consumers understand what they are purchasing.

professional reasoning: A synthesis of occupational reasoning and enablement reasoning, guiding critical reflection and actions with diverse clients in diverse contexts, incorporating narrative, conditional, positivist or other reasoning, and including while extending beyond clinical reasoning (Schön, 1983).CAOT

professional socialization: The personal development/social learning process by which an occupational therapy assistant develops into a fully competent professional.

proficient occupational therapist: Where practitioners demonstrate advanced abilities, their performance is called "proficient"' and where the practitioners demonstrate a recognized level of mastery, they are called "experts." The term *proficient* usually does not describe an occupational therapist in all contexts (e.g., area of practice, setting, etc.); rather, a practitioner may be proficient in one or more areas and competent in the other areas. Proficient infers that the performance expectations for competent are met and exceeded (CAOT, in press).[CAOT]

progesterone: A hormone produced by the ovary responsible for changes in preparing the wall of the uterus for implantation.

prognosis: Prediction of the probable outcome.

program evaluation: Measuring the effectiveness or goal attainment of programs.

programmed cell death: Physiological process in that cells die in the body, thought to be involved in the aging process.

programming: Creating a set of instructions that a computer is able to follow; also a term used to refer to the structuring of activity or influencing of behavior through environmental design, organization, or manipulation.

programming skill use: Prescribing a step-by-step procedure to prepare the consumer to use the skill as needed.[C]

progressive: Compilation of stages that increase in complexity toward maturity (e.g., course of a disease or condition in which signs and symptoms become more prominent and severe over time).

progressive bulbar palsy: A motor neuron disease in which the lowest motor neurons of the brainstem are most affected, causing slurred speech and difficulty chewing and swallowing. There are almost always mildly abnormal signs in the arms and legs.

progressive muscular atrophy: A motor neuron disease that affects only lower motor neurons in the spinal cord. Characterized by muscle weakness, fasciculation, and atrophy.

progressive resistive exercises (PRE): Increase the strength of a weak muscle by gradually increasing the resistance against which the muscle works.

project group: Group whose structure requires two or more people to interact. Some interaction may be forced by having people share materials. The emphasis is on task accomplishment.

projection: A defense mechanism; taking the unacceptable parts of one's self and forwarding them onto the environment.

projective activities: Ambiguous stimuli onto which an individual can project inner needs, thoughts, feelings, and concerns.

projective assessment: Evaluation approach that uses unstructured stimuli to elicit patient responses that suggest personality type, characteristics, and unconscious material.

prolapsed: Any organ that descends and protrudes through an external cavity due to weakness of the supporting structures (e.g., prolapsed uterus, prolapsed bladder).

pronation: Rotation of the forearm so the palm is facing down toward the floor.

prone: Lying with the face down.

prophylactic: Preventive.

proprietary (commercial) facilities: Refers to private profit-making institutions or facilities (e.g., nursing homes).

proprietorship: The most common legal form of business ownership; about 85 percent of all small businesses are proprietorships. The liability of the owner is unlimited in this form of ownership.Small Business Administration

proprioception: Awareness of posture, movement, and changes in equilibrium and the knowledge of position, weight, and resistance of objects in relation to the body.

proprioceptive: Interpreting stimuli originating in muscles, joints, and other internal tissues that give information about the position of one body part in relation to another.UTIII

proprioceptive neuromuscular facilitation (PNF): A form of exercise in which accommodating resistance is manually applied to various patterns of movement for the purpose of strengthening and restraining the muscles guiding joint motion.

propriospinal tract: Contralateral intersegmental tract functioning during reflexes and integration. *Synonym*: spinospinal tract.

prosopagnosia: Inability to identify a familiar face, either by looking at the person or picture.

prospective memory: Remembering to carry out some action in the future.

Prospective Payment System (PPS): Prospective or predetermined rate of payment that the government would make for each inpatient stay by a Medicare beneficiary.

prostaglandins: Lipid-soluble, hormone-like acetic compounds occurring in nearly all tissues, used for inducing labor.

prosthesis: Artificial substitutes, often mechanical or electrical, used to replace missing body parts.

prosthetics: Artificial substitutes for missing body parts.

protective devices: External supports to protect weak or ineffective joints or muscles, including braces, protective taping, cushions, and helmets.

protective extension response: Reflexive act consisting of extending one's arms in front of the head to protect the face and head during forward falling; includes accessibility issues for people with disabilities (not just employees).

proto humans: Early members of the hominidae family such as *Australopithecus* (Greek: protos, proto = first).

protopathic sensation: Gross sensory abilities in the extremities allowing one to detect light moving touch, pain, and temperature but without the ability to make fine discrimination of extent.

Proventil: Inhalant drug for asthma and upper respiratory disorders. *Generic name*: albuterol.

provider: Organization or person who actually provides the health care.

proxemics: Study of humans' use of space and the effects on interpersonal behavior.

proximal: From anatomical position, located nearer to the trunk; near the attachment of an extremity to the trunk.

Prozac: Type of antidepressant and anti–obsessive-compulsive drug. May cause rash, allergic reactions, anxiety, insomnia, and weight loss.

prudence: The ability to govern and discipline one's self through the use of reason.

pruritus vulvae: Disorders marked by severe itching of the external female genitalia.

pseudodementia: Affective disorders, particularly depression, that mimic the signs and symptoms of dementia.

pseudoelastin: A protein found in aging elastin tissue. The essential constituent of yellow elastic connective tissue.

pseudohypertrophic muscular dystrophy: A hereditary disease usually beginning in childhood in which muscular ability is lost. At first there is muscular pseudohypertrophy (growth), followed by atrophy (Thomas & Craven, 1997).

psychiatric rehabilitation services: Services for a person with a psychiatric disability to manage the disability.

psychiatrist: Physician specializing in psychiatry (study, treatment, and prevention of mental disorders).

psychoanalysis: Branch of psychiatry founded by Sigmund Freud using the techniques of free association, interpretation, and dream analysis.

psychoanalytic theory: Approach to the treatment of neuroses that emphasizes unlocking long-repressed feelings and past experiences in order to allow the patient to better understand his or her behavior.

psychodynamic: Any therapy that examines the forces motivating behavior.

psychogenic: Having an emotional or psychological origin.

psychological age: Definition of age based on the functional level of psychological processes rather than on calendar time.

psychological constructs: Psychological concepts; terms (without universal definitions) commonly used to describe mental states.

psychologist: Professional who is trained in psychology (science of mental processes).

psychometric instruments: Apparatus and paper-and-pencil techniques for measuring general intelligence, achievement, abilities, and related characteristics.

psychometric techniques (tests): Methods for measuring personality, interest, and attitude (frequently used in psychology).

psychomotor agitation: Irregular action, unrest, or disquiet.

psychoneuroimmunology: Field of study that links psychological, neural, and immunological processes.

psychopathology: Study of psychological and behavioral dysfunction occurring in mental illness.

psychopharmacotherapy: The study of the action of drugs on psychological function and mental states.

psychosis: A major mental disorder of organic or emotional origin that can cause extreme personality disorganization, loss of reality orientation, and inability to function appropriately in society.

psychosocial: Pertaining to interpersonal and social interactions that influence behavior and development.

psychosocial development: Erikson's theory of human development throughout the lifespan as a progression of stages named according to the possible outcome.

psychosocial disability: Disorder, impairment, or handicap relating to interpersonal relationships and social interactions that influence behavior and development.

psychosocial skills and psychological components: The ability to interact in society and to process emotions.[UTIII]

psychosocial stressor: Psychological and social factors that cause stress.

psychosomatic: Psychological foundation for physiological symptoms.

psychotic: Psychological state characterized by hallucinations and delusions.

psychotropic medications: Drugs that act to relieve psychological symptoms.

ptosis: Drooping of the upper eyelid.

ptyalism: Increased saliva production.

puberty: Period in life when the individual becomes functionally capable of reproduction.

public good: General welfare or benefit to the majority or large contingent of citizens.

public health: Preventing disease, prolonging life, and promoting health and human efficiency through organizing community efforts. Protection of the community or public at large from illness, disease, and epidemics.

puerperium: Period of 6 weeks following childbirth and expulsion of the placenta in which the reproductive organs of the mother return to normal.

pulmonary embolism: An obstruction of the pulmonary artery or one of its branches usually caused by an embolus from a lower extremity thrombosis.

pulmonary postural drainage: Placing the body in a position that uses gravity to drain fluid from the lungs.

pulse rate: Number of heart beats per minute as measured on the radial, carotid, femoral, and pedal arteries.

punishment: Providing an aversive stimulus following an appropriate response.

Purdue Pegboard (PPB): Test used to measure gross motor movements of the upper extremities using a stopwatch to time while rapidly placing pins in the pegboard and assembling pins, washers, and collars.

pure synergism: When a muscle moves several joints simultaneously, its force is divided among them.

pure tone audiogram: Standard method used to determine degree of hearing loss, using a decibel scale of loudness.

Purkinje cells: Large neurons found in the cerebral cortex, which provide the only output from the cerebellar cortex after the cortex processes sensory and motor signals from the rest of the nervous system.

purpose: The desire to engage in behavior to accomplish a goal.

purposeful activity: A goal-directed behavior or activity within a therapeutically designed context that leads to an occupation or occupations. Specifically selected activities that allow the client to develop skills that enhance occupational engagement. OTPF 2008

purposefulness: An individual's plan of action to achieve a goal.

purpura: Hemorrhagic disease that leaves red to purple spots on the body, which then disappear.

purulent: Consisting of or containing pus.

pyosalpinx: Pus in the fallopian tube.

pyrosis: Burning sensation in the epigastric and sternal region with raising of acid liquid from the stomach; heartburn.

quadrigeminal: Four-fold, or in four parts, such as the heart.

quadrilateral: Having four sides.

quadriplegia (QUAD): Paralysis of all four extremities.

qualification: A qualifying skill or being qualified with the skill, knowledge, and experience that fits a person for a position, office, or profession.

qualitative: Subjective elements.

qualitative interviewing: Interviewing that makes use of ethnographic methods to obtain a rich, detailed description of the subject.

qualitative methods: Methods such as interviewing and observation used to gather detailed, extensive, and in-depth information about a situation.

qualitative research: Methods for knowing that consider the unique properties of a natural setting without a reliance on quantitative data.

quality assurance (QA): Maintenance of quality by constant measuring and comparison to set standards. Quality maintenance problems may be identified and corrected through this procedure.

quality improvement (QI): Continuous improvement of performance; sometimes referred to as continuous quality improvement (CQI).

quality of life: Dynamic appraisal of life satisfaction (perception of progress toward identified goals), self-concept (beliefs and feelings about oneself), health and functioning (e.g., health status, self-care capabilities), and socioeconomic factors (e.g., vocation, education, income; adapted from Radomski, 1995).[OTPF 2014]

Jacobs, K., & Simon, L. (Eds.). *Quick Reference Dictionary for Occupational Therapy, Sixth Edition* (pp. 243-244).
© 2015 SLACK Incorporated.

From an occupational perspective, it refers to choosing and participating in occupations that foster hope, generate motivation, offer meaning and satisfaction, create a driving vision of life, promote health, enable empowerment, and otherwise address the quality of life (adapted from CAOT, 1997a, 2002).[CAOT]

quality performance dimensions: Set of nine fundamental elements for change identified by the Joint Commission on Accreditation of Healthcare Organizations: efficacy, appropriateness, availability, timeliness, effectiveness, continuity, safety, efficiency, and respect and caring.

quantitative: Measurable.

Quick Neurology Screening Test: Informal screening for children 5 to 18 years that tests gross motor, praxis, fine motor, visual-motor integration, visual perception, tactile, and vestibular functioning.

race: Group of people united or classified together on the basis of common history, nationality, or geographical distribution.

rachitis: Inflammation of the spinal column due to vitamin D deficiency.

radiator theory: A theory proposed by Dean Falk, an anthropologist, that the evolution of increased brain size was dependent on adequate cooling through heat dispersal. This theory is based on the differences in cranial vessels and drainage patterns (foramen in the skull) between australopithecines and early *Homo* brains. These patterns become increasingly elaborate over evolutionary time.

radical mastectomy: Removal of the entire breast and lymph nodes.

radicular: Pertaining to a radical or root. Commonly associated with a nerve root.

radiographic anatomy: Study of the structures of the body using x-rays.

radiography: Commonly referred to as an x-ray.

rale: *See* crackle.

ramus: A branch; used in anatomical nomenclature as a general term to designate a smaller structure given off by a larger one, such as a blood vessel or a nerve.

Rancho Los Amigos levels: Rancho Los Amigos Hospital described eight progressive levels of cognitive functioning and behavioral response, which are widely observed and referred to: no response/coma; generalized response; localized response; confused and agitated; confused, inappropriate, and nonagitated; confused and appropriate; automatic and appropriate; and purposeful and appropriate.

Jacobs, K., & Simon, L. (Eds.). *Quick Reference Dictionary for Occupational Therapy, Sixth Edition* (pp. 245-258).
© 2015 SLACK Incorporated.

randomization: Process of assigning participants or objects to a control or experimental group on a random basis.

random practice: Tasks practiced in a mixed order.

range of motion (ROM): Moving body parts through an arc[UTIII]; path of motion a joint can move in any one direction, measured in degrees.

rapid eye movement (REM): Sleep state where brain waves show an active pattern; dreaming is occurring. This state is thought to be important for adequate rest and health.

rapport: Harmonious relationship between people.

rate of return: Amount of profit based on the amount of resources used to produce it.[Small Business Administration]

rates under treatment: Needs assessment technique that examines data from service delivery sites such as clinics, hospitals, schools, and mental health centers to ascertain who (sociodemographically) is using what kinds of services.

rating of perceived exertion (RPE): Psychophysical scale for subjective rating of exertion during work.

ratio: Relationships of items within and between financial statements (e.g., current ratio, quick ratio, inventory turnover ratio, and debt/net worth ratios).[Small Business Administration]

rational emotive therapy (RET): Technique used in cognitive behavioral therapy that challenges clients' irrational beliefs of themselves and the world.

ratio scales: Measurement scales that contain values that are equally distant from each other and are characterized by the presence of an absolute zero value.

raw score: Unadjusted score derived from observations of performance; frequently, the arithmetic sum of a subject's responses.

Raynaud's disease: A peripheral vascular disorder characterized by vasoconstriction of the upper extremities usually in response to an emotional disturbance or exposure to cold weather.

reaches: Extends, moves the arm (and when appropriate, the trunk) to effectively grasp or place task objects that are out of reach, including skillfully using a reacher to obtain task objects.[AOTA Framework]

reaction of degeneration: The condition in which a short-duration electrical stimulus (usually less than 1 m/sec) applied to a motor nerve results in a sluggish or absent muscle response rather than the normally brisk contraction. This electrophysiologic reaction can be used as a screening assessment of peripheral nerve integrity.

reaction time: The interval between the application of a stimulus and the detection of a response.

reactivity: Characteristic of assessment instruments whereby the act of administering the assessment changes the behavior of the person being evaluated, thus distorting the representatives of the findings.

reality orientation: Therapeutic technique often used with confused or disoriented clients. Includes both group techniques, to remind the client of facts, and patterned environment, which provides memory cues.

reality testing: Ability to know what is real and what is fantasy, usually accomplished through structured activity.

reality therapy: Form of therapy designed to provide an individual with experience of reasonable consequences of actions.

reappraisal: In coping, reconsideration of a harm, threat, or loss episode after an initial appraisal has taken place. It is thought that during coping, individuals constantly reassess the stressful episode and their resources and alternatives for dealing with it.

reasonable accommodations (RA): In order to allow equal opportunity to a worker with a disability, a company may modify the work environment by doing things such as job restructuring, providing adaptable equipment, or making other such adjustments for modification.

reasoning: The use of one's ability to think and draw conclusions, motives, causes, or justifications, which will form the basis of actions.

rebound phenomenon: Inability to stop a resisted muscle contraction, such that movement of the limb occurs when the resistance is unexpectedly withdrawn from the limb.

recency effect: Tendency for an individual to remember the last items of a list better than those in the middle.

receptive aphasia: Inability to comprehend written or spoken language. *Also known as* Wernicke's aphasia.

receptive field: Receptor area served by one neuron.

receptor: Specific site at which a drug acts through forming a chemical bond.

reciprocal: Present or existing on both sides, expressing mutual, corresponding, or complementary action.

reciprocal innervation: Excitatory innervation of synergists and inhibitory innervation of antagonists. The function is to permit the action of the group of synergists to reinforce one another while eliminating the action of the antagonistic muscles that would oppose the particular movement, either slowing the movement or preventing it.

reciprocal teaching: Instructional procedure used by Brown and Palincsar to develop cognitive monitoring. It requires students to take turns leading a study group in the use of strategies for comprehending and remembering text content.

reciprocity: Mutual exchange between entities. For example, reciprocity between states for licensing of physical therapists whereby one state accepts the licensing qualifications of another state.

recognition: Identifying familiar faces, objects, and other previously presented materials.[UTIII]

reconstruction aides: Individuals who used occupational therapy in World War I with the returning soldiers with disabilities. The use of reconstruction aides ultimately increased the visibility of occupational therapy and resulted in strides in professional education and public policy.

recovery: The process of regaining important life roles, developing healthy relationships with others, and establishing healthy daily routines that support abstinence and sobriety.

rectocele: Herniation of the rectum with protrusion into the vaginal canal or prolapse of the rectum into the perineum.

red nucleus: Large, vascular nucleus found in mesencephalon, involved in transmission of cerebellar communications to the motor cortex and thalamus.

reduction: Realignment of a dislocated bone to its original position.

reductionism: A philosophical stance associated with empiricism and scientific "disciplines" in which understanding is achieved through the study of parts and their effects on each other.

reductionistic: An approach to understanding where the problem is broken into parts and the parts are viewed and managed separately.

re-entry programs: Rehabilitation programs designed to maximize independence; usually the final rehabilitation program after hospitalization and rehabilitation programs are completed. Re-entry programs are often outpatient or community programs.

reevaluation: Reappraisal of the client's performance and goals to determine the type and amount of change that has taken place.[OTPF 2014]

referral: A recommendation that a patient/client seek service from another health care provider or resource.

referred pain: Visceral pain felt in a somatic area away from the actual source of pain.

reflex: Eliciting an involuntary muscle response by sensory input[UTIII]; subconscious, involuntary reaction to an external stimulus.

reflex incontinence: A form of incontinence caused by the inability to inhibit bladder stimulatory reflexes.

reflex sympathetic dystrophy syndrome: Differentiation syndrome with autonomic changes that consists of pain, edema, and sympathetic dysfunction of an extremity following trauma, nerve injury, or central nervous system disorder; usually occurs secondary to a preexisting condition.

reflux: Back flow of any substance (e.g., urine from bladder to ureters or food returning to the esophagus from the stomach).

reformation: A religious movement in 16th-century Europe. Attempts to reform the Roman Catholic church resulted in the establishment of independent Protestant churches.

refractive error: Nearsightedness (myopia), farsightedness (hyperopia), astigmatism, or presbyopia. All conditions are improved with corrective lenses.

regression: A retreat or backward movement in conditions, signs, and symptoms (e.g., returning to behavior patterns that were characteristic of a previous stage of development).

regulation: A process of managing individual conduct by providing normative messages in communication.

rehabilitation: Rehabilitation services are provided to persons experiencing deficits in key areas of physical and other types of function or limitations in participation in daily life activities. Interventions are designed to enable the achievement and maintenance of optimal physical, sensory, intellectual, psychological, and social functional levels. Rehabilitation services provide tools and techniques needed to attain desired levels of independence and self-determination.[OTPF 2014] Helping individuals regain skills and abilities that have been lost as a result of illness, injury, disease, disorder, or incarceration.

Rehabilitation Act (1973): Services were expanded to individuals with severe disabilities, affirmative action provided in employment, and nondiscrimination in facilities by federal contractors and grantees.

rehabilitation frame of reference: Teaches clients to compensate for underlying deficits that cannot be remediated.

rehabilitation planning: Choosing the specific rehabilitation interventions, which will improve the high priority skill and resource deficits.[C]

rehabilitation services: Focus on developing the skills and supports needed for success and satisfaction in specific environments.[C]

reimbursement: Compensation for services provided.

reinforcement: Desired outcome of behavior. In behavior therapy, reinforcement is provided to encourage specific activities; strengthened by fear of punishment or anticipation of reward.

reinforcer: A desirable and rewarding object or activity that can be used to encourage a particular behavior.

relates: Assumes a manner of acting that tries to establish a rapport with others.[AOTA Framework]

relative endurance: Muscular endurance when force of contraction tested is based on percentage of measured strength.

relative mastery: The extent to which the person experiences the occupational response as efficient (use of time and energy), effective (production of the desired result), and satisfying to self and society.

Relative Value Unit (RVU): An index of measure for Medicare resource-based relative value scale.

relaxation: Techniques that increase relaxation by reducing tension (e.g., biofeedback, systematic relaxation exercises).

relaxation techniques: A cognitive treatment technique that addresses muscle tension accompanying pain.

relaxin: A polypeptide ovarian hormone secreted by the corpus luteum; possibly acts on the ligamentous structures of the body, slackening the ligaments to allow greater opening in the pelvic outlet.

release phenomenon: Ongoing action of one part of the central nervous system without modulation from a complementary functional component.

release therapy: Therapy devised by David Levy in which he states that a child will benefit from emotional release if he or she is strong enough to tolerate the emotional upset.

reliability: Predictability of an outcome, regardless of observer. In diagnosis, refers to the probability that several therapists will apply the same label to a given individual.

religious observance: Participating in religion, "an organized system of beliefs, practices, rituals, and symbols designed to facilitate closeness to the sacred or transcendent" (Moreira-Almeida & Koenig, 2006, p. 844).[OTPF 2008]

reminiscence effect: Tendency for the recall of an item to improve for a short period of time after initial learning before being forgotten.

remission: Lessening in severity or abatement of symptoms of a disease.

Renaissance Utopians: Utopians who emerged at the time of the Renaissance in the 14th through 16th centuries. Most were multitalented and interested in humanities. Utopians aimed toward an imagined perfect place, society, or state of things.

renin: A proteolytic enzyme liberated by ischemia of the kidney or by diminished pulse pressure, which changes hypertensinogen into hypertension.

repetition maximum (RM): Maximum weight that can be lifted in isotonic contraction. One RM = maximum that can be lifted one time; two RM = maximum weight that can be lifted twice, etc.

Representative Assembly (RA): Policy-making body of the American Occupational Therapy Association.

reprimand: Expression of disapproval of conduct.

reprivatize: Return responsibility to the private sector as opposed to public responsibility.

research: Systematic investigation, including development, testing, and evaluation design.

Resident Assessment Instrument: Nationwide tool to periodically measure the functional performance of each nursing home resident and identify problem areas that can be open to intervention.

residential treatment facility: Where individuals live temporarily for therapeutic benefit.

resilience: The ability for an individual to overcome trauma or a major life-changing event while maintaining a defined, stable trajectory of healthy functioning (Bonanno & Mancini, 2012). Overcoming an event could be shown in emotional, cognitive-behavioral, social, and/or physical resilience (Sturgeon & Zautra, 2010). This could be measured by an individual's maintaining his or her life's roles and occupational demands.

resistance: Amount of weight to be moved.

resistance development: Adaptation that decreases physiologic response to a chronic stressor.

resistance exercise training: Exercise that applies sufficient force to muscle groups to improve muscle strength.

resonance: The prolongation and intensification of sound produced by the transmission of its vibrations to a cavity, especially a sound elicited by percussion. Decrease in resonance is called dullness; absence of resonance is called flatness.

Resource-Based Relative Value System (RBRVS): A system of reimbursement being developed by Medicare for outpatient service based on assessing the intensity and complexity of a service and assigning a numerical value and dollar amount related to that value.

resource coordination: Linking a consumer to an existing resource in the community.[C]

resource creation: Creating a brand new resource that does not exist in the community.[C]

resource environment: Facilities available to an individual within his or her life space that may meet his or her instruments (survival) or symbolic needs.

resource modification: Modifying an existing resource to better meet the needs of an individual consumer.[C]

respects: Accommodates to other people's reactions and requests. AOTA Framework

respiration: The act or process of breathing; inhaling and exhaling air. The processes by which a living organism or cell takes in oxygen from the air or water, distributes and utilizes it in oxidation, and gives off products of oxidation, especially carbon dioxide.

respiratory exchange ratio (VCO_2/VO_2): The ratio of the volume of carbon dioxide expired and the oxygen consumed.

respiratory failure: Failure of the pulmonary system in which inadequate exchange of carbon dioxide and oxygen occurs between an organism and its environment.

respite care: Short-term health services to the dependent adult or child, either at home or in an institutional setting.

response speed: The time elapsed between presentation of a stimulus and the patient's/client's initiation of movement.

responsivity: Level that the sensory input facilitates reaction or noticing.

rest: "Quiet and effortless actions that interrupt physical and mental activity resulting in a relaxed state" (Nurit & Michel, 2003, p. 227).[OTPF 2008]

resting-pan splint: Splint used to support the wrist, fingers, and thumb in a functional position; can be volar or dorsal design.

restorative aide: A nursing assistant who works in a rehabilitation capacity and assists nursing home residents in carryover of learned functional mobility (i.e., ambulation, transfers) and activities of daily living on the patient/client units.

restores: (a) Puts away tools and materials in appropriate places, (b) restores immediate workspace to original condition (e.g., wiping surfaces clean), (c) closes and seals containers and coverings when indicated, and (d) twists or folds any plastic bags to seal.^{AOTA Framework}

restraints: Devices used to aid in immobilization of patients.

rest/relaxation: Performance during time not devoted to other activity and during time devoted to sleep.

retardation: *See* intellectual disability.

retention: Resistance to movement or displacement.

reticulospinal tract: Pathways that support action of the flexors and extensors of the neck for postural control.

retirement preparation and adjustment: Determining aptitudes, developing interests and skills, and selecting appropriate avocational pursuits.^{AOTA Framework}

retrograde amnesia: The inability to recall events that have occurred during the period immediately preceding a brain injury.

retrospective memory: Remembering information that occurred in the past.

retrospective recording: Waiting until the evaluation is completed to record observations of client function.

retroviruses: A group of RNA viruses causing a variety of diseases in humans. This group of viruses has RNA as their genetic code and are capable of copying RNA and DNA and incorporating them into an infected cell.

Rett syndrome: Disorder characterized by the development of multiple specific deficits following a period of normal functioning at birth. There is a loss of previously acquired purposeful hand skills between ages 5 and 30 months, with the subsequent development of characteristic stereotyped hand movements resembling hand wringing or hand washing. Problems develop in the coordination of gait or trunk movements. There is also severe impairment in expressive and receptive language development, with severe psychomotor retardation.

reverberating loops or circuits: A process by which closed chains of neurons when excited by a single impulse will continue to discharge impulses from collateral neurons back onto the original neuronal pool. The end result may produce a higher level of excitation than the original input itself.

Reye's syndrome: Illness that occurs following a viral infection. It is characterized by vomiting and brain dysfunction, such as disorientation, lethargy, and personality changes, and may progress into coma. Usually affects children and teenagers.

rheumatoid arthritis (RA): Form of joint inflammation that is the second most common rheumatic disease (after osteoarthritis). It typically involves the joints of the fingers, wrists, and ankles, and often the hips and shoulders; the joints are affected symmetrically and there is a considerable range of severity.

Rh factor: Hereditary blood factor found in red blood cells determined by specialized blood tests; when present, a person is Rh positive; when absent, a person is Rh negative.

rhizotomy: Sectioning of the posterior nerve root to relieve pain.

rhonchi: A snoring sound; a rattling in the throat; also a dry, coarse rale in the bronchial tubes due to a partial obstruction.

ribonucleic acid (RNA): Basic genetic material in which a nucleic acid is associated with the control of chemical activities within a cell.

RIC Functional Assessment Scale: Developed by the Rehabilitation Institute of Chicago, a seven-point rating scale used along with a protocol to assess the proficiency of clients with physical disabilities in complex activities of daily living tasks.

rickets: Condition affecting children characterized by soft and deformed bones resulting from inadequate calcium metabolism due to vitamin D deficiency.

righting reactions: Stimuli go through the labyrinths and to tactile receptors in the trunk, neck, and ears to function to keep the upper part of the body upright and to maintain the head and trunk in their proper relationship.

right-left discrimination: Differentiating one side from the other.
UTIII

rights protection services: Focus on upholding moral and legal rights.[C]

right to die: A person's right to die on his or her terms.

right-to-know law: Law that dictates that employers must inform their employees of any chemical hazards or health effects caused by toxic substances used in each workplace.

rigidity: Hypertonicity of agonist and antagonist that offers a constant, uniform resistance to passive movement. The affected muscles seem unable to relax and are in a state of contraction even at rest.

risk factors: Factors that cause a person or group of people to be particularly vulnerable to an unwanted, unpleasant, or unhealthy event.

risk management: Following established policy and procedure regarding risk in the work setting.

risky shift: Type of group polarization of which the post-discussion behaviors of individuals are less safe than before the group discussion.

Ritalin: Central nervous system stimulant used to treat children with attention deficit disorders. *Generic name*: methylphenidate hydrochloride.

rite of passage: Ritual associated with the life cycle of a single individual.

rites of intensification: Rituals resulting from or commemorating changes in the environment designed to confirm, strengthen, or display group membership or identity.

rituals: Sets of symbolic actions with spiritual, cultural, or social meaning contributing to the client's identity and reinforcing values and beliefs. Rituals have a strong affective component (Fiese, 2007; Fiese et al., 2002; Segal, 2004).[OTPF 2014]

robotics: Science of mechanical devices that work automatically or by remote control.

roentgenogram: An x-ray; a film produced by roentgenography.

role competence: Achievement of the behaviors that have some socially agreed-upon function and for which there is an accepted code of behavioral norms or expectations.

role conflict: Occurs when a person encounters pressures within an important role that are in opposition to another valued role.

role dysfunction: Inability to perform and adjust adaptively to social expectations associated with roles of player, student, worker, homemaker, volunteer, or retiree.

role performance: Identifying, maintaining, and balancing functions one assumes or acquires in society (e.g., worker, student, parent, friend, religious participant).[UTIII]

role recovery: Application of the philosophy and technology of the Psychiatric Rehabilitation Approach that has been developed into an implementation model for mental health/behavioral health care organizations and networks.[C]

roles: Sets of behaviors expected by society and shaped by culture and context that may be further conceptualized and defined by the client.[OTPF 2014] From an occupational perspective is a "culturally defined pattern of occupation that reflects particular routines and habits; stereotypical role expectations may enhance or limit persons' potential occupational performance" (CAOT, 1997a, 2002, p. 182).[CAOT]

Rolfing: Technique of massage and deep muscular manipulation designed to realign the body with gravity; structured integration.

Romberg's sign: Inability to maintain body balance with the eyes open and then eyes closed with the feet close together; unsteadiness with eyes closed indicates a loss of proprioceptive control.

Rood: Theory promoting that all motor output is the result of both past and present sensory input.

rooting reflex: This normal reflex in infants up to 4 months of age consists of head turning in the direction of the stimulus when the cheek is stroked gently.

Rosen Method Bodywork: Form of hands-on, nonintrusive somatic bodywork, the goal of which is physical relaxation and emotional awareness to assist and facilitate a client's innate healing capacities.

rotation: Movement about the long axis of a limb, usually resulting from movement of the shoulder or hip.

rotator cuff: The muscle complex of the shoulder that provides stability of the glenohumeral joint inclusive of the supraspinatus, infraspinatus, teres minor, and subscapularis muscles.

rote: Habit performance without meaning.

round ligament: A pair of ligaments that holds the uterus in place, extending laterally from the fundus between the folds of the broad ligaments to the lateral pelvic wall, terminating in the labia majora.

routines: Patterns of behavior that are observable, regular, and repetitive and that provide structure for daily life. They can be satisfying and promoting or damaging. Routines require momentary time commitment and are embedded in cultural and ecological contexts (Fiese et al., 2002; Segal, 2004).[OTPF 2014]

routine supervision: Direct contact at least every 2 weeks at the site of work, with interim supervision occurring by other methods, such as telephone or written communication.

Routine Task Inventory (RTI): Assesses client's performance of routine tasks and behavior while performing the tasks.

RTS: Rehabilitation technology supplier.

rules approach: A method for describing a culture through identification of the ways in which people view reality, make distinctions among categories of things, and make decisions about right courses of action.

rules-oriented style: Main assumption in this style is that people require reinforcement from the manager to function. This manager does things by the book; enforcing policies, rules, and procedures with employees ensures motivation and achievement.

rumination: Repetitive chewing of food; regurgitated after ingestion.

rupture: A bursting, or the state of being broken apart.

S

saccadic eye movement: Extremely fast voluntary movement of the eyes, allowing the eyes to accurately fix on a still object in the visual field as the person moves or the head turns.

saccadic fixation: A rapid change of fixation from one point to another in a visual field.

saccule: Organ in the inner ear that transmits information about linear movement in relation to gravity.

safe position: A more recently used hand position that is thought to be an antideformity position that should be used to prevent stiffness whenever a hand has a tendency to develop stiffness. It calls for immobilization for a certain period of time. The safe position maintains collateral ligament length, decreases the probability of metacarpophalangeal extension development, interphalangeal flexion development, and thumb carpometacarpal adduction contracture development that can occur with immobilization.

safety and emergency maintenance: Knowing and performing preventive procedures to maintain a safe environment, as well as recognizing sudden, unexpected hazardous situations and initiating emergency action to reduce the threat to health and safety.[OTPF 2008]

Safety and Functional ADL Evaluation (SAFE): Evaluates the independence and degree of required supervision in bathing, dressing, feeding, bowel and bladder control, transfers, and mobility.

safety grab bars: Bars mounted on bathtub walls that provide a person with a secure fixture to hold onto and prevent falling.

Jacobs, K., & Simon, L. (Eds.). *Quick Reference Dictionary for Occupational Therapy, Sixth Edition* (pp. 259-289).
© 2015 SLACK Incorporated.

sagittal plane: Divides the body into left and right sections; motion occurs around the coronal axis.

salpingo-oophorectomy: Excision of an ovary and fallopian tube.

sample of behavior: Selected test items chosen because they constitute a subset of the behaviors that need to be assessed.

sandwich generation: Adults who have caregiving responsibilities for their dependent children and their aging parents.

sarcoidosis: A disorder that may affect any part of the body but most frequently involves the lymph nodes, liver, spleen, lungs, eyes, and small bones of the hands and feet; characterized by the presence in all affected organs or tissues of epithelioid cell tubercles, without caseation, and with little or no round-cell reaction, becoming converted, in the older lesions, into a rather hyaline featureless fibrous tissue.

sarcoma: Malignant tissue that originates in connective tissue and spreads through the bloodstream, often attacking bones.

Satisfaction with Performance Scaled Questionnaire (SPSQ): Used to measure a client's satisfaction with performance of independent living skills through a five-point rating questionnaire.

Saturday night palsy: Pressure on radial nerve that causes dorsiflexion of wrist and extension weakness of fingers.

scaffolding: Teaching process that segments a task into separate subgoals in order to allow a child to perform tasks within his or her existing repertoire of skills, while the adult can model the skills and knowledge necessary to complete the entire task.

scanning: Technique for making selections on a device such as a communication aid, computer, or environmental control system. Scanning involves moving sequentially through a given set of choices, and making a selection when the desired position is reached. Types of scanning include automatic, manual, row-and-column, and directed.

scanning speech: An abnormal pattern of speech characterized by regularly recurring pauses.

scapegoat: A symbolic person or thing blamed for other problems.

scapula: Flattened, triangular bone found on the posterior aspect of the body. It is part of the pectoral girdle, which joins the clavicle and humerus.

schemata: Basic units of all knowledge. Each simple organization of experience and knowledge by the mind make up the original "schema," or framework, that represents our everyday experiences. Each experience, thought, and idea is a structural element in an organizational matrix, which integrates a person's experiences and history into a meaningful set of categories, each filled with data from one's memory of prior events.

schema theory: Notion that standard routine performances occur in given situations in a typical sequence and with typical kinds of participants; within the general framework or structure the details of a given performance may vary but the basic structure remains consistent.

schemes: Structural elements of cognition; plans, designs, or programs to be followed.

schizoaffective disorder: A psychotic disorder characterized by significant mood symptoms and symptoms of schizophrenia (Beers, Berkow, & Burs, 1999).

schizophrenia (Sz): Pervasive psychosis that affects a variety of psychological processes involving cognition, affect, and behavior and is characterized by hallucinations, delusions, bizarre behavior, and illogical thinking.

scholarship: Organized inquiry that helps to produce theory and evidence from multiple research paradigms using a dynamic process to move between: (a) knowledge of a specific situation; (b) generalized theories regarding the complex process of engaging or re-engaging people in valued occupations; and (c) emerging knowledge. In client/clinical contexts, the process may include (d) how the client wishes to change or minimize change.[CAOT]

school professionals: School principals, program directors, and directors of special education are committee members who interpret local administrative policies in special education.

sciatica: Nerve inflammation characterized by sharp pains along the sciatic nerve and its branches; area extends from the hip down the back of the thigh and surrounding parts.

science-based: Procedures utilized that have been proven effective via appropriate scientific research methodologies.

scientific-mindedness: A frame of mind that emphasizes generating hypotheses and gathering data to help corroborate or refute the hypotheses.

scissors gait: Gait in which the legs cross midline upon advancement.

scleroderma: Chronic, autoimmune disease of the connective tissue characterized by fibrosis; the skin becomes taut, edematous, and firm, allowing for limited movement. It can also affect internal organs and is usually accompanied by Raynaud's disease.

scoliosis: Abnormal lateral curvature of the spine.

scooter board: Rectangular, flat board with wheels at each corner. It is used to ride on to evoke the pivot prone posture.

scope of practice: Encompassing all of the skills, knowledge, and expertise required to practice a profession, such as physical therapy.

scotoma: "Blind spots"; often occurs as a result of disease or injury.

screening: Review of a client case to determine whether services are necessary.

screening instrument: Assessment device used for purposes of identifying potential problem areas for further in-depth evaluation.

screen time: Time spent in front of an electronic device. This includes television, video games, movies, email, instant messaging, and computer usage.

script: General sequence of events about a common routine or scenario, usually with a common goal.

search engines: Websites or online platforms that allow you to search the Internet for any keywords or topics of interest. Google.com is one of the most well known, but there are others that are specialized for certain purposes, such as PubMed, which indexes scholarly articles.

searches/locates: Looks for and finds tools and materials in a logical manner, including looking beyond the immediate environment (e.g., looking in, behind, on top of).AOTA Framework

seasonal affective disorder (SAD): Mood disorder associated with shorter days and longer nights of autumn and winter. Symptoms include lethargy, depression, social withdrawal, and work difficulties.

seborrhea: Disease of the sebaceous glands marked by the increase in amount and quality of their secretions.

secondary aging: Changes in physical functioning as a result of aging that are not universal or inevitable but are commonly shared by humans as a result of environmental conditions or circumstances.

secondary appraisal: That part of the coping process whereby an individual, having determined the nature of a stressful episode (i.e., harm, threat, or challenge), selects an appropriate strategy for dealing with it.

secondary care: Intervention provided once a disease state has been identified (e.g., treating hypertension).

secondary circular reactions: Repetition of behaviors that bring about pleasing effects on their surrounding world; interest in external results of actions.

secondary conditions: Pathology, impairments, or functional limitations derived from the primary condition. *Also known as* secondary disabilities.

secondary gain: A benefit associated with a mental illness.

secondary market: Those who purchase an interest in a loan from an original lender, such as banks, credit unions, and pension funds.Small Business Administration

secondary prevention: Efforts directed at populations who are considered "at risk" by early detection of potential health problems, followed by the interventions to halt, reverse, or at least slow the progression of that condition.

secretion: The process of elaborating a specific product as a result of the activity of a gland. This activity may range from separating a specific substance of the blood to the elaboration of a new chemical substance.

sedentary work: Exerting up to 10 pounds of force occasionally or a negligible amount of force frequently to lift, carry, push, pull, or otherwise move objects.

seizure disorders: Presence of abrupt irrepressible episodes of electrical hyperactivity in the brain.

selective abstraction: Focusing on one insignificant detail while ignoring the more important features of a situation.

self-actualization: Full humanness; the development of the inner nature and biological potential (destiny) of people. Self-actualizing people are not selfish but altruistic, dedicated, self-transcending, and social.

self-advocacy: Advocating for oneself, including making one's own decisions about life, learning how to obtain information to gain an understanding about issues of personal interest or importance, developing a network of support, knowing one's rights and responsibilities, reaching out to others when in need of assistance, and learning about self-determination.[OTPF 2014]

self-care: The set of activities that comprise daily living, such as bed mobility, transfers, ambulation, dressing, grooming, bathing, eating, and toileting.

self-care activities: Personal activities an individual performs to prepare for and maintain a daily routine.

self-catheterization: Insertion of a flexible plastic tube into the urethra by the patient, permitting the bladder to be emptied and controlled.

self-concept: Developing the value of the physical, emotional, and sexual self[UTIII]; view one has of one's self (e.g., ideas, feelings, attitudes, identity, worth, and capabilities and limitations).

self-control: Modifying one's own behavior in response to environmental needs, demands, constraints, personal aspirations, and feedback from others.[UTIII]

self-deprecator: Type of person who seeks praise by devaluing him- or herself; successful attention-getter initially, but fails over the longer term when other group members become aware of circumstances.

self-determination: Focus on the individual making choices and decisions for him- or herself. Choices and decisions are made through an educational and empowering process.[C]

self-efficacy: An individual's belief that he or she is capable of successfully performing a certain set of behaviors.

self-esteem: An individual's overall feeling of worth.

self-expression: Using a variety of styles and skills to express thoughts, feelings, and needs.[UTIII]

self-fulfilling prophecy: A principle that refers to a belief in or the expectation of a particular outcome is a factor that contributes to its fulfillment.

self-help: Various methods by which individuals attempt to remedy their difficulties without making use of formal care providers (e.g., Alcoholics Anonymous).

self-identity skill: Ability to perceive oneself as holistic and autonomous and to have permanence and continuity over time.

self-image: Internalized view a person holds of him- or herself that usually varies with changing social situations over one's lifespan.

self-monitoring: Process whereby the client records specific behaviors or thoughts as they occur.

self-report: Type of assessment approach where the individual reports on his or her level of function or performance.

self-stimulatory behavior: Actions used to stimulate one's own senses such as body rocking, hand flapping, toe walking, spinning, and echoalia. Often referred to as stimming.

semantic compaction: Technique for reducing the number of selections a user must make to generate a phrase on a voice-output communication aid. Symbols for semantic units are used rather than number or letter codes.

semantic differential: A structured approach to measuring the perceived value of objects or events, developed by Osgood.

semantic memory: Memory for general knowledge.

semantics: The study of language with special attention to the meanings of words and other symbols.

semi-autonomous: Individual is partially dependent upon another for the satisfaction of needs.

semicircular canal: Organ in the inner ear that transmits information about head position.

Semmes-Weinstein monofilaments: Nylon monofilaments used for assessing cutaneous pressure threshold.

senescence: Aging; growing older.

senile dementia: An organic mental disorder resulting from generalized atrophy of the brain with no evidence of cerebrovascular disease.

sensation: Receiving conscious sensory impressions through direct stimulation of the body, such as hearing, seeing, touching, etc.

sensation avoiding: When persons have low thresholds and develop responses to counteract their thresholds, they may appear to be resistant and unwilling to participate.

sensation seeking: When persons have high thresholds but develop responses to counteract their thresholds, they engage in behaviors to increase their own sensory experiences. They add movement, touch, sound, and visual stimuli to every experience.

sense of control: Perception of being able to direct and regulate.

sense of security: Feeling of comfort in being able to trust in knowing that there is predictability in the environment.

sensitivity: Capacity to feel, transmit, and react to a stimulus; rating of how well changes will be measured on subsequent tests to show improvement; the extent to which an assessment instrument detects a disorder when it is truly present.

sensitivity to stimuli: Due to low thresholds, persons who act in accordance with those thresholds tend to seem hyperactive or distracted. They have a hard time staying on tasks to complete them or to learn from their experiences because their low neurologic thresholds keep directing their attention from one stimulus to the next, whether it is part of the ongoing task or not.

sensitization: An acquired reaction; the process of a receptor becoming more susceptible to a given stimulus.

sensorimotor component: The ability to receive input, process information, and produce output.[UTIII]

sensorimotor therapy: Therapy planned to enhance the integration of reflex phenomena and the emergence of voluntary motor behaviors concerned with posture and locomotion.

sensory: Having to do with sensations or the senses; including peripheral sensory processing (e.g., sensitivity to touch) and cortical sensory processing (e.g., two-point and sharp/dull discrimination).

sensory conflict: Situations in which sensory signals that are expected to match do not match, either between systems (vision, somatosensory, or vestibular) or within a system (left versus right sides).

sensory defensiveness: Constellation of symptoms that are the result of adverse or defensive reactions to non-noxious stimuli across one or more sensory modalities.

sensory deprivation: An involuntary loss of physical awareness caused by detachment from external sensory stimuli, which can result in psychological disturbances.

sensory diet: A carefully designed and personalized activity plan that provides targeted sensory input and controls exposure to specific sensations for individuals with sensory integration dysfunction. Designed to minimize negative behaviors and improve function by scheduling specific activities to produce calm or develop new sensory skills.

sensory environment: The conditions that exist in the world around us that impact balance (i.e., darkness, visual movement, complaint surfaces, etc.).

sensory integration (SI): Ability of the central nervous system to process sensory information to make an adaptive response to the environment; also refers to therapeutic intervention, which uses strong kinesthetic and proprioceptive stimulation to attempt to better organize the central nervous system.

Sensory Integration and Praxis Test (SIPT): Evaluates children ages 4 to 8 years 11 months in the areas of form and space, somatosensory and vestibular processing, bilateral integration and sequencing, and praxis. The test consists of 17 subtests that require integration of bilateral function in either gross, fine, and oral motor movements, as well as tactile perception.

sensory integrative dysfunction: A disorder or irregularity in brain function that makes sensory integration difficult. Many, but not all, learning disorders stem from sensory integrative dysfunctions.

sensory integrative therapy: Therapy involving sensory stimulation and adaptive responses to it according to a child's neurologic needs.

sensory memory: Memory store that holds sensory input in its uninterpreted sensory form for a brief period of time.

sensory modulation: The ability to maintain an alert and focused state.

sensory neuron: Nerve cell that sends signals to the spinal cord or brain.

sensory or body disregard: Condition characterized by lack of awareness of one side of the body.

sensory-perceptual skills: Actions or behaviors a client uses to locate, identify, and respond to sensations and to select, interpret, associate, organize, and remember sensory events via sensations that include visual, auditory, proprioceptive, tactile, olfactory, gustatory, and vestibular sensations.^OTPF 2008

sensory registration: The brain's ability to receive input and select what will receive attention and what will be inhibited from consciousness.

sensory stimulation: Therapeutic intervention that makes use of patterned sensory input.

sensory testing: Evaluation of sensory system.

sensory training: General term for therapy aimed at enabling a person to regain contact with his or her environment; usually offered in groups, sensory training includes social introductions among the group, body awareness exercises, and sensory activities utilizing objects.

separation anxiety disorder: Excessive anxiety that occurs when a child is separated from home or caregiver.

sepsis: Poisoning that is caused by the products of a putrefactive process; infection.

septicemia: Systemic disease associated with the presence and persistence of pathogenic microorganisms or toxins in the blood.

sequela: Morbid condition resulting from another condition or event.

sequestrum: Fragment of necrosed bone that has become separated from the surrounding tissue.

serial casting: Process of applying casts of increasing degrees of joint position every few days to stretch a limb progressively away from a contracted spastic posture.

serial speech: Overlearned speech involving a series of words such as counting and reciting the days of the week.

serology: Study of blood serum.

Service Corps of Retired Executives (SCORE): Both retired and working business persons who volunteer to provide assistance in counseling, training, and guiding small business clients.Small Business Administration

service delivery model: Set of methods for providing services to or on behalf of clients.OTPF 2014

service entrance: An entrance intended primarily for delivery of goods or services.

Servicemen's Readjustment Act (GI Bill) of 1944: U.S. federal legislation that provides for the education and training of individuals whose education or career had been interrupted by military service.

service operations: Departmental/facility management.

service team: Client-centered service teams include clients, professionals, and other members/stakeholders. Teams work closely together at one site or are extended groups working across multiple settings and in the broader community (CAOT, in press).CAOT

set: A belief or expectation one has about a person, place, or thing.

setting an overall rehabilitation goal: Choosing a preferred environment in which the consumer intends to live, learn, work, or socialize within the next 6 to 24 months.C

severe retardation: Within an IQ range of 20 to 34.

sex identification: Assigning of a masculine or feminine connotation to a given activity.

sexual activity: Engaging in activities that result in sexual satisfaction.OTPF 2008

sexual dimorphism: The male and female of a species are distinctly different (e.g., in size or shape).

sexuality: The behaviors that relate psychological, cultural, emotional, and physical responses to the need to reproduce.

sexually transmitted disease (STD): A contagious disease usually acquired by sexual intercourse or genital contact.

sexual orientation: A person's emotional, sexual, and/or relational attraction to others. Sexual orientation is usually classified as heterosexual, bisexual, and homosexual (i.e., lesbian and gay) (Substance Abuse and Mental Health Services Administration, 2014).

shaken baby syndrome: A condition of whiplash-type injuries, ranging from bruises on the arms and trunk to retinal hemorrhages or convulsions, as observed in infants and children who have been violently shaken; a form of child abuse that often results in intracranial bleeding from tearing of cerebral blood vessels.

shaman: A type of specialized healer commonly found in many traditional cultures in North and South America.

shamanic path: A way of seeing and knowing that which is hidden from ordinary members of a community but revealed to a shaman.

shearing: Pressure exerted against the surface and layers of the skin as tissues slide in opposite but parallel planes.

sheltered housing: Living arrangements (e.g., group homes) that provide structure and supervision for individuals who do not require institutionalization but are not fully capable of independent living.

shingles: Viral disease of the peripheral nerves with the eruption of skin vesicles along the path of the nerve.

shock therapy: Induced by delivering an electric current through the brain; a procedure used for treating depression.

shopping: Preparing shopping lists (grocery and other); selecting and purchasing items; selecting method of payment; and completing money transactions. AOTA Framework

short opponens: Splint that maintains thumb in abduction and partial rotation under the second metacarpal.

short-term memory: Limited capacity memory store that holds information for a brief period of time; the "working memory."

shoulder dystocia: Occurs when the presenting part in the pelvic inlet is the fetal shoulder during delivery, thereby arresting normal progression of labor.

shoulder hand syndrome: A neurovascular disorder characterized by shoulder pain; stiffness, swelling, and pain in the hand; trophic changes; and vasomotor instability, which results in limited range of motion on that side (Hansen & Atchison, 2000). *Synonym:* reflex sympathetic dystrophy.

shoulder separation: Separation of the acromioclavicular joint due to trauma, injury, or disease.

shoulder subluxation: Incomplete downward, usually partial, dislocation of the humerus out of the glenohumeral joint caused by weakness, stretch, or abnormal tone in the scapulohumeral and/ or scapular muscles.

shower seat: Chair placed in the shower, allowing a bather to sit.

Shroeder-Black-Campbell: Sensory integration evaluation, used to assess sensory integrative function in the adult psychiatric population.

shunt: Passage between two natural channels, especially blood vessels.

side effect: Having a result other than the desired action (e.g., effect produced by a drug).

signage: Displayed verbal, symbolic, tactile, or pictorial information.

signal risk factors: Workers exposed to these factors are at greater risk for developing work-related musculoskeletal disorders. The factors are the following: fixed or awkward work posture for more than 2 hours, performance of the same motion or motion pattern every few seconds for more than a total of 2 hours, use of vibrating or impact tools or equipment for more than a total of 1 hour, and unassisted frequent or forceful manual handling for more than 1 hour.

sign of behavior: Clients' responses that are viewed as "indirect manifestations" (or signs) of one's underlying personality.

simple fracture: Bone that is broken internally but does not pierce the skin so that it can be seen.

simple reflex: Reflex with a motor nerve component that involves only one muscle.

simultaneous consumption: Concurrently performing several activities (e.g., commuting to school and listening to an audiotape of an anatomy lecture).

single trait sample: Evaluation that focuses on the assessment of a single worker trait.

situational assessment: Assesses the person's performance under each circumstance of a realistic work situation by systematically altering variables such as production demands and stress factors.

situation-specific: In psychosocial assessment, those behaviors and tasks that must be mastered to function every day in a particular environment.

skeletal demineralization: The loss of bone mass due to loss of minerals from the bone, as seen in conditions like osteoporosis.

skeletal system: Supporting framework for the body that is composed of the axial and appendicular divisions.

skilled nursing facility (SNF): Institution or part of an institution that meets criteria for accreditation established by the sections of the Social Security Act that determine the basis for Medicaid and Medicare reimbursement.

skin fold measurement: Method for estimating the percentage of body fat by measuring subcutaneous fat with skin fold calipers.

Skype: An online Voice Over Internet Protocol (VoIP) program that allows users to speak directly with each other, video conference, and instant message at no charge.

slate and stylus: Method of writing in Braille in which the paper is held in a slate while the stylus is pressed through openings to make indentations in the paper.

sleep: "A natural periodic state of rest for the mind and body, in which the eyes usually close and consciousness is completely or partially lost, so that there is a decrease in bodily movement and responsiveness to external stimuli. During sleep the brain in humans and other mammals undergoes a characteristic cycle of brain-wave activity that includes intervals of dreaming" (*The Free Dictionary*, 2007). A series of activities resulting in going to sleep, staying asleep, and ensuring health and safety through participation in sleep involving engagement with the physical and social environments.OTPF 2008

sleep apnea: Disorder characterized by period of an absence of attempts to breathe; person is momentarily unable to move respiratory muscles or maintain air flow through nose and mouth.

sleep paralysis: Temporary inability to talk or move when falling asleep or waking up.

sleep participation: Taking care of personal need for sleep such as cessation of activities to ensure onset of sleep, napping, dreaming, sustaining a sleep state without disruption, and nighttime care of toileting needs or hydration. Negotiating the needs and requirements of others within the social environment. Interacting with those sharing the sleeping space such as children or partners, providing nighttime caregiving such as breast feeding, and monitoring the comfort and safety of others such as the family while sleeping.OTPF 2008

sleep preparation: (1) Engaging in routines that prepare the self for a comfortable rest, such as grooming and undressing, reading or listening to music, saying goodnight to others, and meditation or prayers; determining the time of day and length of time desired for sleeping or the time needed to wake; and establishing sleep patterns that support growth and health (patterns are often personally and culturally determined). (2) Preparing the physical environment for periods of unconsciousness, such as making the bed or space on which to sleep; ensuring warmth/coolness and protection; setting an alarm clock; securing the home, such as locking doors or closing windows or curtains; and turning off electronics or lights.OTPF 2008

small business health care tax credits: Although the Affordable Care Act does not require that businesses provide health insurance, it does offer tax credits for eligible small businesses that choose to provide insurance to their employees for the first time or maintain the coverage they already have. To qualify for a small business health care tax credit of up to 35%, the business must have fewer than 25 full-time equivalent employees, pay average annual wages below $50,000, and contribute 50% or more toward the employees' self-only health insurance premiums. In 2014, this tax credit goes up to 50% (Olafson, 2013).

SOAP (subjective, objective, assessment, plan): The four parts of a written account of a health problem.

sobriety: Describes a new way of living without alcohol and drugs.

social access activities: Tasks involving interaction.

social age: Definition of age emphasizing the functional level of social interaction skills rather than calendar time.

social change: Lies on a continuum and is interconnected with individual change, looks beyond psychological or other individualized explanations for human behavior, and targets social structures, systems, culture, and the built and natural environment.[CAOT]

social climate: Combined variables in the social environment that directly or indirectly influence individual behavior and are influenced by individual behavior.

social clock: Set of internalized beliefs that forms the standards that individuals use in assessing their conformity to age-appropriate expectations.

social construction: Social construct or social concept is an institutionalized entity or artifact in a social system "invented" or "constructed" by participants in a particular culture or society that exists because people agree to behave as if it exists or agree to follow certain conventional rules or behave as if such agreement or rules existed (Answers.com).[CAOT]

social constructivists: Those who believe in a psychological relativism suggesting that perceptions of individuals and individuality are culturally defined rather than biologically dictated.

social Darwinism: A largely discredited doctrine of the late 19th and early 20th centuries that applied (mostly erroneously) Darwin's theory of biological evolution to societies.

social disadvantage or handicap: Results when an individual is not able to fulfill a role that he or she expects or is required to fill.

social environment: Presence of, relationships with, and expectations of persons, groups, and populations with whom clients have contact (e.g., availability and expectations of significant individuals, such as spouse, friends, and caregivers).[OTPF 2014]

social identity theory: Social psychologist Henry Taifel's theory that when individuals are assigned to a group, they invariably think of that group as an in-group for them. This occurs because individuals want to have a positive image.

social indicators: An approach to needs assessment that examines data from public records—census, county health department, police records, and housing offices.

social interaction skills: "Occupational performance skills observed during the ongoing stream of a social exchange" (Boyt Schell et al., 2014a, p. 1241).[OTPF 2014]

socialization: Development of the individual as a social being and a participant in society that results from a continuing, changing interaction between a person and those who attempt to influence him or her.[OTPF 2008]

social justice: "Ethical distribution and sharing of resources rights and responsibilities between people recognizing their equal worth as citizens. [It recognizes] 'their equal right to be able to meet basic needs, the need to spread opportunities and life chances as widely as possible, and finally the requirement that we reduce and where possible eliminate unjustified inequalities'" (Commission on Social Justice, 1994, p. 1). "The promotion of social and economic change to increase individual, community, and political awareness, resources, and opportunity for health and well-being" (Wilcock, 2006, p. 344).[OTPF 2008] A "vision and an everyday practice in which people can choose, organize, and engage in meaningful occupations that enhance health, quality of life, and equity in housing, employment and other aspects of life" (CAOT, 1997a, 2002, p. 182).[CAOT]

social learning theory: View of psychologists who emphasize behavior, environment, and cognition as the key factors for development.

social media: A broad term used to describe the tools and platforms people use to publish, converse, and share content online. Includes but is not limited to Facebook, blogs, wikis, podcasts, and sites to share photos and bookmarks.

social modeling theory: Maintains that learning is accomplished through observing others. A person may learn a behavior or its consequences by watching another person experience that behavior.

social participation: "Interweaving of occupations to support desired engagement in community and family activities as well as those involving peers and friends" (Gillen & Boyt Schell, 2014, p. 607) or involvement in a subset of activities that involve social situations with others (Bedell, 2012) and that support social interdependence (Magasi & Hammel, 2004). Social participation can occur in person or through remote technologies such as telephone calls, computer interaction, and video conferencing.[OTPF 2014]

social phobia: Intense fear of social situations, stemming from fear of negative judgment by others. Social phobics feel scrutinized and tend to be overly critical of themselves.

social referencing: Communicating behavior in which babies keep a watchful eye on their caregiver's expression to see how they should interpret unusual events.

social role: The behavior expected as appropriate for a specific status position in a particular situation.

Social Security Acts and Amendments (1935): U.S. federal legislation that provided financial support for workers with disabilities and retirement income for the elderly.

Social Security Amendments of 1972: U.S. federal legislation that provided for the establishment of Professional Standard Review Organizations to ensure that federally funded programs were used in an efficient and effective manner.

social skills: Behaviors include greeting, taking turns, listening, and maintaining a topic during social interactions; one of the skills of social competence that refers to the ability to produce mutually reciprocal interactions with others.

social skills training: Cognitive/behavioral approach to teaching skills basic to social interaction.

social structure: The relationship of various status positions in a society.

social support: Social relatedness and interactions with others that are perceived by the individual as supplying emotional, physical, and social resources.

social systems: Organized interactions among individuals, as within marriages, families, communities, and organizations, both formal and informal.

societal limitations: When societal policy, attitudes, and actions (or lack of actions) create a physical, social, or financial barrier to access health care, housing, or vocational/avocational opportunities.

society: An organization of people.

sociobiology: The study of animal behavior, especially social behavior, from the perspective of evolution by natural selection.

sociodramatic play: Imaginary or make-believe play involving two or more children enacting various social roles.

sociological aging: Age-specific roles a person adopts within his or her context of society and individual environment. It includes the changes of a person's roles and functions, and the reflected behavior of these changes within society throughout life.

socket: The part of a prosthesis into which a stump of the remaining limb fits.

soft end feel: Movement stops secondary to one muscle belly hitting another (e.g., elbow flexion).

soft neurological signs: Mild or slight neurological abnormalities that are difficult to detect.

software: Programs that run on computers.

solitary play: Play in which a child is completely involved in the activity and blocks out the surroundings both physically and psychologically.

soma: Cell body of a nerve that contains the nucleus.

somatic complaints: Complaints focused on bodily functions such as loss of energy and reduced sleep.

somatic nervous system: Portion of the nervous system composed of a motor division that excites skeletal muscles and a sensory division that receives and processes sensory input from the sense organs.

somatization: Refers to the tendency to report physical symptoms when a person is experiencing psychological distress.

somatoform disorders: Group of mental disorders characterized by (a) loss or alteration in physical functioning for which there is no physiological explanation, (b) evidence that psychological factors have caused the physical symptoms, (c) lack of voluntary control over physical symptoms, and (d) indifference by the patient to the physical loss.

somatosensory evoked potential (SEP): Peripheral nerve stimulation produces potentials that can be recorded from the scalp, over the spine, or the periphery.

somatotopagnosia: Lack of awareness of the relationship of one's own body parts or the body parts of others.

somatotopic: Organization of cells in the somatosensory system that enables one to identify the exact skin surface touched.

spasm: An involuntary muscle contraction.

spastic diplegia: An increase in postural tonus that is distributed primarily in the lower extremities and the pelvic area.

spastic gait: Stiff movement, toes drag, legs held together, and hip and knee joints are slightly flexed.

spasticity: Increase in the muscle tone and stretch reflex of a muscle resulting in increased resistance to passive stretch of the muscle and hyperresponsivity of the muscle to sensory stimulation.

spastic quadriplegia: An increase in postural tonus that is distributed throughout all four extremities. These findings are often coexistent with relatively lower tone in the trunk and severe difficulty in controlling posture.

spatial awareness: Ability to orient oneself in space, to visualize what an object looks like from all angles, to know where sounds are coming from, and to know where body parts are in space.

spatial relations: Ability to perceive the self in relation to other objects.[OTPF 2008]

speaks: Makes oneself understood through use of words, phrases, and sentences.[AOTA Framework]

special interest groups: Collectives of individuals and organizations who are bound by beliefs about specific issues or populations and who seek to influence decisions about the allocation of resources.

specialize: A key enablement skill to use specific techniques in particular situations, examples being therapeutic touch and positioning, the use of neurodevelopmental techniques to enable children to participate in occupations, or psychosocial rehabilitation techniques to engage adults in their own empowerment. In *Profile of Occupational Therapy Practice in Canada* (CAOT, in press), specialize is a composite of enablement skills that contributes to the competency role of expert in enabling occupation.[CAOT]

specialized battery: Tests that measure a specific component (e.g., cognitive functioning, such as attention or language).

specificity: Instrument's ability to accurately identify subjects possessing a specific trait.

specific needs: Activities the patient or client requires in daily life.

speculum: An instrument used to hold open and dilate the vagina during inspection.

speech: The meaningful production and sequencing of sounds by the speech sensorimotor system (e.g., lips, tongue) for the transmission of spoken language.

speech-language pathology and audiology: Science that specializes in the investigation of the scientific bases of the normal processes of communication and its disorders.

sphygmomanometer: Instrument used to measure arterial blood pressure indirectly.

spina bifida: Congenital malformation of the spine in which the walls of the spinal canal do not develop typically due to the lack of union between vertebrae; the degree of impairment depends on the location of the malformation.

spinal: An injection of anesthesia into the spinal fluid to produce numbness.

spinal cord injury (SCI): Injury to the spinal cord that results in temporary or permanent paralysis of the muscles of the limbs and the autonomic nervous system. Usually manifested below the level of injury. Temporary symptoms usually result from compression of the cord; permanent paralysis is generally caused by fractures or dislocations that puncture or transect the cord.

spinal fusion: Joining together of spinal vertebrae to prevent damage to the bones or spinal cord from disease processes.

spinal muscular atrophy (SMA): A genetic disease caused by the progressive loss of motor neurons, resulting in muscle weakness and atrophy. There are four types that vary in severity with the most severe type (SMA Type I) being the most common among children. SMA is an autosomal recessive disease that has been linked to a gene called the SMN gene. An individual must receive a defective copy of the gene from both parents in order to be affected. Most children are diagnosed at a young age when they fail to hit developmental milestones such as sitting up, rolling over, and walking.

spinal nerve: Nerve extending from the spinal cord.

spinocerebellar tracts: Dorsal—afferent ipsilateral ascending tract to cerebellum serving mostly lower extremities for touch, pressure, and proprioception. Ventral—afferent contralateral ascending tract to cerebellum serving lower extremities for proprioception.

spinothalamic tract: Afferent contralateral and ipsilateral ascending tract to thalamus for sensation of pain, temperature, and light (erude) touch. *Also known as* the anterolateral system.

spiritual activities: Religion- or spirituality-based tasks.

spirituality: "Aspect of humanity that refers to the way individuals seek and express meaning and purpose and the way they experience their connectedness to the moment, to self, to others, to nature, and to the significant or sacred" (Puchalski et al., 2009, p. 887).[OTPF 2014] Sensitivity to the presence of spirit (McColl, 2000), a "pervasive life force, manifestation of a higher self, source of will and self-determination, and a sense of meaning, purpose and connectedness that people experience in the context of their environment" (CAOT, 1997a, 2002, p. 182); "spirituality resides in persons, is shaped by the environment, and gives meaning to occupations" (CAOT, 1997a, 2002, p. 33).[CAOT]

spiritual meaning: Meaning, usually symbolic, related to one's concerns with matters that transcend physical life.

splint: Supportive device used to immobilize, fix, or prevent deformities or assist in motion.

Splint Classification System (SCS): System created by a specifically appointed committee of splinting experts, either internationally or nationally recognized, that classifies splints in a manner that is logical, practical, and organized. In this system, splints are not classified according to whether static or dynamic components are present.

splinter skills: Skills learned by rote that are not intended to be generalized into other situations.

splint evaluation criteria list: List of guidelines that creates an organized approach or method to evaluating splints. This list involves both the evaluation of the splint as a whole as well as its individual components.

spondylitis: Inflammation of the vertebrae.

spondylolisthesis: Forward displacement of one vertebra over another, usually of the fifth lumbar vertebra over the body of the sacrum or the fourth lumbar over the fifth.

spontaneous remission: Unusual occurrence (e.g., when cancer cells revert back to normal without aid or apparent cause).

Spork: Utensil that combines the bowl of a spoon and the tines of a fork and eliminates the need to change utensils.

spot reading: Reading a few words at a time, such as a sign or label.

sprain: Injury to a joint that causes pain and disability, with the severity depending on the degree of injury to ligaments or tendons.

spreadsheet: Type of computer software organized in section or table format used in financial management and accounting systems.

sputum: Substance expelled by coughing or clearing the throat.

stabilizer: Any muscle that acts to fix one attachment of a prime mover or hold a bone steady to provide a foundation for movement; equipment or device used to maintain a particular position.

staff development: Various educational resources for professionals that are used to attain new skills and knowledge.

staging: Classification of tumors by their spread through the body.

standard assessment: Tests and evaluation approaches with specific norms, standards, and protocol.

standard deviation: Mathematically determined value used to derive standard scores and compare raw scores to a unit normal distribution; measure that demonstrates how scores in a distribution deviate from the mean.

standard error: Possible range in the variability of a person's "true" score in a test; a number that recognizes the amount by which a score might vary on different days or in different situations.

standard error of the mean: Standard deviation of the entire distribution of random sample means, successively selected from a single population.

standardization: Method by which test scores of a typical population are derived, thus allowing subsequent test scores to be analyzed in light of that broad population; standardization requires a rigorous process of data collection and comparison.

standardized battery: A battery of tests in which the testing and scoring procedures are well defined and fixed, and the interpretation involves the use of standardized norms.

Standards and Ethics Commission (SEC): Body of the American Occupational Therapy Association that is responsible for the Code of Ethics and the Standards of Practice of the profession.

standard scores: Raw scores mathematically converted to a scale that facilitates comparison.

Standards of Practice for Occupational Therapy: Guidelines assembled to assist occupational therapy practitioners in the delivery of occupational therapy services.

Stanford-Binet Intelligence Scales: One of the most widely used intelligence tests.

static equilibrium: Ability of an individual to adjust to displacements of the center of gravity while maintaining a constant base of support.

static flexibility: Range of motion in degrees that a joint will allow.

statics: Study of objects at rest.

static splint: Rigid orthosis used for the prevention of movement of a joint or for the fixation of a displaced part.

static strength: Holding the lengthened position without movement.

status: A position in society with certain rights and obligations.

steatorrhea: Fatty stools, seen in pancreatic diseases; increased secretion of the sebaceous glands.

stent: Any material used to hold in place or to provide a support for a graft or anastomosis while healing takes place.

step test: Graded exercise test in which a person is required to rhythmically step up and down steps of gradually increasing heights.

stereognosis: Ability to identify sizes, shapes, and weights of familiar objects without the use of vision.^{OTPF 2008}

stereopsis: Quality of visual fusion.

stereotype: A generalization or categorization about a particular group based on some common feature like gender or physical appearance.

stereotypic behavior: Repeated, persistent postures or movements, including vocalizations.

stereotyping: Applying generalized and oversimplified labels of characteristics, actions, or attitudes to a specific socioeconomic, cultural, religious, or ethnic group. Often used to belittle or discount a particular group.

stertorous: Respiratory effort that is strenuous and struggling; sounds like snoring.

stethoscope: Instrument used to listen to heart and lung sounds.

stigma: An undesirable difference that becomes a basis for separating an individual bearing such traits from the rest of society.

stimulation: Arousal of attention, interest, or tension.

stimulus-arousal properties: Alerting potential of various sensory stimuli, generally thought to be related to their intensity, pace, and novelty.

stochastic: Any process in which there is a random variable.

storage fat: Adipose tissue found primarily subcutaneously and surrounding the major organs.

strabismus: Weakness of eye muscles allowing the eyes to cross.

strain: Usually a muscular injury caused by the excessive physical effort that leads to a forcible stretch.

strategic compliance: A decision to comply with demands in the environment but retain different views concerning appropriate treatment strategies.

strategic planning: Goals that are essential, basic, or critical to the continuation of an institution or organization. It involves the use of resources to achieve long-range goals.

strength: Nonspecific term relating to muscle contraction, often referring to the force generated by a single maximal isometric contraction.[OTPF 2008]

strengthening: Active—A form of strength-building exercise in which the physical therapist applies resistance through the range of motion of active movement. Assistive—A form of strength-building exercise in which the physical therapist assists the patient/client through the available range of motion. Resistive—Any form of active exercise in which a dynamic or static muscular contraction is resisted by an outside force. The external force may be applied manually or mechanically.

streptokinase: An enzyme produced by streptococci that catalyzes the conversion of plasminogen to plasmin.

stress: Individual's general reaction to external demands or stressors. Stress results in psychological as well as physiological reactions.

stress incontinence: A type of urinary incontinence that occurs when the bladder pressure exceeds urethral resistance and sphincter activity is weak or absent.

stress management techniques: Methods of relieving or controlling chronic stress by interrupting reflexive neurologic stress reactions.

stressors: External events that place demands on an individual above the ordinary.

stretch: Temporary lengthening of tissues that is not maintained for a sufficient period of time to encourage collagen remodeling.

stretching: A sense of overcoming cultural stereotypes after encountering diverse individuals.

striae gravidae: Stretch marks appearing on the distended skin caused by the rupture of elastic fibers due to excessive distention.

stridor: A harsh, high-pitched respiratory sound such as the inspiratory sound often heard in laryngeal or bronchial obstruction. Sometimes heard through a tracheostomy tube.

stripping and ligation: Removal and tying off of a vein.

stroke: Syndrome characterized by a sudden onset in which blood vessels in the brain have become narrowed or blocked. *Synonym*: cerebrovascular accident.

stroke volume: Amount of blood pumped out of the heart on each beat.

structural theory: Dividing of the mind into three structures: the id, the ego, and the superego.

structured activities: Activities that have rules and can be broken down into manageable steps that have been preplanned and preorganized.

Structured Assessment of Independent Living Skills (SAILS): Assessment procedure in which the client is observed performing 50 tasks and is scored on the quality of his or her motor and cognitive skills used in performing the task. The 10 areas of daily activities include fine motor skills, dressing, eating, expressive language, receptive language, time, orientation, money-related skills, instrumental activities, and social interaction.

stupor: A condition of unconsciousness or lethargy with suppression of feeling or sense.

sty, stye: Localized circumscribed inflammatory swelling of one of the sebaceous glands of the eyelid. *Synonym*: hordeolum.

subacute care: Short-term, comprehensive inpatient level of care.

subacute patient: Medically complex cases requiring a longer period of rehabilitation and recovery, usually from 1 to 4 weeks.

sub-ASIS bar: Orthotic bar included in seating and positioning systems placed snugly below the anterior superior iliac spine of the pelvis to maintain a forward tilt of the pelvis and better postural alignment.

subcortical: Region beneath the cerebral cortex.

subculture: Ethnic, regional, economic, or social group exhibiting characteristic patterns of behavior sufficient to distinguish it from others within an embracing culture or society. Does not usually include rejection of the larger culture. Most people are members of several subcultures.

subjective measure: Assessment designed to identify the client's own view of problems and performance.

subjective well-being: Individual perceptions of positive events and level of happiness based on personal, internal experience.

subjugation to nature: A value orientation found in some cultures that suggests that humans are controlled by the natural world.

sublingual: Under the tongue.

subluxation: Partial or incomplete dislocation (e.g., shoulder of client with cerebrovascular accident).

substance abuse: "A maladaptive pattern of behavior in regard to the use of chemically active agents that lead to clinically significant impairment or distress" (Thomas & Craven, 1997, p. 1856).

substance dependence: An essential feature is a cluster of cognitive, behavioral, and physiologic symptoms within the 12-month period as substance abuse.

substantia nigra: Movement control center in the brain where loss dopamine-producing nerve cells triggers symptoms of Parkinson's disease.

sudden infant death syndrome (SIDS): Rare form of death in infants from ages 2 to 6 months in which the child dies mysteriously without cause.

sudomotor: Stimulating the sweat glands.

suffix: Word element of one or more syllables added to the end of a combining form in order to change its meaning.

sundowning: Condition in which frail elderly persons tend to become more confused or disoriented at the end of the day.

sunrise syndrome: Condition of unstable cognitive ability on arising in the morning.

superego: In psychoanalytic theory, one of three personality components. It houses one's values, ethics, standards, and conscience; an analytic concept that equates roughly to the conscience.

superficial: Area of the body that is located closest to the surface.

superior: Toward the head or upper portion of a part or structure. *Synonym*: cephalad.

supervisor: Any person having authority in the interests of the employer to hire, transfer, layoff, recall, promote, assign, reward, or discipline other employees.

supination (Sup): Rotation of the forearm so the palm is facing up toward the ceiling.

supine: Lying on the spine with the face up.

support: Focus on providing assistance for as long as it is needed and wanted.[C]

supported employment: Paid employment for people with disabilities without employment or for those whose employment has been interrupted as a result of a severe disability and who need support services to perform job-related tasks.

supportive devices: External supports to protect weak or ineffective joints or muscles. Supportive devices include supportive taping, compression garments, corsets, slings, neck collars, serial casts, elastic wraps, and oxygen.

supportive personnel: Aides and technicians other than occupational therapy assistants.

supportive services: Those that enable and empower an individual to function more independently within a community or facility.

suppression: Ability of the central nervous system to screen out certain stimuli so that others may be attended to more carefully.

surfactant: A surface agent.

surrogate: Person or thing that replaces another (e.g., substitute parental figure).

sustains: Keeps up speech for appropriate duration.[AOTA Framework]

swan neck deformity: Condition of the hand characterized by hyperextension of the proximal interphalangeal joint and flexion of the distal interphalangeal joint.

symbolic associations: Object's broader, cultural connotations and its narrower, idiosyncratic associations for individuals or families.

symbolic deficit hypothesis: Lack of representational skills.

symbolic play: Imagining or assigning roles to objects or other people (e.g., playing house).

symbols: Abstract representations of perceived reality.

symmetrical: Equal in size and shape; very similar in relative placement or arrangement about an axis.

sympathetic nervous system: Autonomic nervous system that mobilizes the body's resources during stressful situations.

sympatholytic: Opposing the effects of impulses conveyed by adrenergic postganglionic fibers of the sympathetic nervous system. An agent that opposes the effects of impulses conveyed by adrenergic postganglionic fibers of the sympathetic nervous system.

sympathomimetic: Mimicking the effects of impulses conveyed by adrenergic postganglionic fibers of the sympathetic nervous system. An agent (drug) may be used to do this.

symptom (Sx): Subjective indication of a disease or a change in condition as perceived by the individual.

synapse: Minuscule space that exists between the end of the axon of one nerve cell and the cell body or dendrite of another.

synaptogenesis: The process of forming "synaptic connections" between nerve cells or between nerve cells and muscle fibers; the basis of neuronal communication.

synarthrodial joint: A nonsynovial joint; bony surfaces are connected by fibrous tissue (e.g., suture of the skull).

synchronous: Occurring at regular intervals. Objects, events, or electronic data transmission coordinated in time.

syncope: Fainting or brief lapse in consciousness caused by transient cerebral hypoxia.

syndactyly: Webbing of the fingers (or toes) involving only the skin or in complex cases the fusing of adjacent bones. It is usually seen in children and can be surgically corrected.

syndrome: Combination of symptoms resulting from a single course or commonly occurring together that they constitute a distinct clinical picture.

synergism: Action of two or more substances, organs, or organisms to achieve an effect of which each is not individually capable.

synergist: Any muscle that functions to inhibit extraneous action from a muscle that would interfere with the action of prime mover.

synergy: Fixed set of muscles contracting with a present sequence and time of contraction.

synovectomy: Excision of the synovial membrane (e.g., as in the knee joint).

synthetic Darwinism: A modern synthesis of Charles Darwin's arguments of natural selection with Gregor Mendel's mechanisms of heredity. This was accomplished in the 1940s by a group of evolutionists and geneticists and accounts for the origin of genetic variation as mutations in DNA as well as rearrangement of genetic structures in a process known as recombination. *Synonym:* neo-Darwinism.

syringomyelia: Chronic progressive degenerative disorder of the spinal cord characterized by the development of an irregular cavity within the spinal cord.

systematic desensitization: Behavioral procedure that uses relaxation paired with an anxiety-provoking stimulus in an attempt to reduce the anxiety response.

systemic: Involving the whole system such as in systemic rheumatoid arthritis.

systems interactions: The ways the various central nervous systems affect or interact with each other in order to provide a more integrative and functional nervous system.

systems model: A conceptual representation that incorporates a set of major functional divisions or systems within the central nervous system, which interlock and interrelate to create the functional whole. Although each division may be considered a whole in and of itself, with multiple subsystems interlocking to form its entire division, each major component or division influences and is influenced by all others, and thus the totality of the central nervous system is based on the summation of interactions, not individual function.

systole: Contraction of the heart, especially of the ventricles, during which blood is forced into the aorta and pulmonary artery.

tachycardia: Rapid heartbeat.

tachypnea: Excessively rapid respiration marked by quick, shallow breathing.

tacit: Implied understanding that is not verbalized.

tactile: Pertaining to the sense of touch; tangible.

tactile defensiveness: Adverse reaction to being touched.

tactile discrimination: Ability to discriminate among objects by the sense of touch.

tactile fremitus: A thrill or vibration that is perceptible on palpation. A thrill, as in the chest wall, that may be felt by a hand applied to the thorax while the patient is speaking.

talipes: Deformities of the foot, especially those congenital in origin. *Synonym*: clubfoot.

tamponade: Acute compression of the heart that is due to effusion of fluid into the pericardium or to the collection of blood in the pericardium from rupture of the heart or a coronary vessel.

target site: Desired site for a drug's action within the body.

task: What individuals do or have done (e.g., drive, bake a cake, dress, make a bed; A. Fisher, personal communication, December 16, 2013).^OTPF 2014 A set of actions having an end point or a specific outcome; simple or compound actions involving tool use, such as printing a report (adapted from Polatajko et al., 2004; Zimmerman et al., 2006).^CAOT Work assigned to, selected by, or required of a person that is related to the development of occupational performance skills; collection of activities related to the accomplishment of a specific goal.

Tax Equity and Fiscal Responsibility Act (TEFRA) (1982): U.S. federal act that put limits on Medicare and Medicaid reimbursements (including occupational therapy); also limits items such as inpatient hospital costs.

taxonomy: Laws and principles for classification of living things and organisms; also used for learning objectives.

Tay-Sachs disease: Genetic progressive disorder of the nervous system that causes profound mental retardation, deafness, blindness, paralysis, and seizures; life expectancy is 5 years old.

T cell: A heterogeneous population of lymphocytes comprising helper/inducer T cells and cytotoxic/suppressor T cells.

technology: *See* high technology, low technology.

Technology-Related Assistance for Individuals with Disabilities Act of 1988: U.S. federal legislation that requires assistive technology be made available to persons with disabilities to enhance their functional capabilities.

technology transfer: In occupational therapy, the process by which knowledge is applied; occupational therapy knowledge is technology that is transferred by administering evaluation and treatment.

Tegretol: Drug used to treat bipolar disorders that has some neurotoxic side effects. *Generic name*: carbamazepine.

telecommunication device for the deaf (TDD) or teletype-writer (TTY): Device connected to a telephone by a special adapter that allows telephone communication between a hearing person and a person with impaired hearing.

tele-ergonomics: A form of health care that allows ergonomic specialists to assess, evaluate, and provide interventions to clients long distance using telecommunication and information technologies (term coined by occupational therapists Nancy Baker and Karen Jacobs).

telehealth: The application of evaluative, consultative, preventative, and therapeutic services delivered through telecommunication and information technologies (AOTA, 2014a).

Telehealth: A form of health care that allows physicians, nurses, and health care specialists to assess, diagnose, and provide interventions to clients without requiring both individuals to be physically located in the same place.

telemedicine: Provision of consultant services by off-site physicians to health care professionals on the scene using closed-circuit television.

telereceptive: The exteroceptors of hearing, sight, and smell that are sensitive to distant stimuli.

telerehabilitation: The application of telecommunication and information technologies for the delivery of rehabilitation services.

temporal: "Location of occupational performance in time" (Neistadt & Crepeau, 1998, p. 292). The experience of time as shaped by engagement in occupations. The temporal aspects of occupations "which contribute to the patterns of daily occupations" are "the rhythm. . .tempo. . .synchronization. . .duration . . .and sequence" (Larson & Zemke, 2003, p. 82; Zemke, 2004, p. 610). It includes stages of life, time of day, duration, rhythm of activity, or history.[OTPF 2008]

temporal context: Experience of time as shaped by engagement in occupations. The temporal aspects of occupations that "contribute to the patterns of daily occupations" include "rhythm . . . tempo . . . synchronization . . . duration . . . and sequence" (Larson & Zemke, 2003, p. 82; Zemke, 2004, p. 610). The temporal context includes stage of life, time of day, duration and rhythm of activity, and history.[OTPF 2014]

temporal environment: Manner in which social and cultural expectations influence behavior by organizing the time during which activities occur and the amount of time devoted to them.

temporality: Of time (Latin: tempus, por = time).

tendon: Bands of strong fibrous tissue that attach muscles to bones.

tendon injuries: Lacerations, avulsion-type injuries, and crash injuries to the flexor or extensor tendons of the hand; frequently work or sports related.

tenodesis: Surgical fixation of a tendon.

tenodesis splint: Orthosis fabricated to allow pinch and grasp movements through use of wrist extensors in substitution for finger flexors.

tenotomy: Surgical section of a tendon used in some cases to treat spasticity and contractures.

TENS (transcutaneous electrical nerve stimulation): Application of mild electric stimulation to skin electrodes placed over the region of pain to cause interference with the transmission of painful stimuli.

tensile force: Resistive force generated within a tissue in response to elongation or stretching.

tensiometer: Device used to measure force produced from an isometric contraction.

teratogen: Any agent that causes malformation in a developing embryo (e.g., radiation, chemicals, drugs, alcohol, pollutants).

teratogenic: Substances that harm the developing fetus, causing birth defects.

tertiary care: Rehabilitation of disabilities resulting from disease/pathology to optimize and maximize an individual's functional status (e.g., hypertension leading to stroke, tertiary care would prevent progression of disability).

tertiary circular reaction: Child's repetition of behavior with adaptations to make a new or different behavior.

tertiary prevention: Efforts that attempt to maximize function and minimize the detrimental effects of illness or injury.

Testing, Orientation, and Work Evaluation in Rehabilitation (TOWER): First work sampling system developed in 1936 for individuals with physical disabilities. It is now used for all types of people, including those with emotional disabilities.

Test of Playfulness Skills (TOPS): Sixty-item observational assessment of playfulness in young clients.

Test of Visual Perceptive Skills (TVPS) (non-motor): Norm-referenced test for children 4 to 12 years that assesses visual perception.

test protocol: Specific procedures that must be followed when assessing a patient; formal testing procedures.

test-retest reliability: Extent to which repeated administrations of a test to the same people produce the same results.

tests and measures: Specific standardized methods and techniques used to gather data about the patient/client after the history and systems review have been performed.

test sensitivity: An instrument's ability to detect change within a measured variable.

tetany: A syndrome manifested by sharp flexion of joints (especially the wrist and ankle joints), muscle twitching, cramps, and convulsions and sometimes by attacks of difficult breathing.

tetraplegia: Impairment or loss of motor and/or sensory function in the cervical segments of the spinal cord due to damage of neural elements within the spinal cord.

text-to-speech synthesis: Translation of written communication into speech sounds and messages.

thalamic pain: Central nervous system pain caused by injury to the thalamus and characterized by contralateral and sometimes migratory pain brought on by peripheral stimulation.

thalamus: "The largest subdivision of the diencephalon on either side, consisting chiefly of an ovoid gray nuclear mass in the lateral wall of the third ventricle. All sensory stimuli, with the exception of olfactory, are received by the thalamus" (Thomas & Craven, 1997, p. 1931).

theoretical base: The theory that supports a frame of reference.

theoretical rationale: Reason, based on theory or empirical evidence, for using a particular intervention for a specific person.

theory: Set of interrelated concepts used to describe, explain, or predict phenomena.

therapeutic activities: Activities within the limits of the patient's physical, social, or cognitive capacity.

therapeutic communication: Verbal and nonverbal interaction that occurs within a therapeutic relationship.

therapeutic community: Structured inpatient environment designed to provide a rehabilitative experience.

therapeutic environment: Organizing all aspects of the environment in a systematic way so that they enhance a patient's/client's abilities to perform desired tasks and activities (mental, emotional, functional).

therapeutic exercise: Exercise interventions directing toward maximizing functional capabilities. A broad range of activities intended to improve strength, range of motion (including muscle length), cardiovascular fitness, or flexibility or to otherwise increase a person's functional capacity.

therapeutic horseback riding (THR): Use of horseback riding as form of therapy.

therapeutic horsemanship (TH): Interaction with horses as a method of therapy. Can include horse care such as grooming and tacking, education about horse anatomy and horse health, learning about showing procedures and traditions, and learning to lunge horses and use the round pen.

therapeutic mechanisms of change (therapeutic interventions): Interventions that include learning, development of therapeutic rapport, and purposeful activity.

therapeutic play programs: Hospital-based programs offering children play materials as a means of confronting fear, anxiety, and hostility.

therapeutic potential: The degree of likelihood that a therapeutic goal can be achieved.

therapeutic riding (TR): *See* therapeutic horseback riding.

therapeutic touch: The exchange of energy from one person to another for the purpose of healing.

therapeutic use of occupations and activities: Occupations and activities selected for specific clients that meet therapeutic goals. To use occupations/activities therapeutically, context or contexts, activity demands, and client factors should be considered in relation to the client's therapeutic goals. Use of assistive technologies, application of universal-design principles, and environmental modifications support the ability of clients to engage in their occupations.[OTPF 2008]

there-and-then experience: Past experience used as a means to understand present conflicts.

thermistor: An electrical resistor that uses a semiconductor whose resistance varies sharply in a known manner with the ambient temperature; used in determining temperature.

thermoplastic: Plastic-based material that is soft and pliable when warmed and hard when cooled.

thermotherapy: Intervention through the application of heat, causing vasodilatation to enhance the healing process. The use of heat or cold for therapeutic purposes.

third-party payer: An insurance company or health maintenance organization paying for occupational therapy services.

third-party payment: Payment for services by someone other than the person receiving them.

thoracic (Th): Pertaining to the chest.

thoracocentesis: Surgical puncture of the chest wall to drain fluid.

Thorazine: Drug administered for psychotic disorders (e.g., manic-depression). Also given to children with behavior problems (e.g., hyperactivity, aggression). May cause drowsiness, jaundice, anemia, hypertension, and agranulocytosis. *Generic name:* chlorpromazine hydrochloride.

thought disorder: Disturbance in thinking, including distorted content (e.g., ideas, beliefs, sensory interpretation) and distorted written and spoken language (e.g., word salad, loose associations, echolalia).

thought form: Pattern or flow of ideas; the way thoughts take form.

threat minimization: Psychological coping strategy whereby emotions are managed through "playing down" the importance or significance of a stressor.

three-point pressure splints: Type of splint in which the middle force is directed opposite to the two distal or end forces. These splints operate through a series of reciprocal forces. Most splints incorporate the three-point pressure design.

threshold: Level at which a stimulus is recognized by sensory receptors.

thrombin: The enzyme derived from prothrombin, which converts fibrinogen to fibrin.

thrombocytopenia: A condition in which the blood platelets are destroyed, causing severe bleeding if injury occurs.

thrombolytic: Dissolving or splitting up a thrombus.

thrombophlebitis: Inflammation of a vein associated with thrombus formation.

thromboplastin: Enzyme that assists in the process of blood clotting.

thrombosis: Coagulation of the blood in the heart or a blood vessel forming a clot.

thumb carpometacarpal (CMC) stabilization splint: "Short, static splint that slips over the first metacarpal to relieve thumb pain and increase hand function" (Trombly, 1995, p. 558).

thyrotropin-releasing hormone: A hormone of the anterior pituitary gland having an affinity for and specifically stimulating the thyroid gland.

tibial torsion: Rotation occurring inherently in the shaft of the tibia from proximal to distal ends.

tic: Spasmodic muscular contraction, usually involving the face, head, and neck.

time management: Planning and participating in a balance of self-care, work, leisure, and rest activities to promote satisfaction and health.[UTIII]

time-related measures: Assessment in which the client records the thoughts, feelings, and/or behaviors that occur during a specific time period; time sampling and duration are included.

Tinel's sign/test: A test used to assess the rate of nerve recovery; a positive test is a tingling sensation.

tinnitus: Subjective ringing or tinkling sound in the ear.

titer: The required quantity of a substance needed to produce a reaction to a given amount of another substance. Titer is synonymous with level.

Title VII of the Medicare Prospective Payment Legislation (1983): U.S. federal legislation that provides incentives for cost containment and better management of resources by a reimbursement structure based on client's diagnosis rather than direct cost of care.

Title XVIII and Title XIX of the Social Security Act (1965): U.S. federal legislation that established reimbursement based on reasonable cost for medical services for the elderly and through state grants to the poor.

titration: Volumetric determinations by means of standard solutions of known strength.

Toglia Category Assessment (TCA): Assessment that examines the ability of adults who have brain injury or psychiatric illness to establish categories and switch conceptual sets.

toilet hygiene: Obtaining and using supplies; clothing management; maintaining toileting position; transferring to and from toileting position; cleaning body; and caring for menstrual and continence needs (including catheters, colostomies, and suppository management).^{AOTA Framework}

token economy: Providing tokens as rewards for appropriate behavior, which may be redeemed for specific reinforcers unique to each person's taste.

tolerance: Physiological and psychological accommodation or adaptation to a chemical agent over time.

tone: State of muscle contraction at rest, may be determined by resistance to stretch.

tongue-thrust swallow: An immature form of swallowing in which the tongue is projected forward instead of retracted during swallowing.

tonic-clonic: Muscle stiffening and falling into unconsciousness followed by rhythmic jerking, breathing problems, drooling, loss of bladder control, and finally, confusion and sleepiness.

tonic labyrinthine reflex (TLR): A normal postural reflex in animals, abnormally accentuated in decerebrate humans, characterized by extension of all four limbs when the head is positioned in space at an angle above the horizontal in quadrupeds or in the neutral, erect position in humans. *Synonym*: decerebrate rigidity.

tonic neck reflex: A normal response in newborns to extend the arm and the leg on the side of the body to which the head is quickly turned while the infant is supine and to flex the limbs of the opposite side; integrated at 3 to 4 months of age; absence or persistence of the reflex may indicate central nervous system damage. *Synonym*: asymmetric tonic neck reflex.

tonotopic: Organization of cells within the auditory system that enables one to identify the exact sound heard.

tool use: Enables the performance of compound tasks, which can be broken into task segments and units, where a task unit is an action involving tool use and a task segment is a set of task units (Polatajko et al., 2004).CAOT

top-down processing: When processing starts with higher order stored knowledge and depends on contextual information or is "conceptually driven."

topobiology: A term used by Edelman in his theories about brain evolution because many transactions leading to shape are place dependent (topo = place).

topographic: Organization of cells in the visual system that enables one to identify the exact location and features of the stimulus.

topographic orientation: Determining the location of objects and settings, and the route to the location.UTIII

torque: Rotating tendency of force; equals the product of force and the perpendicular distance from the axis of a lever to the point of application of the same force.

torsion dystonia: A condition in which twisting occurs in the alignment of body parts due to a lack of normal muscle tone secondary to infection or disease of the nervous system.

torticollis: Spasm of the neck muscles that causes such persistent turning of the head that eventually the head is held continually to one side. The spasm of the muscles is often painful, and this condition may be caused by a birth injury to the sternocleido-mastoid muscle. *Synonym:* wryneck.

total hip arthroplasty: Type of hip surgery involving the removal of the head and neck of the femur and replacement with a pros-thetic appliance.

total lymphoid irradiation (TLI): Radiation therapy targeted to the body's lymph nodes; the goal is to suppress immune system functioning (reduce the number of lymphocytes in the blood).

total quality management (TQM): Paradigm for management developed by Deming; emphasized three themes: continuous quality improvement, empowerment of workers at all levels, and having a standard to do things right the first time.

toxicology: Branch of pharmacology that examines harmful chem-icals and their effects on the body.

tracheotomy: Incision of the trachea through the skin and muscles of the neck for establishment of an airway, exploration, removal of a foreign body, or obtaining a biopsy specimen or removal of a local lesion.

trachoma: Chronic infectious eye disease of the conjunctiva and cornea.

trackball: Control device used to move and operate the cursor on the computer screen.

traction: Act of drawing or pulling.

training effect: As a result of exercise, heart rate and blood pressure become less than previously required for the same amount of work.

tranquilizer: Drug that produces a calming effect, relieving tension and anxiety.

transaction: Process that involves two or more individuals or elements that reciprocally and continually influence and affect one another through the ongoing relationship (Dickie, Cutchin, & Humphry, 2006).OTPF 2014

transcutaneous electrical nerve stimulation (TENS): Application of mild electrical stimulation via the skin.

transcutaneous nerve stimulation: *See* TENS.

transdisciplinary: An integrated team collaborates and often shares treatments.

transfer: The process of relocating a body from one object or surface to another (e.g., getting into or out of bed, moving from a wheelchair to a chair).

transfer-appropriate processing: The concept that the cognitive processes used while learning determine the type of criteria task on which one will best perform when evaluated for what has been learned.

transference: Redirection of feeling and desires, especially those unconsciously retained from childhood trauma, toward a new object.

transfer of learning: Practice and learning of one task can influence the learning of another task.

transfer of training: The ability to take a learned skill or behavior and transfer it to other life needs.

transformative learning: A process of getting beyond gaining factual knowledge alone to instead become changed by what one learns in some meaningful way. It involves questioning assumptions, beliefs, and values and considering multiple points of view, while always seeking to verify reasoning (Mezirow, 2000). CAOT

transgender: A person whose gender identity and/or expression is different from that typically associated with their assigned sex at birth (Substance Abuse and Mental Health Services Administration, 2014).

transient ischemic attack (TIA): Episode of temporary cerebral dysfunction caused by impaired blood flow to the brain. TIAs have many symptoms, such as dizziness, weakness, numbness, or paralysis of a limb or half of the body. TIAs may last only a few minutes or up to 24 hours but do not have any persistent neurologic deficits.

transparent access: Complete emulation usable with all or an entire major class of software (e.g., a successful keyboard emulating interface provides transparent access to standard software using alternate keyboards).

transsexual: A person whose gender identity differs from their assigned sex at birth (Substance Abuse and Mental Health Services Administration, 2014).

Transtheoretical Model: The core constructs are the stages of change, which are ordered categories along a continuum of readiness to change behavior. The main focus is on emotions, cognitions, and behavior.

transudate: A fluid substance that has passed through a membrane or been extruded from a tissue, sometimes as a result of inflammation. A transudate, in contrast to an exudate, is characterized by high fluidity and a low content of protein, cells, or solid materials derived from cells.

transverse plane: The body is divided at midsection forming a top and bottom portion; motion occurs around the vertical axis. *Synonym:* horizontal plane.

trapezius: The kite-shaped muscle mass that originates from the occipital bone of the skull down the vertebral column to the end of the thoracic vertebrae. The trapezius fibers insert on the

spine of the scapula and the clavicle. It is responsible for elevation, retraction, and depression of the scapula.

traumatic brain injury (TBI): Injury caused by impact to the head.

traveling notebook: System of communication in which "messages" are written; the notebook accompanies the individual in
his or her activities of daily living.

treatment (Tx): The sum of all interventions provided by the therapist to a patient/client during an episode of care. Application of
or involvement in activities/stimulation to effect improvement
in abilities for self-directed activities, self-care, or maintenance
of the home.

treatment plan: Legal document that outlines the map of treatment.

treatment services: Focus on alleviating emotional distress and
symptoms of illness.[C]

tremor: Involuntary shaking or trembling.

Trendelenburg's gait: A gait pattern that can be the result of weakness of the hip abductor muscles.

Trendelenburg's position: A position with the patient/client lying
on his or her back on a plane inclined 30 to 40 degrees, with the
legs and feet hanging over the end of the table.

trephination: Process of making a circular hole in the skull.

treppe: Type of muscle contraction in which the first few contractions increase in strength when a rested muscle receives
repeated stimuli.

Tri-Alliance of Health and Rehabilitation Professions: Created in
September 1991 between the American Occupational Therapy
Association, American Physical Therapy Association, and
American Speech-Language-Hearing Association as a forum to
represent and address the concerns of health and rehabilitation
professions.

trial use: An established period of time when equipment may be
applied and evaluated as to its effectiveness.

triangulation: A mechanism by which various information sources
are checked against each other to confirm interpretations.

triaxial joint: Movement occurs in three planes along three axes,
allowing for three degrees of freedom (e.g., hip and shoulder).

tricyclic: Commonly used family of antidepressants whose classification is based on the drug's chemical make-up. Some drugs in this category are Sinequan/doxepin, Elavil/amitriptyline, and Tofranil/imipramine (trade/generic names).

trigeminal neuralgia: A neurologic condition of the trigeminal facial nerve characterized by brief but frequent flashing, stabbing pain radiating usually throughout mandibular and maxillary regions. Caused by degeneration of the nerve or pressure on it. *Synonym:* tic douloureux.

trigeminy: The condition of occurring in threes, especially the occurrence of three pulse beats in rapid succession.

triglyceride: Any of a group of esters derived from glycerol and three fatty acid radicals; the chief component of fats and oils.

trigonal: Relating to a triangular shape.

trimipramine: Tricyclic antidepressant drug that also possesses sedative properties. Common side effects include drowsiness, dry mouth, and a decrease in blood pressure. *Trade name:* Surmontil.

trophotropic: Combination of parasympathetic nervous system activity, somatic muscle relaxation, and cortical beta rhythm synchronization. Resting or sleep state.

truncal ataxia: Uncoordinated movement of the trunk.

trustworthiness: When referring to qualitative data, the dependability, credibility, transferability, and applicability of the information gathered.

truth: Faithful to facts and reality.

T score: Converted standard score where the mean equals 50 and the standard deviation equals 10.

t-test: Parametric statistical test comparing differences of two data sets.

tuberculosis (TB): Respiratory disease caused by the tubercle bacilli.

tuberosity: Medium-sized protrusion on a bone.

tunnel vision: The visual field is limited to one side; the peripheral fields are lost, usually due to damage to the optic chiasm.

Turner's syndrome: Absence of an X chromosome in females resulting in lower amounts of estrogen produced and tendencies to be shorter in height, have fertility problems, and have mild mental retardation or learning difficulties.

turnover (business): The number of times that an average inventory of goods is sold during a fiscal year or some designated period._{Small Business Administration}

Twitter: An online service that allows friends, family, and strangers to stay connected through quick text updates called "tweets," which are limited to 140 characters.

two-tail (nondirectional) test: A test of the null hypothesis where both tails of the distribution are utilized.

tympany: A tympanic, or bell-like, percussion note. A modified tympanitic note heard on percussion of the chest in some cases of pneumothorax.

Type A behavior: A cluster of personality traits that includes high achievement motivation, drive, and a fast-paced lifestyle.

Type B behavior: A cluster of personality traits that include low achievement motivation, laziness, and a laid-back sort of lifestyle. Associated with inactivity, lack of exercise, and sedentary-related diseases such as heart disease.

ulcer: An open sore on the skin or some mucous membrane characterized by the disintegration of tissue and, often, the discharge of serous drainage.

ultrasound (US): A diagnostic or therapeutic technique using high-frequency sound waves to produce heat. **pulsed:** The application of therapeutic ultrasound using predetermined interrupted frequencies.

ultraviolet (UV): A form of radiant energy using light rays with wavelengths beyond the violet end of the visible spectrum.

unconditional positive regard: Unconditional love and acceptance.

unconscious proprioceptive pathways: Pathways in the side portion of the spinal cord that transmit body position information to the cerebellum.

underground practice: A mechanism by which health care professionals adhere to organizational dicta while finding ways to meet client needs that do not conform to those dicta (Mattingly, 1998).

uniaxial joint: Movement occurs in one plane with one axis and one degree of freedom (e.g., elbow).

Uniform Terminology: Published by the American Occupational Therapy Association, ensured that health professions use common language when completing required documents.

universal: Pertaining to any group, need, or environment.

universal access design: Concept of designing the built environment to permit access regardless of physical or sensory capability.

universal assessments: Used to evaluate the environmental needs of any group using all sizes and types of settings.

Jacobs, K., & Simon, L. (Eds.). *Quick Reference Dictionary for
Occupational Therapy, Sixth Edition* (pp. 305-307).
© 2015 SLACK Incorporated.

universal cuff: Device used on the dominant hand to hold tools such as a pencil or brush.

universal goniometer: Instrument used to measure joint motion. It consists of a protractor, an axis, and two arms.

universal hemiplegic sling: Sling that is used to support a nonfunctional shoulder and prevent shoulder subluxation by restricting active motion and keeping the humerus in adduction and internal rotation.

universal precautions: An approach to infection control designed to prevent transmission of blood-borne diseases such as HIV and hepatitis B; includes specific recommendations for use of gloves, protective eye wear, and masks.

unobtrusive observation: Observation for assessment that minimizes reactivity.

unstructured activities: Activities that are not preplanned or broken down into steps.

upper motor neuron (UMN): Neurons of the cerebral cortex that conduct stimuli from the motor cortex of the brain to motor nuclei of cerebral nerves of the ventral gray columns of the spinal cord.

urbanization: Fundamental belief and societal attitude that men were to provide financial support and women were to care for their families. This is a 19th-century concept.

uremia: Toxic condition associated with renal insufficiency in which urine is present in the blood.

urethrocele: Prolapse of the urethra with bulging into the vaginal opening.

urgency: Need to excrete urine immediately.

urogenital diaphragm: The perineal membrane, the deep muscle layer of the deep fascial layer that supports the pelvic organs.

urokinase: A substance found in the urine of mammals, including humans, that activates the fibrinolytic system, acting enzymatically by splitting plasminogen.

usury: Interest that exceeds the legal rate charged to a borrower.

uterine inversion: When the uterus loses its shape and comes out toward its opening.

uterus: The pear-shaped organ in which the fetus grows. *Synonym*: womb.

utilization review (UR): Assessment of the appropriateness and economy of an admission to a health care facility or continued hospitalization.

vaginismus: Painful spasms of the vagina from contraction of the muscles surrounding the vagina.

valgus: A limb deformity in which the extremity is moved away from the midline.

validity: Degree to which a test measures what it is intended to measure.

Valium: Drug administered for moderate or severe anxiety disorders, as well as some seizures; relieves anxiety. *Generic name*: diazepam.

Valsalva's maneuver: Forced exhalation against a closed glottis.

value orientation: A predisposition toward a particular set or kind of values.

values: Acquired beliefs and commitments, derived from culture, about what is good, right, and important to do (Kielhofner, 2008); principles, standards, or qualities considered worthwhile or desirable by the client who holds them (Moyers & Dale, 2007).OTPF 2014

valvuloplasty: Replacement of a cardiac valve with a prosthetic valve.

valvulotomy: Incision of a valve, such as a valve of the heart.

vantage: Any observing mind's specific point of view with physical, psychological, and cultural dimensions that restrict how much can be observed at any moment.

vantage effects: The ways in which vantage alters one's perception of reality.

variance: Measure that demonstrates how scores in a distribution deviate from the mean.

varicocele: Enlargement of the veins in the spermatic cord.

Jacobs, K., & Simon, L. (Eds.). *Quick Reference Dictionary for Occupational Therapy, Sixth Edition* (pp. 308-314). © 2015 SLACK Incorporated.

varicose veins: Refers to the enlargement of veins when the valves in the veins become swollen and have retrograde flow within them.

vasomotor center: A regulatory center in the lower pons and medulla oblongata that regulates the diameter of blood vessels, especially the arterioles.

vasopneumatic compression device: A device to decrease edema by using compressive forces that are applied to the body part.

vasopressor: Stimulating contraction of the muscular tissue of the capillaries and arteries. An agent that stimulates the contraction of the muscular tissue of the capillaries and arteries.

vector: Arrow that indicates direction and magnitude of a force.

ventilation: The circulation of air; to aerate (blood); oxygenate. Mechanical ventilation is the use of equipment to circulate oxygen to the respiratory system.

ventilatory equivalent (VE/VO$_2$): The ratio of minute ventilation to oxygen consumption. The normal ratio is 25:1, meaning that for 25 L of air breathed, 1 L of oxygen has been consumed.

ventilatory pump: Thoracic skeleton and skeletal muscles and their innervation responsible for ventilation. The muscles include the diaphragm; the intercostal, scalene, and sternocleidomastoid muscles; accessory muscles of ventilation; and the abdominal, triangular, and quadratus lumborum muscles.

ventilatory pump dysfunction: Abnormalities of the thoracic skeleton, respiratory muscles, airways, or lungs that interrupt or interfere with the work of breathing or ventilation.

ventral: From anatomical position, located toward the front or the belly.

venture capital: Money used to support new or unusual commercial undertakings; equity, risk or speculative capital. This funding is provided to new or existing firms that exhibit above-average growth rates, a significant potential for market expansion and the need for additional financing for business maintenance or expansion.Small Business Administration

veracity: Authenticity.

verbal communication: Process of interpreting another's words and expressing one's own thoughts and emotions through words.

verbal cues: Verbal hints given to the client by the occupational therapy assistant to trigger desired behavior.

verbal rating scale (VRS): A pain intensity measurement in which patients/clients rate pain on a continuum that is subdivided from left to right into gradually increasing pain intensities.

verbal therapies: Any therapy in which talk and discussion are the primary modes of intervention.

vergence: Movement of the two eyes in the opposite direction.

vermis: Forms the unpaired medial region of the cerebellum.

versions: Movement of the two eyes in the same direction.

vertical or job enrichment: Used as an administrative control in ergonomics, the job content includes taking over some responsibilities that were previously assigned to a supervisor.

vertigo: One's sensation of revolving in space or of having objects move around him or her.

vestibular: The sensory system that responds to head position and movement; coordinates eye, head, and body movements; and maintains posture and a stable visual field. Vestibular receptors are located within the inner ear (Sensory Solutions, 2014).

vestibular-bilateral disorder: A sensory integrative dysfunction characterized by shortened duration nystagmus, poor integration of the two sides of the body and brain, and difficulty in learning to read or compute. The disorder is caused by underreactive vestibular responses.

vestibular function: Pertaining to the sense of balance.

vestibulocochlear nerve: Combined portions of the eighth cranial nerve.

vestibulo-ocular reflex: A normal reflex in which eye position compensates for movement of the head, induced by excitation of vestibular apparatus.

vicarious reinforcement: Idea that one person's observation of another person experiencing a positive consequence as a result of a particular behavior increases the probability that the observer will exhibit that behavior.

videofluoroscopy: Radiological study that allows visualization of the pharyngeal and esophageal phases of swallowing.

vigorometer: Alternative measurement of hand strength that requires the person to squeeze a rubber bulb.

virtual: Environment in which communication occurs by means of airways or computers and an absence of physical contact. Includes simulated or real-time or near-time existence of an environment, such as chat rooms, email, video conferencing, and radio transmissions.[OTPF 2008]

virtual context: Environment in which communication occurs by means of airwaves or computers in the absence of physical contact. The virtual context includes simulated, real-time, or near-time environments such as chat rooms, email, video conferencing, and radio transmissions; remote monitoring via wireless sensors; and computer-based data collection.[OTPF 2014]

virtual reality: Term describing any optical or sensory simulation of something real, to the point of confounding the senses into accepting that simulation.

virtual worlds: Online communities or virtual games that are created to mimic real-life situations or places, such as Second Life. The users are able to develop characters and interact with other users. Disability organizations are now using these as places to hold virtual support groups and meetings and to facilitate socialization and networking.

viscosity: Describes the extent to which a tissue's resistance to deformation is dependent on the rate of the deforming force.

vision screening: Can include distance and near visual acuities, oculomotilities, eye alignment or posture, depth perception, and visual fields.

visions of possibility: Are grounded in particular values, beliefs, and ideals about hope and the value and potential of persons to use diverse abilities to engage in life in mind, body, and spirit not limited to usual expectations in particular contexts.[CAOT]

visual: Interpreting stimuli through the eyes, including peripheral vision and acuity, and awareness of color and pattern.[UTIII]

visual acuity: Measure of visual discrimination of fine details of high contrast.

visual agnosia: Inability to name objects as viewed.

visual analog scale (VAS): A tool used in a pain examination that allows the patient/client to indicate degree of pain by pointing to a visual representation of pain intensity.

visual-closure: The ability to recognize a whole word/item when only partial information is given (e.g., the process of filling in a missing letter in a word).

visual defensiveness: Hypersensitivity to visual information.

visual evoked response (VER): Presentation of a particular visual stimulus evokes consistent electrocortical activity that can be recorded from electrodes placed on the scalp.

visual field defect or hemianopia: Blindness in one-half of the field of vision in one or both eyes.

visual fields: Areas/angles of vision that are seen without moving the head or eyes.

visualization: An effective means of deepening relaxation and desensitizing a real-life situation that is generally met with stress and tension.

visual motor coordination: The ability to coordinate vision with the movements of the body or parts of the body.

visual motor function: The ability to draw or copy forms or to perform constructive tasks.

visual motor integration: Coordinating the interaction of information from the eyes with body movement during activity.[UTIII]

visual neglect: Inattention to visual stimuli occurring in the space on the involved side of the body.

visual orientation: Awareness and location of objects in the environment and their relationship to each other and to oneself.

visual perception: Brain's ability to understand sensory input to determine size, shape, distance, and form of objects.

visual perceptual dysfunction: May include deficits in any of the areas of visual perception: figure-ground, form constancy, or size discrimination. Distinct from deficits in functional visual skills and tested separately.

vital capacity (VC): Measurement of the amount of air that can be expelled at the normal rate of exhalation after a maximum inspiration, representing the greatest possible breathing capacity.

vital signs (VS): Measurements of pulse rate, respiration rate, and body temperature.

vocational activities: Participating in work-related activities.[UTIII]

vocational exploration: Determining aptitudes; developing interests and skills; and selecting appropriate vocational pursuits. [UTIII]

vocational maturity: Scale along which people are placed during their working lives. Maturity is reached when occupational activities are aligned with what is expected of the corresponding age group.

Vocational Rehabilitation Act and Amendments (1943): U.S. federal legislation that brought about a change to include payment for medical services, thus allowing occupational therapy services to be covered as a legitimate service.

Voice Over Internet Protocol (VoIP): Programs that enable use of a computer or other Internet device for phone calls and video chat without additional charge, including conference calls and teleconferences. Most also have instant messaging components.

volar: Palm of the hand or the sole of the foot.

volar splint: Splint that runs from the lower third of the forearm to the individual's fingertips with the thumb extended and abducted. The phalangeal joint should be slightly flexed, thus enabling this type of splint construction to prevent stiffening of the phalangeal joints in extension. This splint is often used as a night splint for inpatients.

volitional postural movements: Movement patterns under volitional control that relate specifically to controlling the center of gravity, as in skating, ballet, gymnastics, etc.

volition subsystem: Concept in the Model of Human Occupation that includes one's values, interests, and feelings of personal causation.

Volkmann's contracture: Permanent contracture of a muscle due to replacement of destroyed muscle cells with fibrous tissue that lacks the ability to stretch. Destruction of muscle cells may occur from interference with circulation caused by a tight bandage, splint, or cast.

volume measurement: The amount of fluid that has been displaced from a container (of any size) following the introduction of part or all of the body.

voluntary movement: A simple voluntary muscle or mental activation, such as flexion, extension, adduction, abduction, rotation, supination, pronation, blinking, memory, attention, focusing, scanning, etc. (adapted from Polatajko et al., 2004 and Zimmerman et al., 2006).CAOT

voluntary muscle: Type of muscle tissue that can be controlled by the brain to produce movement.

volunteer exploration: Determining community causes, organizations, or opportunities for unpaid "work" in relationship to personal skills, interests, location, and time available.AOTA Framework

volunteer participation: Performing unpaid "work" activities for the benefit of identified selected causes, organizations, or facilities.AOTA Framework

volvulus: Twisting of the bowel upon itself.

waddling gait: Gait pattern in which the feet are wide apart, resembling that of a duck.

wallerian degeneration: The physical and biochemical changes that occur in a nerve because of the loss of axonal continuity following trauma.

wandering cells: Connective cells usually involved with short-term activities such as protection and repair.

warm-up: Exercise that prepares the person for the experience to follow.

waxy rigidity: Symptom of catatonia in which an individual will assume any position in which he or she is placed and remain there until moved again.

wear-and-tear theory: Theory that describes the biological effects of aging as the body deteriorates.

wearing schedule: Amount of time the splint is to be worn and when it should be removed.

Wechsler Adult Intelligence Scale—Revised (WAIS-R): Test of general intelligence.

Wechsler Preschool and Primary Scale of Intelligence (WPPSI): Individual intelligence test of children aged 4 to 6½.

weight (wt): Measure of matter that incorporates the effect of gravity on an object; a kinematic measurement.

weight shift: Bearing the body's weight from one leg to another; shifting the center of gravity.

well-being: "General term encompassing the total universe of human life domains, including physical, mental, and social aspects" (WHO, 2006, p. 211).[OTPF 2014] Experienced when people engage in occupations that they perceive: (a) are consistent with their values and preferences; (b) support their abilities to competently perform valued roles; (c) support their occupational identities; and (d) support their plans and goals (Caron Santha & Doble, 2006; Christiansen, 1999; Doble et al., 2006). CAOT

wellness: "Perception of and responsibility for psychological and physical well-being as these contribute to overall satisfaction with one's life situation" (Boyt Schell et al., 2014a, p. 1243).OTPF 2014

wellness programs: A program intended to improve and promote health and fitness that is typically offered through the workplace, although insurance plans can offer them directly to their enrollees. The program allows employers or plans to offer employees premium discounts, cash rewards, gym memberships, and other incentives to participate. The Affordable Care Act creates new incentives to promote employer wellness programs and encourage opportunities to support healthier workplaces (Olafson, 2013).

Welsh-Clark Act (World War II Disabled Veterans Rehabilitation Act): U.S. federal legislation that provided vocational rehabilitation for veterans of World War II.

Wernicke-Korsakoff syndrome: Caused by a thiamine deficiency; found in chronic alcoholism, it is characterized by dementia and ataxia.

Wernicke's aphasia: Infarct to a specific area of the brain that severely affects the person's level of comprehension. The person is able to visualize but is frequently nonfunctional.

wheelchair pushing cuffs: Soft gloves worn to protect the hands and to provide traction when pushing a wheelchair.

wheeze: A whistling sound made in breathing resulting from constriction and/or partial obstruction of the airways. Heard on auscultation; however, in severe cases of asthma and COPD, it can often be audible without the use of a stethoscope.

whey proteins: The protein content of mother's milk.

whiplash injury: Caused by sudden hyperextension and flexion of the neck, traumatizing cervical ligaments; common in rear-end car accidents.

white matter: Area of the central nervous system that contains the axons of the cells.

wiki: A website or group of associated pages that allows users to add, edit collaboratively, and consolidate information about any given topic. The most well-known wiki is Wikipedia. Efforts are made to verify information and provide references; however, the information is often not considered correct and valid unless verified by a third party or backed by evidence-based practice.

Wilbarger Deep Pressure and Proprioceptive Technique (DPPT) and Oral Tactile Technique (OTT): *Also known as* the Wilbarger Brushing Protocol, these terms refer to the specific sensory modulation techniques developed by Patricia Wilbarger, MEd, OTR, FAOTA. DPPT uses a specific pattern of stimulation delivered using a special type of brush and gentle joint compressions. It is believed to facilitate the coordination of mind-brain-body processes in a manner that influences positive change and reduces tactile defensiveness. OTT is used similarly to desensitize the mouth and is believed to help facilitate oral care.

Williams syndrome: Syndrome caused by a genetic defect, characterized by cardiovascular problems, high blood calcium levels, mental retardation, developmental delays, and a "little pixie face" with puffy eyes and a turned-up nose.

Wilma L. West Library: Located in the American Occupational Therapy Foundation, it contains over 3,600 volumes of occupational therapy related subjects.

within normal limits (WNL): The normal range of motion at a given joint.

word prediction: Technique used in software to guess the current word or next word when beginning letters or the previous word, respectively, is typed.

word processing: Type of application software that is used to enter, edit, manipulate, and format text.

word salad: A jumble of extremely incoherent speech; sometimes observed in schizophrenia.

work: "Labor or exertion; to make, construct, manufacture, form, fashion, or shape objects; to organize, plan, or evaluate services or processes of living or governing; committed occupations that are performed with or without financial reward" (Christiansen & Townsend, 2010, p. 423).[OTPF 2014]

work behaviors: Behaviors that are necessary for successful participation in a job or independent living (e.g., cooperative behavior). *Synonyms*: prevocational readiness or personal skills.

work capacity evaluation: Comprehensive process that systematically uses work, real or simulated, to assess and measure an individual's physical abilities to work.

work conditioning: An intensive work-related, goal-oriented conditioning program designed specifically to restore systemic neuromuscular functions (e.g., strength, endurance, movement, flexibility, motor control) and cardiopulmonary functions. The objective of a work conditioning program is to restore physical capacity and function to enable the patient/client to return to work.

work/education: Skill and performance in purposeful and productive activities in the home, employment, school, and community.

Workers' Compensation: State-mandated form of insurance covering workers injured in job-related accidents. In some states, the state is the insurer; in other states, insurance must be acquired from commercial insurance firms. Insurance rates are based on a number of factors, including salaries, firm history, and risk of occupation.[Small Business Administration]

work hardening: Type of treatment program that is graded work simulation to increase an individual's productivity to an acceptable level to be able to function in a work environment.

work or job performance: Performing job tasks in a timely and effective manner; incorporating necessary work behaviors.[UTIII]

work practice controls: Techniques used to improve worker safety, such as education and training in safe and proper work techniques.

work rehabilitation: Structured rehab; uses a graded program of exercise, education.

work samples: Well-defined work activity involving tasks, materials, and tools that are identical or similar to those in an actual job or cluster of jobs. It is used to access an individual's vocational aptitude, worker characteristics, and vocational interests.

work setting: Any environment in which an individual performs productive activity.

work site analysis: Formal assessment of the relationship between worker habits, specific work tasks, and the work environment.

work space: Physical area in which one performs work.

work tolerance: Refers to how a person deals with his or her work environment. This includes being able to handle the stress and pressures that are part of the job and to maintain one's productivity, quality, and effort, time after time.

work-up: The process of performing a complete evaluation of an individual including history, physical examination, laboratory test, and radiographs or other diagnostic procedures to acquire an accurate database on which a diagnosis and treatment plan may be established.

World Occupational Therapy Day: First launched on October 27, 2010, by the World Federation of Occupational Therapists, World Occupational Therapy Day is an opportunity to heighten the visibility of the profession's development work, promote the field, and celebrate the profession internationally.

wound care: Procedures used to achieve a clean wound bed, promote a moist environment or facilitate autolytic débridement, and absorb excessive exudation from a wound complex.

wound management: Comprehensive physical therapy intervention to reduce pressure points and manage the interdisciplinary efforts to facilitate wound care and healing.

wrist system: Computerized glove that measures range of motion.

Xanax: Anti-anxiety drug in the benzodiazepine class. *Generic name:* alprazolam.

xenophobia: Fear and/or hatred of any person or thing that is strange or foreign.

xeroderma: Condition of rough and dry skin.

X-linked recessive: Trait transmitted by a gene located on the X chromosome. These traits are passed on by a carrier mother to an affected son.

Jacobs, K., & Simon, L. (Eds.). *Quick Reference Dictionary for Occupational Therapy, Sixth Edition* (p. 320).
© 2015 SLACK Incorporated.

yarn cone: Object used to measure thumb abduction and extension and can also be adapted to measure the first web space of burned hands. There are no norms for this measurement. It is used to measure a patient's progress over time.

young old: Persons between 60 and 75 years of age.

YouTube: A video-sharing website on which users can upload, share, and view videos.

Z

zar: Possession by spirits.

Zoloft: Oral antidepressant. One contraindication is that it may cause serotonin syndrome with the interaction of other medicines. *Generic name*: sertraline hydrochloride.

zone of proximal development: Difference between what a child can do alone and what he or she can do with the assistance of a more skilled helper.

z-plasty: Surgical incision made in the shape of a Z that is used to lengthen a burn scar.

z score (standard score): Numerical value from the transformation of a raw score into units of standard deviation.

zygote: Single cell formed at conception by the union of the 23 chromosomes of the sperm and the 23 chromosomes of the ovum.

References

Abate, F. (Ed.). (1996). *The Oxford dictionary and thesaurus: The ultimate language reference for American readers.* Oxford, UK: Oxford University Press.

Aliseda, A. (2006). *Abductive reasoning: Logical investigations into discovery and explanation.* Dordrecht, The Netherlands: Springer Publishing Co.

American Occupational Therapy Association. (1994). Uniform terminology for occupational therapy (3rd ed.). *American Journal of Occupational Therapy, 48,* 1047-1054.

American Occupational Therapy Association. (2002a). Broadening the construct of independence [Position Paper]. *American Journal of Occupational Therapy, 56,* 660.

American Occupational Therapy Association. (2002). Occupational therapy practice framework: Domain and process. *American Journal of Occupational Therapy, 56,* 609-639.

American Occupational Therapy Association. (2007b). Specialized knowledge and skills in feeding, eating, and swallowing for occupational therapy practice. *American Journal of Occupational Therapy, 61,* 686-700.

American Occupational Therapy Association. (2008). Occupational therapy practice framework: Domain and process (2nd ed.). *American Journal of Occupational Therapy, 62,* 625-668.

American Occupational Therapy Association. (2010). Standards of practice for occupational therapy. *American Journal of Occupational Therapy, 64*(Suppl.), S106-S111. http://dx.doi.org/10.5014/ajot.2010.64S106

American Occupational Therapy Association. (2011). *Definition of occupational therapy practice for the AOTA Model Practice Act.* Retrieved from www.aota.org/~/media/Corporate/Files/Advocacy/State/Resources/PracticeAct/Model%20Definition%20of%20OT%20Practice%20%20Adopted%2041411.ashx

American Occupational Therapy Association. (2013a). Guidelines for documentation of occupational therapy. *American Journal of Occupational Therapy, 67*(Suppl.), S32-S38. http://dx.doi.org/10.5014/ajot.2013.67S32

Jacobs, K., & Simon, L. (Eds.). *Quick Reference Dictionary for Occupational Therapy, Sixth Edition* (pp. 323-332).
© 2015 SLACK Incorporated.

American Occupational Therapy Association. (2013b). Occupational therapy in the promotion of health and well-being. *American Journal* of *Occupational Therapy, 67*(Suppl.), S47-S59. http://dx.doi.org/10.5014/ajot.2013.67S47

American Occupational Therapy Association. (2014a). *Emerging niche: Telehealth.* Retrieved from www.aota.org/en/Practice/Rehabilitation-Disability/Emerging-Niche/Telehealth.aspx

American Occupational Therapy Association. (2014). Occupational therapy practice framework: Domain and process (3rd ed.). *American Journal of Occupational Therapy, 68*(Suppl. 1), S1-S48. http://dx.doi.org/10.5014/ajot.2014.682006

American Physical Therapy Association. (2003). *Guide to physical therapist practice* (rev. 2nd ed.). Alexandria, VA: Author.

Angelman Syndrome Foundation. (2014). *What is Angelman syndrome?* Retrieved from www.angelman.org/understanding-as/

Answers.com. *Online dictionary.* Retrieved from www.answers.com/

Apert International. (2014). *What is Apert syndrome?* Retrieved from www.apert.org/apert.htm

Association of Canadian Occupational Therapy Regulatory Organizations, Association of Canadian Occupational Therapy University Programs, Canadian Association of Occupational Therapists, Canadian Occupational Therapy Foundation, & Presidents' Advisory Committee. (2006). *Welcome to the OT education finder.* Retrieved from www.caot.ca/default.asp?pageid=1296

Atherton, J. S. (2002). Tools: Frames of reference: On learning to "see." *Doceo.* Retrieved from www.doceo.co.uk/tools/frame.htm

Ayres, A. J. (1985). *Developmental dyspraxia and adult onset apraxia.* Torrance, CA: Sensory Integration International.

Bedell, G. M. (2012). Measurement of social participation. In V. Anderson & M. H. Beauchamp (Eds.), *Developmental social neuroscience and childhood brain insult: Theory and practice* (pp. 184-206). New York: Guilford Press.

Beers, H., Berkow, R., & Burs, M. (Eds.). (1999). *Merck manual diagnosis and therapy* (17th ed.). Whitehouse Station, NJ: Merck.

Bendixon, H. J., Kroksmark, U., Magnus, E., Jakobsen, K., Alsaker, S., & Nordell, K. (2006). Occupational pattern: A renewed definition of the concept. *Journal of Occupational Science, 13*(1), 3-10.

Bergen, D. (Ed.). (1988). *Play as a medium for learning and development: A handbook of theory and practice.* Portsmouth, NH: Heinemann Educational Books.

Blanche, E. I., & Parham, L. D. (2002). Praxis and organization of behavior in time and space. In S. Smith Roley, E. I. Blanche, & R. C. Schaaf (Eds.), *Understanding the nature of sensory integration with diverse populations* (pp. 183-200). San Antonio, TX: Therapy Skill Builders.

Bonanno, G., & Mancini, A. (2012). Beyond resilience and PTSD: Mapping the heterogeneity of responses to potential trauma. *Psychological Trauma: Theory, Research, Practice, and Policy, 4*(1), 74-83.

Bottomley, J. (Ed.). (2003). *Quick reference dictionary for physical therapy* (2nd ed.). Thorofare, NJ: SLACK Incorporated.

Boyt Schell, B. A., Gillen, G., & Scaffa, M. (2014a). Glossary. In B. A. Boyt Schell, G. Gillen, & M. Scaffa (Eds.), *Willard and Spackman's occupational therapy* (12th ed., pp. 1229-1243). Philadelphia, PA: Lippincott Williams & Wilkins.

Brown, L. (Ed.). (1993). *The new shorter Oxford English dictionary on historical principles* (vol. 1). Oxford, UK: Oxford University Press.

Bruce, M. A., & Borg, B. (2001). *Psychosocial occupational therapy: Frames of reference for intervention: Core for occupation-based practice* (3rd ed.). Thorofare, NJ: SLACK Incorporated.

Buring, S., Bhushan, A., Broeseker, A., Conway, S., Duncan-Hewitt, W., Hansen, L., & Westberg, S. (2009). Interprofessional education: Definitions, student competencies, and guidelines for implementation. *American Journal of Pharmacy Education, 73,* 59.

Canadian Association of Occupational Therapists. (1991). *Occupational therapy guidelines for client-centred practice.* Toronto, Ontario, Canada: CAOT Publications ACE.

Canadian Association of Occupational Therapists. (1997a). *Enabling occupation: An occupational therapy perspective.* Ottawa, Ontario, Canada: CAOT Publications ACE.

Canadian Association of Occupational Therapists. (2002). *Enabling occupation: An occupational therapy perspective* (rev. ed.). Ottawa, Ontario, Canada: CAOT Publications ACE.

Canadian Association of Occupational Therapists. (in press). *Profile of occupational therapy practice in Canada.* Ottawa, Ontario, Canada: Author.

Canadian Association of Occupational Therapists, Association of Canadian Occupational Therapy University Programs, Association of Canadian Occupational Therapy Regulatory Organizations, & Presidents' Advisory Committee. (1999). Joint position statement on evidence-based occupational therapy. *Canadian Journal of Occupational Therapy, 66,* 267-269. Retrieved from www.caot.ca/default.asp?pageid=156

Canadian Institute of Health Research. (2002). *Knowledge translation framework.* Retrieved from www.cihr-irsc.gc.ca/e/193.html

Caron Santha, J., & Doble, S. (2006). *Development and measurement properties of the Occupational Well-Being Questionnaire.* Canadian Association of Occupational Therapy Conference 2006; Montreal, Canada; June 2006.

Christiansen, C. H. (1999). Occupation as identity: Competence, coherence and the creation of meaning: 1999 Eleanor Clarke Slagle lecture. *American Journal of Occupational Therapy, 53,* 547-558.

Christiansen, C. H., & Baum, M. C. (Eds.). (1997). *Occupational therapy: Enabling function and well-being* (2nd ed.). Thorofare, NJ: SLACK Incorporated.

Christiansen, C. H., & Hammecker, C. L. (2001). Self care. In B. R. Bonder & M. B. Wagner (Eds.), *Functional performance in older adults* (pp. 155-175). Philadelphia, PA: F. A. Davis.

Christiansen, C. H., & Townsend, E. A. (2010). *Introduction to occupation: The art and science of living* (2nd ed.). Cranbury, NJ: Pearson Education.

Clark, F. A., Azen, S. P., Carlson, M., Mandel, D., LaBree, L., Hay, J., . . . Lipson, L. (2001). Embedding health-promoting changes into the daily lives of independently-living older adults: Long-term follow-up of occupational therapy intervention. *Journals of Gerontology: Psychological Sciences, 56B*(1), 60-63.

Commission on Social Justice. (1994). *Social justice: Strategies for national renewal. The report of the Commission on Social Justice.* London, England: Vintage.

Craik, J. (2003). *Enhancing research utilization in occupational therapy.* Unpublished master's thesis, Graduate Department of Rehabilitation Science, University of Toronto, Ontario, Canada.

Crepeau, E. (2003). Analyzing occupation and activity: A way of thinking about occupational performance. In E. Crepeau, E. Cohn, & B. A. Boyt Schell (Eds.), *Willard and Spackman's occupational therapy* (10th ed., pp. 189-198). Philadelphia, PA: Lippincott Williams & Wilkins.

Davis, J. A., & Polatajko, H. J. (2006). The occupational development of children. In S. Rodger, & J. Ziviani (Eds.), *Occupational therapy with children: Understanding children's occupations and enabling participation* (pp. 136-157). Oxford, UK: Blackwell Science.

Dewey, J. (1900). *The school and society.* Chicago, IL: University of Chicago Press.

Dewey, J., & Bentley, A. F. (1949). *Knowing and the known.* Boston, MA: Beacon Press.

Dickie, V., Cutchin, M., & Humphry, R. (2006). Occupation as transactional experience: A critique of individualism in occupational science. *Journal of Occupational Science, 13*, 83-93. http://dx.doi.org/10.1080/14427591.2006.9686573

Doble, S., Caron Santha, J., Theben, J., Knott, L., & Lall-Phillips, J. (2006). *The Occupational Well-Being Questionnaire: The development of a valid outcome measure.* World Federation of Occupational Therapy Congress 2006; Sydney, Australia; July 2006.

Dubouloz, C., Egan, M., Vallerand, J., & von Zweck, C. (1999). Occupational therapists' perceptions of evidence-based practice. *American Journal of Occupational Therapy, 53*, 445-453.

Dunn, W. (2000a). *Best practice in occupational therapy in community service with children and families.* Thorofare, NJ: SLACK Incorporated.

Dunn, W. (2000b). Habit: What's the brain got to do with it? *OTJR: Occupation, Participation and Health, 20*(Suppl. 1), 6S-20S.

Dyck, I. (1998). Multicultural society. In D. Jones, S. E. Blair, & J. T. Hartery (Eds.), *Sociology and occupational therapy: An integrated approach* (pp. 67-80). London, England: Harcourt Brace.

Fearing, V. G., & Clark, J. (2000). *Individuals in context: A practical guide to client centered practice.* Thorofare, NJ: SLACK Incorporated.

Fearing, V. G., Law, M., & Clark, M. (1997). An occupational performance process model: Fostering client and therapist alliances. *Canadian Journal of Occupational Therapy, 64*(1), 7-15.

Fetzer, J. K. (1990). *Artificial intelligence: Its scope and limits.* Dordrecht, The Netherlands: Kluwer Academic Publishers.

Fiese, B. H. (2007). Routines and rituals: Opportunities for participation in family health. *OTJR: Occupation, Participation and Health, 27*, 41S-49S.

Fiese, B. H., Tomcho, T. J., Douglas, M., Josephs, K., Poltrock, S., & Baker, T. (2002). A review of 50 years of research on naturally occurring family routines and rituals: Cause for celebration. *Journal of Family Psychology, 16*, 381-390. http://dx.doi.org/10.1037/0893-3200.16.4.381

Filley, C. M. (2001). *Neurobehavioral anatomy.* Boulder, CO: University Press of Colorado.

Fisher, A. (2006). Overview of performance skills and client factors. In H. Pendleton & W. Schultz-Krohn (Eds.), *Pedretti's occupational therapy: Practice skills for physical dysfunction* (pp. 372-402). St. Louis, MO: Mosby/Elsevier.

Fisher, A. G. (2009). *Occupational Therapy Intervention Process Model: A model for planning and implementing top-down, client-centered, and occupation-based interventions.* Fort Collins, CO: Three Star Press.

Fisher, A. G., & Griswold, L. A. (2014). Performance skills: Implementing performance analyses to evaluate quality of occupational performance. In B. A. Boyt Schell, G. Gillen, & M. Scaffa (Eds.), *Willard and Spackman's occupational therapy* (12th ed., pp. 249-264). Philadelphia, PA: Lippincott Williams & Wilkins.

Fisher, A., & Kielhofner, G. (1995). Skill in occupational performance. In G. Kielhofner (Ed.), *A model of human occupation: Theory and application* (2nd ed., pp. 113-128). Philadelphia, PA: Lippincott Williams & Wilkins.

Freidson, E. (1970). *Profession of medicine: A study in the sociology of applied knowledge.* Chicago, IL: University of Chicago Press.

Freidson, E. (1986). *Professional powers: A study of the institutionalization of formal knowledge.* Chicago, IL: University of Chicago Press.

Freidson, E. (1994). *Professionalism reborn: Theory, prophecy and policy.* Cambridge, UK: Polity Press.

Freidson, E. (2001). *Professionalism: The third logic.* Chicago, IL: The University of Chicago Press.

Gillen, G., & Boyt Schell, B. (2014). Introduction to evaluation, intervention, and outcomes for occupations. In B. A. Boyt Schell, G. Gillen, & M. Scaffa (Eds.), *Willard and Spackman's occupational therapy* (12th ed., pp. 606-609). Philadelphia, PA: Lippincott Williams & Wilkins.

Hansen, R. A., & Atchison, B. (2000). *Conditions in occupational therapy: Effect on occupational performance* (2nd ed). Philadelphia, PA: Lippincott Williams & Wilkins.

Heilman, K. M., & Rothi, L. J. G. (1993). *Clinical neuropsychology* (3rd ed.). New York, NY: Oxford University Press.

Hillman, A., & Chapparo, C. J. (1995). An investigation of occupational role performance in men over sixty years of age, following a stroke. *Journal of Occupational Science, 2*(3), 88-99.

Houghton Mifflin Company. (2004). *The American heritage dictionary of the English language* (4th ed.). Retrieved from www.answers.com

International Coach Federation. (2006). *What is coaching?* Retrieved from www.coachfederation.org

International Spectrum. (2014). Retrieved from http://internationalspectrum.umich.edu/life/definitions

Iwama, M. (2005). Occupation as a cross-cultural construct. In G. Whiteford & V. Wright-St. Clair (Eds.), *Occupation & practice in context* (p. 8). Marickville, NSW, Australia: Churchill Livingstone.

James, A. B. (2008). Restoring the role of independent person. In M. V. Radomski & C. A. Trombly Latham (Eds.), *Occupational therapy for physical dysfunction* (pp. 774-816). Philadelphia, PA: Lippincott Williams & Wilkins.

Jonsson, H. (in press). Occupational transitions in retirement. In C. Christiansen & E. A. Townsend (Eds.), *Introduction to occupation: The art and science of living* (2nd ed.). Upper Saddle River, NJ: Pearson Education.

Kielhofner, G. (2008). *The model of human occupation: Theory and application* (4th ed.). Philadelphia, PA: Lippincott Williams & Wilkins.

Kielhofner, G., Mallinson, T., Forsyth, K., & Lai, J. (2001). Psychometric properties of the second version of the occupational performance history interview (OPHI-II). *American Journal of Occupational Therapy, 55,* 260-267.

Kronenberg, F., & Pollard, N. (2005). Overcoming occupational apartheid: A preliminary exploration of the political nature of occupational therapy. In F. Kronenberg, S. Simo Algado, & N. Pollard (Eds.), *Occupational therapy without borders: Learning from the spirit of survivors* (pp. 58-86). London, England: Elsevier Churchill Livingstone.

Larson, E., & Zemke, R. (2003). Shaping the temporal patterns of our lives: The social coordination of occupation. *Journal of Occupational Science, 10,* 80-89. http://dx.doi.org/10.1080/14427591.2003.9686514

Law, M., Cooper, B., Strong, S., Stewart, D., Rigby, P., & Letts, L. (1996). Person–Environment–Occupation Model: A transactive approach to occupational performance. *Canadian Journal of Occupational Therapy, 63,* 9-23. http://dx.doi.org/10.1177/000841749606300103

Levine, R., Walsh, C., & Schwartz, R. (1996). *Pharmacology: Drug actions and reactions* (5th ed.). London, England: CRC Press-Parthenon Publishers.

Liepmann, H. (1920). Apraxie. *Ergebnisse der Gesamten Medizin, 1,* 516-543.

Linden, R. (2003). The discipline of collaboration. *Leader to Leader, 29,* 41-47.

Lurye, L. E., Zosuls, K. M., & Ruble, D. N. (2008). Gender identity and adjustment: Understanding the impact of individuals and normative differences in sex typing. In M. Azmitia, M. Syed, & K. Radmacher (Eds.), *The intersections of personal and social identities: New directions for child and adolescent development* (no. 120, pp. 31-46). San Francisco, CA: Jossey-Bass.

Maciejewski, M., Kawiecki, J., & Rockwood, T. (1997). Satisfaction. In R. L. Kane (Ed.), *Understanding health care outcomes research* (pp. 67-89). Gaithersburg, MD: Aspen.

Magasi, S., & Hammel, J. (2004). Social support and social network mobilization in African American woman who have experienced strokes. *Disability Studies Quarterly, 24*(4). Retrieved from http://dsq-sds.org/article/view/878/1053

Mattingly, C. (1998). *Healing dramas and clinical plots: The narrative structure of experience.* New York, NY: Cambridge University Press.

McColl, M. (2000). Muriel Driver Memorial Lecture: Spirit, occupation and disability. *Canadian Journal of Occupational Therapy, 67,* 217-228.

McColl, M., Law, M. C., & Stewart, D. (2002). *Theoretical basis of occupational therapy: An annotated bibliography of applied theory in the professional literature* (2nd ed.). Thorofare, NJ: SLACK Incorporated.

McKee, P., & Morgan, L. (1998). *Orthotics in rehabilitation: Splinting the hand and body.* Philadelphia, PA: F. A. Davis.

Meltzer, P. J. (2001). Using the self-discovery tapestry to explore occupational careers. *Journal of Occupational Science, 8*(2), 16-24.

Merriam-Webster. (2003). *Merriam-Webster's collegiate dictionary* (11th ed.). Retrieved from www.m-w.com/dictionary

Mezirow, J. A. (2000). *Learning as a transformation: Critical perspectives on theory in progress.* San Francisco, CA: Jossey-Bass Publishers.

Molineux, M., & Whiteford, G. (1999). Prisons: From occupational deprivation to occupational enrichment. *Journal of Occupational Science, 6,* 124-130.

Moreira-Almeida, A., & Koenig, H. G. (2006). Retaining the meaning of the words religiousness and spirituality: A commentary on the WHOQOL SRPB group's "A cross-cultural study of spirituality, religion, and personal beliefs as components of quality of life" (62: 6, 2005, 1486-1497). *Social Science and Medicine, 63,* 843-845.

Mosey, A. C. (1986). *Psychosocial components of occupational therapy.* New York, NY: Raven Press.

Mosey, A. C. (1996). *Applied scientific inquiry in the health professions: An epistemological orientation* (2nd ed.). Bethesda, MD: American Occupational Therapy Association.

Moyers, P. A., & Dale, L. M. (2007). *The guide to occupational therapy practice* (2nd ed.). Bethesda, MD: AOTA Press.

Neistadt, M. E., & Crepeau, E. B. (Eds.). (1998). *Willard and Spackman's occupational therapy* (9th ed.). Philadelphia, PA: Lippincott Williams & Wilkins.

New York State Education Law. Section 6731. *Definition of physical therapy.*

Nilsson, I., & Townsend, E. (2010). Occupational justice—Bridging theory and practice. *Scandinavian Journal of Occupational Therapy, 17,* 57-63. http://dx.doi.org/10.3109/11038120903287182

Nurit, W., & Michel, A. B. (2003). Rest: A qualitative exploration of the phenomenon. *Occupational Therapy International, 10,* 227-238.

Office of Communications and Public Liaison. (2013, December 30). *NINDS Pervasive Developmental Disorders Information Page.* Retrieved from www.ninds.nih.gov/disorders/pdd/pdd.htm

Olafson, M. K. (2013, April 23). 7 key terms in the affordable care act that small businesses should know. *U.S. Small Business Association.* Retrieved from www.sba.gov/community/blogs/7-key-terms-afford-able-care-act-small-businesses-should-know

Parham, L. D., & Fazio, L. S. (Eds.). (1997). *Play in occupational therapy for children.* St. Louis, MO: Mosby.

Polatajko, H. J., Davis, J. A., Hobson, S., Landry, J. E., Mandich, A. D., Street, S. L., . . . Yee, S. (2004). Meeting the responsibility that comes with the privilege: Introducing a taxonomic code for understanding occupation. *Canadian Journal of Occupational Therapy, 71,* 261-264.

Primeau, L., & Ferguson, J. (1999). Occupational frame of reference. In P. Kramer & J. Hinojosa (Eds.), *Frames of reference for pediatric occupational therapy* (pp. 469-516). Philadelphia, PA: Lippincott Williams & Wilkins.

Puchalski, C., Ferrell, B., Virani, R., Otis-Green, S., Baird, P., Bull, J., . . . Sulmasy, D. (2009). Improving the quality of spiritual care as a dimension of palliative care: The report of the Consensus Conference. *Journal of Palliative Medicine, 12,* 885-904. http://dx.doi.org/10.1089/jpm.2009.0142

Radomski, M. V. (1995). There is more to life than putting on your pants. *American Journal of Occupational Therapy, 49,* 487-490. http://dx.doi.org/10.5014/ajot.49.6.487

Rand, K. L., & Cheavens, J. S. (2009). Hope theory. In S. J. Lopez & C. R. Snyder (Eds.), *The Oxford handbook of positive psychology* (2nd ed., pp. 323-334). Oxford, England: Oxford University Press.

Rebeiro, K. L., Day, D. G., Semeniuk, B., O'Brien, M. C., & Wilson, B. (2001). Northern initiative for social action: An occupation-based mental health program. *American Journal of Occupational Therapy, 55,* 493-500.

Reed, K. L., & Sanderson, S. N. (1983). *Concepts of occupational therapy* (2nd ed.). Baltimore, MD: Williams & Wilkins.

Rogers, J. C., & Holm, M. B. (1994). Assessment of self-care. In B. R. Bonder & M. B. Wagner (Eds.), *Functional performance in older adults* (pp. 181-202). Philadelphia, PA: F. A. Davis.

Schaeffer, J. (2002). *Community and communication in a diverse society.* Chicago, IL: University of Chicago Press.

Schkade, J. K., & Schultz, S. (1992). Occupational adaptation: Toward a holistic approach for contemporary practice: Part 1. *American Journal of Occupational Therapy, 46*, 829-837.

Schön, D. A. (1983). *The reflective practitioner: How professionals think in action.* New York, NY: Basic Books.

Segal, R. (2004). Family routines and rituals: A context for occupational therapy interventions. *American Journal of Occupational Therapy, 58*, 499-508. http://dx.doi.org/10.5014/ajot.58.5.499

Sensory Solutions. (2014). *Definitions.* Retrieved from www.sensorysolutions.org/definitions.html

Stadnyk, R., Townsend, E. A., & Wilcock, A. A. (in press). Occupational justice. In C. Christiansen, & E. A. Townsend (Eds.), *Introduction to occupation: The art and science of living* (2nd ed.). Upper Saddle River, NJ: Prentice Hall.

Sturgeon, J. A., & Zautra, A. J. (2010). Resilience: A new paradigm for adaptation to chronic pain. *Current Pain and Headache Reports, 14*(2), 105-112.

Substance Abuse and Mental Health Services Administration. (2014). Retrieved from www.samhsa.gov

The Free Dictionary. Retrieved from www.thefreedictionary.com

Thomas, C., & Craven, R. (Eds.). (1997). *Taber's cyclopedic medical dictionary* (18th ed.). Philadelphia, PA: F. A. Davis.

Townsend, E., & Polatajko, H. (2007). *Enabling occupation II: Advancing an occupational therapy vision for health, well-being & justice through occupation.* Ottawa, Ontario, Canada: Canadian Association of Occupational Therapists.

Townsend, E. A., & Wilcock, A. A. (2004). Occupational justice and client-centred practice: A dialogue in progress. *Canadian Journal of Occupational Therapy, 71*(2), 75-87.

Trombly, C. A. (1995). *Occupational therapy for physical dysfunction* (4th ed.). Baltimore, MD: Williams & Wilkins.

Uniform Data System for Medical Rehabilitation. (1996). *Guide for the uniform data set for medical rehabilitation (including the FIM instrument).* Buffalo, NY: Author.

Upshur, R. E. G. (2001). The status of qualitative research as evidence. In J. M. Morse, J. M. Swanson, & A. J. Kuzel (Eds.), *The nature of qualitative evidence* (pp. 5-27). Thousand Oaks, CA: Sage Publications.

Weiner, N. (2012). *Limb apraxia: A treatment guide for occupational therapists. Today in OT*, 22-27. Retrieved from ce.todayinot.com/course/ot19/limb-apraxia/

Wells, S. (1994). Valuing diversity. In *A multicultural education and resource guide for occupational therapy educators and practitioners* (pp. 9-11). Bethesda, MD: American Association of Occupational Therapy.

Whiteford, G. (1997). Occupational deprivation and incarceration. *Journal of Occupational Science: Australia, 4*, 126-130.

Whiteford, G. (2000). Occupational deprivation: global challenge in the new millennium. *British Journal of Occupational Therapy, 63,* 200-204.

Whiteford, G. (2004). When people cannot participate: Occupational deprivation. In C. Christiansen & E. A. Townsend (Eds.), *Introduction to occupation: The art and science of living* (pp. 221-242). Upper Saddle River, NJ: Prentice Hall.

Wilcock, A. A. (1996). *The relationship between occupation and health. Implications for occupational therapy and public health.* Adelaide, Australia: University of Adelaide.

Wilcock, A. A. (2006). *An occupational perspective on health* (2nd ed.). Thorofare, NJ: SLACK Incorporated.

Wilcock, A. A., & Townsend, E. A. (2000). Occupational justice: Occupational terminology interactive dialogue. *Journal of Occupational Science, 7*(2), 84-86.

Wilcock, A. A., & Townsend, E. A. (2008). Occupational justice. In E. B. Crepeau, E. S. Cohn, & B. B. Schell (Eds.), *Willard and Spackman's occupational therapy* (11th ed., pp. 192-200). Baltimore, MD: Lippincott Williams & Wilkins.

World Health Organization. (1986, November 21). *The Ottawa Charter for Health Promotion. (First International Conference on Health Promotion, Ottawa.)* Retrieved from www.who.int/healthpromotion/conferences/previous/ottawa/en/print.html

World Health Organization. (2001). *The international classification of functioning, disability and health—Towards a common language for functioning, disability and health.* Geneva, Switzerland: Author.

World Health Organization. (2006). *Constitution of the World Health Organization* (45th ed.). Retrieved from www.afro.who.int/index.php?option=com_docman&task=doc_download&gid=19&Itemid=2111 WHO2006

Zemke, R. (2004). Time, space, and the kaleidoscopes of occupation (Eleanor Clarke Slagle Lecture). *American Journal of Occupational Therapy, 58,* 608-620. http://dx.doi.org/10.5014/ajot.58.6.608

Zemke, R., & Clark, F. (1996). *Occupational science: An evolving discipline.* Philadelphia, PA: F. A. Davis.

Zimmerman, D., Purdie, L., Davis, J., & Polatajko, H. (2006, June). *Examining the face validity of the taxonomic code of occupational performance.* (Presented at the Thelma Cardwell Research Day, Faculty of Medicine, University of Toronto, ON.) Retrieved from www.ot.utoronto.ca/research/research_day/documents/rd_06_proceedings.pdf

Bibliography and Suggested Readings are located at www.healio.com/books/qrdappendices6th

List of Appendices

**Additional appendices are located at
www.healio.com/books/qrdappendices6th**

Acronyms and Abbreviations: General

A: accommodation

A: anterior

a.: artery

(A): assisted, assistance

AAROM: active assistive range of motion

AAT: animal-assisted therapy

ABA: Applied Behavioral Analysis (*formerly known as* behavior modification)

ABD: abduction

ABNORM: abnormal

ABR: absolute bedrest

AC: acromioclavicular

ACA: Affordable Care Act (*also known as* ObamaCare, PPACA)

ACCE: Academic Coordinator of Clinical Education

ACLF: adult congregate living facility

ACT: adaptive control of thoughts

ACTH: adrenocorticotrophic hormone

ACVD: acute cardiovascular disease

AD: admitting diagnosis

AD: Alzheimer's disease

AD: autogenic drainage

ADA: Americans with Disabilities Act

ADAAA: Americans with Disabilities Act Amendments Act

ADD: adduction

Jacobs, K., & Simon, L. (Eds.). *Quick Reference Dictionary for Occupational Therapy, Sixth Edition* (pp. 336-359). © 2015 SLACK Incorporated.

ADD: attention deficit disorder

ADH: antidiuretic hormone

ADHD: attention deficit hyperactivity disorder

ADL: activities of daily living

ad lib: as desired

ADM: administration

ADP: adenosine diphosphate

ADS: alternative delivery system

AE: above elbow

AFDC: Aid to Families with Dependent Children

AFO: ankle foot orthosis

AI: autistic impaired

AIDS: acquired immunodeficiency syndrome

AJOT: *American Journal of Occupational Therapy*

AJPT: *American Journal of Physical Therapy*

AK: above knee

AKA: above knee amputation

ALOS: average length of stay

ALS: amyotrophic lateral sclerosis

AMA: against medical advice

Am't: amount

ANCOVA: analysis of covariance

ANOVA: analysis of variance

ANS: autonomic nervous system

Ant: anterior

Ant-THP: anterior total hip precautions

AP: anterior-posterior

APG: ambulatory patient (payment) group

Approx: approximately

AROM: active range of motion

ART: active resistive training

AS: Angelman syndrome

ASA: aspirin

ASAP: as soon as possible

ASCII: American Standard Code for Information Interchange

ASD: autism spectrum disorder

ASHD: arterial sclerotic heart disease

ASL: American Sign Language
ASO: arteriosclerosis obliterans
ASROM: assistive range of motion
AT: assistive technology
ATNR: asymmetrical tonic neck reflex
ATP: adenosine triphosphate

(B): both, bilateral
BADL: basic activities of daily living
Ba Enema: barium enema
BBA: Balanced Budget Act
BBS: bulletin board system
BE: base equivalent
BE: below elbow
BG: blood glucose
bid: twice a day
Bilat: bilateral
BK: below knee
BKA: below knee amputation
Bl: blood
BLT: bilateral lung transplant
bm: body mechanics
BM: bowel movement
BMD: bone mineral density
BMI: body mass index
BMR: basal metabolic rate
BOS: base of support
BP: blood pressure
BPM: beats per minute
BR: bedrest
BRP: bathroom privileges
BS: blood sugar
BSA: body surface area
BSF: benign senescent forgetfulness
BT: brain tumor
BTB: back to bed
BUN: blood urea nitrogen

C: centigrade, Celsius
C: cervical
C: coefficient of contingency
Ca: calcium
Ca: cancer
Cal: calorie
CART: classification and regression trees
CAT: computer-assisted tomography
CAT: computer axial tomography
CBC: complete blood count
CBI: closed brain injury
CBR: community-based rehabilitation
CBR: complete bedrest
CBS: chronic brain syndrome
CC: chief complaint
cc: cubic centimeter(s)
CCCE: clinical coordinator of clinical education
C-Collar: cervical collar
CCS: Certified Cardiopulmonary Specialist
CCU: coronary care unit
CD: cardiovascular disease
CDC: Centers for Disease Control and Prevention
CDM: Charge Description Master (HCFA)
CE: continuing education
CEO: chief executive officer
CF: cystic fibrosis
CFR: Code of Federal Regulations
CHAMPUS: Civilian Health and Medical Program of the Uniformed Services
CHD: coronary heart disease
CHF: congestive heart failure
CHI: closed head injury
CHT: Certified Hand Therapist
CI: cardiac index
CI: clinical instructor
CICU: coronary intermediate care unit

CINAHL: Cumulative Index to Nursing and Allied Health Literature

CK: creatine kinase

Cl: chloride; chlorine

cm: centimeter(s)

CMCE: Canadian Model of Client-Centred Enablement

CMOP-E: Canadian Model of Occupational Performance and Engagement

CMP: competitive medical plan

CNS: central nervous system

c/o: complains of

CO: carbon monoxide

CO$_2$: carbon dioxide

COB: coordination of benefits

COE: Commission on Education

COG: center of gravity

COJ: *Classification of Jobs According to Worker Trait Factors*

COLA: cost of living adjustment

COLD: chronic obstructive lung disease

COM: center of mass; center of motion

CONTRA: contraindication

COPD: chronic obstructive pulmonary disease

CORF: comprehensive outpatient rehabilitation facility

COTA™: from NBCOT—Certified Occupational Therapy Assistant; will be referred to as OTA in this text

CP: cerebral palsy

CP: certified professional

CP: chest pain

CPE: Certified Professional Ergonomist

CPE: continuing professional education

CPEF: Clinical Performance Evaluation Form (developed by the New England Consortium of Academic Coordinators of Clinical Education)

CPI: consumer price index

CPM: continuous passive motion

CPMM: continuous passive motion machine

CPPF: Canadian Practice Process Framework

CPR: cardiopulmonary resuscitation
CPT: Current Procedural Terminology
CPU: central processing unit
CQI: continuous quality improvement
CRI: chronic renal insufficiency
CSF: cerebrospinal fluid
CSHN: children with special health needs
CSM: Combined Sections Meeting (APTA)
CST: cranial sacral therapy
CT: computed tomography
CTS: carpal tunnel syndrome
cu: cubic
CV: cardiovascular
CV: coefficient of variation
CVA: cardiovascular accident
CVA: cerebrovascular accident
CVD: cardiovascular disease
CVP: central venous pressure
CXR: chest x-ray

D: distal
d/c: discharge
D&C: dilation and curettage
DD: developmental disability
Dep: dependent
Derm: dermatology
DFF: directions for the future
dia: diameter
DIP: distal interphalangeal joint
DJD: degenerative joint disease
DKA: diabetic ketoacidosis
dL: deciliter (= 100 mL)
DM: diabetes mellitus
DME: durable medical equipment
DMEPOS: durable medical equipment, prosthetics, orthotics, and
   supplies
DMERC: durable medical equipment regional carrier (HCFA)

DMG: dimethylglycine
DNA: deoxyribonucleic acid
DNR: do not resuscitate
DOA: dead on arrival
DOB: date of birth
DOE: dyspnea on exertion
doff: take off clothing
DOMS: delayed onset muscle soreness
don: put on clothing
DOT: *Dictionary of Occupational Titles*
DPT: Doctor of Physical Therapy
DRG: diagnosis-related groups
DRS: disability rating scale
DSM-5: *Diagnostic and Statistical Manual of Mental Disorders* (5th ed.)
DSR: dynamic spatial reconstructor
DT: delirium tremens
DTP: diphtheria-tetanus-pertussis (vaccine)
DTR: deep tendon reflex
DVT: deep vein thrombosis
Dx: diagnosis
DZ: disease

EAP: employee assistance program
EBV: Epstein-Barr virus
ECF: extended care facility
ECF: extracellular fluid
ECG: electrocardiogram
ECT: electroconvulsive therapy
ECU: environmental control unit
EDM: extensor digitorum minimi
EEG: electroencephalogram
EENT: eye, ear, nose, and throat
EKG: electrocardiogram
EMA: external moment arm
EMG: electromyelogram
EMG: electromyogram

EMG: electromyograph
EMI: educable mentally impaired
EMS: electrical muscle stimulation
EMS: emergency medical service
ENT: ear, nose, and throat
EOB: end of bed, edge of bed
EOB: explanation of benefits
EOM: edge of mat
EPL: extensor pollicis longus
EPSDT: early and periodic screening, diagnostic, and treatment
ER: emergency room
ER: external rotation
ERV: expiratory reserve volume
ESR: erythrocyte sedimentation rate
ESRD: end-stage renal disease
ESTR: electrical stimulation for tissue repair
ETIOL: etiology
EVAL: evaluation; evaluate
Ex: example
EX: exercise
EXT: extension

F: Fahrenheit
F-: fair (40%)
F: fair (50%)
F+: fair (60%)
F: female
FAOTA: Fellow of the American Occupational Therapy Association
FAPTA: Fellow of the American Physical Therapy Association
FAS: fetal alcohol syndrome
FCU: flexor carpi ulnaris
FEMS: functional electrical muscle stimulation
FES: functional electrical stimulation
FET: force expiratory technique
FEV1: forced expiratory volume
FH: family history
FLEX: flexion

FOR: frame of reference

FRG: functional-related groups

FSH: follicle-stimulating hormone

ft: foot; feet

FTM: a person who transitions from female-to-male (meaning a person who was assigned the female sex at birth but identifies and lives as a male)

FUNC: function

FUO: fever undetermined origin

FWB: full weight bearing

FWC: fieldwork coordinator (COE-AOTA)

FWE: fieldwork evaluation

FWE: fieldwork experience

FWS: fieldwork supervisor

FWW: front-wheeled walker

FY: fiscal year

Fx: fracture

G-: good (70%)

G: good (80%)

G+: good (90%)

GABA: gamma-aminobutyric acid

GAS: General Adaptation Syndrome

GAU: geriatric assessment unit

GBS: Guillain-Barré syndrome

GCRC: General Clinical Research Center

GCS: Geriatric Certified Specialist

GDP: gross domestic product

GEC: geriatric education center

GED: general educational development

GER: gerontology

GFR: glomerular filtration rate

GI: gastrointestinal

gm: gram(s)

GME: graduate medical education

GNP: gross national product

GOE: *Guide for Occupational Exploration*

Gr: grain
GSR: galvanic skin response
GSW: gunshot wound
GTO: Golgi tendon organ
GU: genitourinary
GYN: gynecology

H2: histamine
H/A: headache
HCFA: Health Care Finance Administration
HCG: human chorionic gonadotropin
HCO$_3$: bicarbonate
H&CP: hospital and community psychiatry
HCPCS: Healthcare Common Procedure Coding System
HCS: Health Communication Services
Hct: hematocrit
HCVD: hypertensive cardiovascular disease
HDL: high-density lipoprotein
HEA: Higher Education Act
hemi: hemiplegia
HEP: home exercise program
HF: heart failure
Hg: mercury
Hgb: hemoglobin
HHA: home health agency
HHE: home health equipment
HI: head injury
HI: hearing impaired
HI: hospital insurance
HIV: human immunodeficiency virus
HL: human leukocyte
HMO: health maintenance organization
HOB: head of bed
H&P: history and physical
HP: hot pack
HPI: history of present illness
HR: heart rate

Hr: hour
HS: high school
HS: hours of sleep
HSA: health systems agency
HSN: hospital satellite network
HTN: hypertension
HVPS: high-voltage pulsed stimulation
Hx: history
HYPO: hypodermic
Hz: hertz (cycles/second)

I: independent
IADL: instrumental activities of daily living
IAT: interagency transfer
IC: inspiratory capacity
IC: integrated circuit
ICC: intraclass correlation coefficient
ICD: International Classification of Diseases
ICF: International Classification of Function, Disability and Health
ICF: intermediary care facility
ICF: intracellular fluid
ICIDH: International Classification of Impairments, Disabilities, and Handicaps
ICU: intensive care unit
IDDM: insulin-dependent diabetes mellitus
IDEA: Individuals with Disabilities Education Act
IDT: interdepartmental transfer
IEP: individualized education plan
IFSP: individualized family service plan
IgA, etc.: immunoglobulin A, etc.
ILC: independent living center
IM: intramuscular
IME: indirect medical education
IMP: impression (tentative diagnosis)
in: inch(es)
IND: indications
Indep: independent

inf: inferior
Inhal: inhalation
Inj: injection
IP: interphalangeal joint
IPA: independent practice association
IPPB: inspiratory positive pressure breathing
IR: incidence rate
IR: internal rotation
IRV: inspiratory reserve volume
ITC: information technology and communications
ITP: individual transition plan
IU: international unit(s)
IV: intravenous
IVDU: intravenous drug user
IVP: intravenous pyelogram

JOTS: *Journal of Occupational Therapy Students*
JRA: juvenile rheumatoid arthritis
JROM: joint range of motion

K: potassium
KAFO: knee ankle foot orthosis
KB: kilobyte
kcal: kilocalorie (food calorie)
kg: kilogram(s)
KJ: knee jerk
KO: knee orthosis
KUB: kidney, ureter, bladder

(L): left
L: liter(s); lumbar
LAD: language acquisition device
Lat: lateral
lb: pound
LBP: low back pain
LBQC: large base quad cane
LC: locus coeruleus

LCR: lifetime clinical record
LCST: lateral corticospinal tract
LD: learning disability
LDH: lactic dehydrogenase
LDL: low-density lipoprotein
LDRP: labor, delivery, recovery, postpartum
LE: lower extremity
LE: lupus erythematosus
LH: luteinizing hormone
LLB: long leg brace
LLD: leg length discrepancy
LLE: left lower extremity
LLQ: left lower quadrant (of abdomen)
LMN: lower motor neuron
LMP: last menstrual period
LOA: leave of absence
LOC: loss of consciousness
LOS: length of stay
LP: lumbar puncture
LRP: long-range plan (AOTA)
LS: lumbosacral
LTC: long-term care
LTG: long-term goals
LUE: left upper extremity
L&W: living and well

M: male
m: meter(s)
m.: muscle
MA: mechanical advantage
ma: milliampere(s)
MAO: monoamine oxidase
MAS: mobile arm support
Max: maximum
max VO$_2$: maximal oxygen consumption
MBD: minimal brain damage
MC: metacarpal

MCC: medical center computing
MCE: medical care evaluation
mcg: microgram(s)
MCH: maternal and child health
MCH: mean corpuscular hemoglobin
MCHC: mean corpuscular hemoglobin concentration
MCO: managed care organization
MCP: metacarpophalangeal
MCV: mean corpuscular volume
MD: muscular dystrophy
Mdn: median
med: medium; medial; median
MED: minimum effective dose
MEP: motor evoked potential
mEq: milliequivalent(s)
MET: metabolic equivalent level
MFR: myofascial release
MFT: muscle function test
Mg: magnesium
mg: milligram(s)
MG: myasthenia gravis
MH: mental health
MHB: maximum hospital benefit
MHC: myosin heavy chain
MI: myocardial infarction
MIN: minimal
min: minute
MIS: Medical Information System
mL: milliliter(s)
MLF: medial longitudinal fasciculus
mm: millimeter(s)
MMT: manual muscle testing
MNE: motor neuron excitability
Mo: mode
mo: month
MOC: military occupational classification
Mod: moderate

MOHO: Model of Human Occupation

MP: metacarpophalangeal joint

mph: miles per hour

MPSMS: materials, products, subject matter, or services

MRI: magnetic resonance imaging

MRSA: methicillin-resistant *Staphylococcus aureus*

MS: mitral stenosis

MS: multiple sclerosis

MSM: men who have sex with men

MSP: Medicare secondary payer

MSQ: mental status questionnaire

MTEWA: machines, tools, equipment, and work aids used

MTF: a person who transitions from male-to-female (meaning a person who was assigned the male sex at birth but identifies and lives as a female)

MUP: motor unit potential

MVA: motor vehicle accident

MVC: maximum voluntary contraction

MVE: maximum voluntary effort

MVV: maximal voluntary ventilation

n.: nerve

N: nitrogen

N: normal

N/A: not applicable; not available

Na: sodium

NaC: normal saline

NBCOT: National Board for Certification in Occupational Therapy

NCS: Neurology Certified Specialist

ND: new drugs

NDT: Neurodevelopmental Treatment

Neg: negative

ng: nanogram

NG tube: nasogastric tube

NICU: neonatal intensive care unit

NIDDM: non–insulin-dependent diabetes mellitus

NK: natural killer (cell)

NKA: no known allergy
NKDA: no known drug allergy
NORC: Naturally Occurring Retirement Community
NP: neuropsychiatry
NP: nursing procedure
NPH: neutral protein Hagedorn (insulin)
NPN: nonprotein nitrogen
NPO: nothing by mouth
NPTE: National Physical Therapy Examination
NREM: nonrapid eye movement
NSAID: nonsteroidal anti-inflammatory drug
NSG: nursing
NWB: non-weight bearing

O$_2$: oxygen
O$_2$ Sat: oxygen saturation
OA: osteoarthritis
OB: obstetrics
OBRA '87: Omnibus Budget Reconciliation Act of 1987
OBS: observation
OCS: Orthopedic Certified Specialist
OD: once daily
OD: right eye
OHT: orthotopic heart transplant
OI: occupational issues
OLPR: online patient record
OLT: orthotopic liver transplant
OOB: out of bed
OOT: outpatient occupational therapy (Medicare)
OPD: outpatient department
OPG: occupational performance goal
OPI: occupational performance issue
OPM: occupational performance model
OPPM: occupational performance process model
OR: operating room
Orth: orthopedic
OS: left eye

OSHA: Occupational Safety and Health Administration

OT: occupational therapy; occupational therapist

OTA-FWEF: occupational therapy assistant fieldwork evaluation form

OTAS: occupational therapy assistant student

OTC: over-the-counter

OT-FWEF: professional level student fieldwork evaluation form

OTIP: occupational therapist in independent practice (Medicare)

OTIS: occupational therapy information system (AOTA)

OTJR: *Occupational Therapy Journal of Research*

OTR™: from NBCOT—Occupational Therapist, Registered; will be referred to as OT in this text

OTS: occupational therapy student

OU: both eyes

oz: ounce

P: phosphorus; pressure

P-: poor (10%)

P: poor (20%)

P+: poor (30%)

PA: posterior anterior

PaCO$_2$: arterial carbon dioxide pressure

PADL: personal activities of daily living

PAO$_2$: alveolar oxygen pressure

PaO$_2$: arterial oxygen pressure

PAM: physical agent modality

PARA: paraplegia

PATH: pathology

PATRA: professional and technical role analysis

PCA: personal care attendant

PCO$_2$: carbon dioxide pressure (or tension)

PCS: Pediatric Certified Specialist

PCS: post-concussion syndrome

PCT: periarticular connective tissue

PD: physical disabilities

PDD: pervasive developmental disorder

PDR: *Physicians' Desk Reference*

PE: physical examination
Ped: pediatric
PES: Professional Examination Service
PET: positron emission tomography
PFS: patient financial services
PFT: pulmonary function test
Phy Dys: physical disabilities
PHYS: physical; physiology
PI: present illness
PI: proactive interference
PICU: pediatric intensive care unit
PID: pelvic inflammatory disease
PIP: proximal interphalangeal joint
PKU: phenylketonuria
PMH: previous medical history
PMR: physical medicine and rehabilitation
PMT: premotor time
PNF: proprioceptive neuromuscular facilitation
PNS: peripheral nervous system
PO: by mouth
PO: postoperative
PO$_2$: oxygen pressure (or tension)
POHI: physically or otherwise health impaired
POMR: problem-oriented medical record
Postop: postoperative
Post-THP: posterior total hip precautions
PPACA: Patient Protection and Affordable Care Act (*also known as* ACA, ObamaCare)
PPE: personal protective equipment
PPI: preprimary impaired
ppm: parts per million
PPO: preferred provider organization
PPS: Prospective Payment System (Medicare)
PRE: progressive resistive exercises
Preop: preoperative
PRN: whenever necessary
PRO: peer review organization

PROG: prognosis
PROM: passive range of motion
PROSTUD: Prospective Student Program Database
PT: physical therapy; physical therapist
pt: pint(s)
PTA: physical therapist assistant
PTA: prior to admission
PTB: patella tendon bearing
PTSD: post-traumatic stress disorder
PVD: peripheral vascular disease
PVE: prevocational evaluation
PWA: person with AIDS
PWB: partial weight bearing
Px: physical examination

q: every
q2h: every 2 hours
QA: quality assurance
qd: every day
qh: every hour
QI: quality improvement
qid: four times daily
qn: every night
qod: every other day
qt: quart
QUAD: quadriplegia

(R): right
R, r: roentgen(s)
RA: reasonable accommodations
RA: rheumatoid arthritis
RAIS: registered apprenticeship information system
RAM: random access memory
RAP: resident assessment protocol
RAS: reticular activating system
RBC: red blood count
RBRVS: Resource-Based Relative Value Scale (Medicare)

RC: rehabilitation counselor
RD: retinal detachment
Rehab: rehabilitation
REM: rapid eye movement
RET: rational emotive therapy
RF: renal failure
RF: rheumatoid factor; rheumatic fever
RHC: rural health clinic
RHD: rheumatic heart disease
RLE: right lower extremity
RM: repetition maximum
RNA: ribonucleic acid
RO: rule out
ROH: roster of honor
ROM: range of motion
ROS: review of systems
ROTE: Role of Occupational Therapist with the Elderly (AOTA)
RPCH: rural primary care hospital
RPE: rating of perceived exertion
RPT: registered physical therapist
RPTA: registered physical therapist assistant
RROM: resistive range of motion
RTS: rehabilitation technology supplier
RUE: right upper extremity
RUG: resource utilization grouping
RV: residual volume
RVU: Relative Value Unit
RW: rolling walker
Rx: prescription

S: sacral
S: social history
SAD: seasonal affective disorder
SaO$_2$: arterial oxygen saturation
SAQ: short arc quad
sat: saturated
SB: sliding board

SBQC: small base quad cane
SBE: subacute bacterial endocarditis
SBF: skin blood cell flux
SC: straight cane
s.c.: subcutaneous(ly)
SCI: spinal cord injury
SCORE: service corps of retired executives
SCS: Splint Classification System
SCS: Sports Certified Specialist
SE: side effects
sec: second(s)
SED: seriously emotionally disturbed
SEFWF: student evaluation of fieldwork form
SEP: somatosensory evoked potential
SGOT: serum glutamic oxaloacetic transaminase
SGPT: serum glutamic pyruvic transaminase
SHUR: System for Hospital Uniform Reporting
SI: sensory integration
SICU: surgical intensive care unit
SIDS: sudden infant death syndrome
SIMS: Strategic Integrated Management System (AOTA)
SLB: short leg brace
SLE: systemic lupus erythematosus
SLH: state and local hospitalization
SLP: speech language pathologist
SLR: straight leg raise
SMA: spinal muscular atrophy
SMI: severely mentally impaired
SMI: supplemental medical insurance
SMS: shared medical systems
SNF: skilled nursing facility
SOAP: subjective, objective, assessment, plan
SOB: shortness of breath
SOC: Standard Occupational Classification
soln: solution
SOP: standard operating procedure
SOS: if necessary

SP: speech
s/p: status post
SPEM: smooth pursuit eye movement
sp. gr.: specific gravity
SPO$_2$: pulse oxygen saturation
SPT: student physical therapist
SPSS: Statistical Package for Social Sciences
sq: square
SR: systematic review
SSI: supplemental security income
SSLI: severe speech and language impaired
Stat: at once
STD: sexually transmitted disease
STG: short-term goals
STNR: symmetrical tonic neck reflex
SUDS: single-use diagnostic system
sup: superior
Sup: supination
SVP: specific vocational preparation
SW: standard walker
Sx: symptom
SXI: severely multi-impaired
SYM: symptom
Sz: schizophrenia
Sz: seizure

t1/2: half-life
T: trace (5%)
T&A: tonsils and adenoids
TAB: temporarily abled body
TAP: turning and positioning program
TB: tuberculosis
TBG: thyroxin-binding globulin
TBI: traumatic brain injury
TDD: telecommunication device for the deaf
TDWB: touch down weight bearing
TEFRA: Tax Equity and Fiscal Responsibility Act

TENS: transcutaneous electrical nerve stimulation
Th: thoracic
THR: total hip replacement
TIA: transient ischemic attack
tid: three times daily
TKR: total knee replacement
TLI: total lymphoid irradiation
TLR: tonic labyrinthine reflex
TLSO: thoracic lumbar sacral orthosis
TMI: trainable mentally impaired
TOTEMS: Training: Occupational Therapy Educational Management in Schools (AOTA)
TPR: temperature, pulse, respiration
TQM: total quality management
TSH: thyroid-stimulating hormone
TTWB: toe touch weight bearing
TTY: teletypewriter
TV: tidal volume
Tx: treatment

u: unit(s)
UAP: university-affiliated programs
UE: upper extremity
UMN: upper motor neuron
Un: unable
UR: utilization review
URI: upper respiratory infection
US: ultrasound
USA: unstable angina
UTI: urinary tract infection
UV: ultraviolet

VC: vital capacity
VER: visual evoked response
VE/VO$_2$: ventilation equivalent
VI: visually impaired
VI: volume index

VO: verbal order
VO$_2$: maximum oxygen consumption
VS: vestibular stimulation
VS: vital signs

WBAT: weight bearing as tolerated
WBC: white blood cell count
WBQC: wide-base quad cane
W/C or WC: wheelchair
WD: well developed
WFL: within functional limits
WIC: special supplemental nutrition program for women, infants, and children
Wk: week
WMSDs: work-related musculoskeletal disorders (NIOSH)
WN: well nourished
WNL: within normal limits
WORK: *Work: A Journal of Prevention, Assessment & Rehabilitation*
WSW: women who have sex with women
wt: weight

x: times

y/n: yes/no
y/o: years old
yrs: years

Acronyms: Evaluations

A/A Index: Ankle/Arm Index
ABI: Ankle Brachial Index
ABS: Adaptive Behavior Scale
ACL: Allen Cognitive Level Test
ADAPT: Additive Activities Profile Test
AIMS: Alberta Infant Motor Scale
ALSR: Assessment of Living Skills and Resources
AMPS: Assessment of Motor and Process Skills
APIB: Assessment of Premature Infant Behavior

BaFPE: Bay Area Functional Performance Evaluation
BCT: Boston Cancellation Test
BDI: Battelle Developmental Inventory
BDI: Beck Depression Inventory
BIT: Behavioral Inattention Test
BOMC: Blessed Orientation Memory Test
BOTMP: Bruininks-Oseretsky Test of Motor Proficiency
BP: blood pressure
BSID-II: Bayley Scales of Infant Development (2nd ver.)
BTE: Baltimore Therapeutic Equipment (work simulator)
BVRT: Benton Visual Retention Test

Jacobs, K., & Simon, L. (Eds.). *Quick Reference Dictionary for Occupational Therapy, Sixth Edition* (pp. 360-366). © 2015 SLACK Incorporated.

CAM: Cognitive Assessment of Minnesota
CARS: Childhood Autism Rating Scale
CBDI: Cognitive Behavioral Driver's Index
CBRS: Cognitive Behavior Rating Scales
CEBLS: Comprehensive Evaluation of Basic Living Skills
CES-D: Center for Epidemiological Studies Depression Scale
CFA: Comprehensive Functional Assessment
CHART: Craig Handicap Assessment and Reporting Technique
CIQ: Community Integration Questionnaire
CMCE: Canadian Model of Client-Centred Enablement
CMT: Contextual Memory Test
COPM: Canadian Occupational Performance Measure
COTE: Comprehensive Occupational Therapy Evaluation
CPT: Cognitive Performance Test
CRS-R: JFK Coma Recovery Scale–Revised
CVMT: Continuous Visual Memory Test

DDS: Descriptor Differential Scale (pain scale)
DDST-R: Denver Developmental Screening Test–Revised
DPQ: Dallas Pain Questionnaire
DPT: Driver Performance Test
DRS: Dementia Rating Scale
DSM-5: *Diagnostic and Statistical Manual of Mental Disorders* (5th ed.)
DTVP-2: Developmental Test of Visual Perception (2nd ed.)

EAE: Eligibility and Agency Evaluation (ED)
ECG: electrocardiogram
EDPA: Erhardt Developmental Prehension Assessment
EDSS: Kurtzke Expanded Disability Status Scale
EIDP: Early Intervention Developmental Profile
ELC: EPIC Lift Capacity
EMG: electromyograph
EPESE: Established Populations for Epidemiologic Studies of the Elderly

FAP: Functional Ambulation Profile
FAQ: Functional Activities Questionnaire
FCE: Functional Capacity Evaluation
FDS: Framingham Disability Scale
FHS: Functional Health Scale
FIM: Functional Independence Measure
FMA: Fugl-Meyer Assessment (stroke)
FSI: Functional Status Index
FSQ: Functional Status Questionnaire

GARS: Gait Abnormality Rating Scale
GAS: Goal Attainment Scale
GDS: Geriatric Depression Scale
GMFM: Gross Motor Function Measure
GOAT: Galveston Orientation and Amnesia Test

HAOF: Hospice Assessment of Occupational Function
HELP: Hawaii Early Learning Profile
HHD: hand-held dynamometer
HR: heart rate

ILSE: Independent Living Skills Evaluation
INFANIB: Infant Neurological International Battery
IQ: intelligence quotient

JPSA: Jacobs Prevocational Skills Assessment

KELS: Kohlman Evaluation of Living Skills
KSHQ: Knickerbocker Sensorimotor History Questionnaire

LAP-R: Learning Accomplished Profile–Revised Edition
LCFS: Levels of Cognitive Function Scale
LCL: Low Cognitive Level Test
LNNB: Luria Nebraska Neuropsychological Battery
LOTCA: Loewenstein Occupational Therapy Cognitive Assessment

MAI: Multilevel Assessment Instrument; Movement Assessment of Infants

MAI-ST: Movement Assessment of Infants Screening Test

MAP: Miller Assessment for Preschoolers

MAS: Carr and Sheperd's Motor Assessment Scale

MAS: Modified Ashworth Scale

MBHI: Million Behavioral Health Inventory

MDI: Maryland Disability Index (most commonly referred to as the Barthel Index)

MDS: McCarron-Dial System

MDS: Minimum Data Set

MEAMS: Middlesex Elderly Assessment of Mental State

MEAP: Multiphasic Environmental Assessment Procedure

MEDLS: Milwaukee Evaluation of Daily Living Skills

MFAQ: Multidimensional Functional Assessment Questionnaire

MMPI: Minnesota Multiphasic Personality Inventory

MMSE: Mini-Mental State Exam

MMT: manual muscle test

MOHOST: Model of Human Occupation Screening Tool

MOS-36: Measure of Self-Functioning

MPQ: McGill Pain Questionnaire

MRMT: Minnesota Rate of Manipulation Test

MSQ: Mental Status Questionnaire

MVAS: Million Visual Analog Scale (pain)

MVPT: Motor-Free Visual Perception Test

NAPFI: Neurological Assessment of the Pre-Term and Full-Term Infant

NBAS: Neonatal Behavioral Assessment Scale

NCS: Nerve Conduction Studies

NCSE: Neurobehavioral Cognitive Status Examination

NCSSE: Neurobehavioral Cognitive Status Screening Examination

NDDG: National Diabetes Data Group

NHANES: National Health and Nutrition Examination Survey

NIDCAP: Neonatal Individualized Developmental and Care Assessment Profile (also referred to as NONB)

NLTCS: National Long-Term Care Survey

NMES: National Medical Expenditure Survey
NNE: Neonatal Neurobehavioral Evaluation
NNHS: National Nursing Home Survey
NOMAS: Neonatal Oral-Motor Assessment Scale
NONB: Naturalistic Observation of Newborn Behavior (also referred to as NIDCAP)
NRS: numerical rating scale

OARS: Older American Resources and Services—Multidimensional Functional Assessment Questionnaire
OASIS: Outcomes and Assessment Information Set (Medicare)
OGA: observational gait assessment (amputee)
OTFACT: Occupational Therapy Functional Assessment Compilation Tool

PACE: Program of All-Inclusive Care for the Elderly
PADL: Performance Activities of Daily Living
PAPL: Pizzi Assessment of Productive Living
P-CTSIB: Pediatric Clinical Test of Sensory Integration for Balance
PDMS: Peabody Developmental Motor Scales
PDS: pain discomfort scale
PECS: Patient Evaluations Conference System
PEDI: Pediatric Evaluation of Disability Inventory
PFMAI: Posture and Fine Motor Skills Assessment of Infant
PFT: pulmonary function test
PGC: Philadelphia Geriatric Center Scale
PGCII: Philadelphia Geriatric Center Scale II
POE: Post-Occupancy Evaluation
PPB: Purdue Pegboard Battery
PPS: Preschool Play Scale
PPT: physical performance test
PST: postural stress test
PULSES: physical condition, upper limb function, lower limb function, sensory components, excretory function, support factors

QST: Quantitative Somatosensory Thermostat
QUEST: Quality of Upper Extremity Skills Test

RAI: resident assessment instrument
RAP: resident assessment protocol
RBMT: Rivermead Behavioral Memory Test
RCFT: Rey Complex Figure Test
REG: Rapid Exchange of Grip
RER: Respiratory Exchange Ratio
RNL: Reintegration to Normal Living Index
ROM: range of motion
RPM: Raven Progressive Matrices
RR: respiratory rate
RT: reach test
RTI: Routine Task Inventory

SAFE: Safety and Functional ADL Evaluation
SAFER: Safety Assessment of Function and the Environment for Rehabilitation
SAILS: Structured Assessment of Independent Living Skills
SAQ: Services Assessment Questionnaire
SCOPE: Strategies, Concepts, and Opportunities for Program Development
SCT: Short Category Test
SCWT: Stroop Color and Word Test
SDMT: Symbol Digit Modalities Test
SDS: Zung Self-Rating Depression Scale
SF-36: Self-Functional Assessment (36 items)
SIB: Severe Impairment Battery
SIP: Sickness Impact Profile
SIPT: Sensory Integration and Praxis Test
SIT: Sensory Integration Test
SM: sphygmomanometer
SMAF: Functional Autonomy Measurement System
SOA: National Health Interview Survey: Supplement on Aging
SOT: Sensory Organization Test
SOTOF: Structured Observational Test of Function
SPA: Sensorimotor Performance Analysis
SPMSQ: Short Portable Mental Status Questionnaire
SPSQ: Satisfaction with Performance Scaled Questionnaire

TCA: Toglia Category Assessment
TIE: Touch Inventory for Elementary School-Aged Children
TIME: Toddler and Infant Motor Evaluation
TIP: Touch Inventory for Preschoolers
TMP: timed manual performance
TOPS: Test of Playfulness Skills
TORP: Test of Orientation for Rehabilitation Patients
TOWER: Testing, Orientation, Work, Evaluation, and Rehabilitation
TQSB: Teacher Questionnaire on Sensorimotor Behavior
TSI: Test of Sensory Integration (also called the DeGangi-Berk Test)
TVMS: Test of Visual Motor Skills
TVPS: Test of Visual Perceptual Skills (non-motor)

ULTT: Upper Limb Tension Test

VAS: visual analog scale
VCWS: VALPAR Component Work Samples
VMI: Berry-Buktenica Developmental Test of Visual-Motor Integration
VOSP: Visual Object and Space Perception Test
VRS: verbal rating scale (pain scale)

WAIS: Wechsler Adult Intelligence Scale
WAIS-R: Wechsler Adult Intelligence Scale–Revised
WCST: Wisconsin Card Sorting Test
WeeFIM: Functional Independence for Children
WEST: Work Evaluation Systems Technology
WIRE: Work and Industrial Rehabilitation Evaluation
WPPSI: Wechsler Preschool and Primary Scale of Intelligence

Acronyms: Organizational

AA: Alcoholics Anonymous

AAA: Area Agencies on Aging

AAACE: American Association of Adult and Continuing Education

AAAS: American Association for the Advancement of Science

AACHP: American Association for Comprehensive Health Planning

AAFP: American Academy of Family Practitioners

AAHPERD: American Alliance for Health, Physical Education, Recreation, and Dance

AAMR: American Association on Mental Retardation

AAOT: Australian Association of Occupational Therapists, Inc.

AAP: American Academy of Pediatrics

AAPC: American Association of Pastoral Counselors

AAPD: American Academy of Pediatric Dentists

AAPH: American Association of Partial Hospitalization

AARP: American Association for Retired Persons

AART: American Association for Respiratory Therapy

AART: Association for the Advancement of Rehabilitation Technology

ABPTS: American Board of Physical Therapy Specialists

ACA: American Counseling Association

ACALD: Association for Children and Adults with Learning Disabilities

ACCD: American Coalition of Citizens with Disabilities

Jacobs, K., & Simon, L. (Eds.). *Quick Reference Dictionary for Occupational Therapy, Sixth Edition* (pp. 367-377). © 2015 SLACK Incorporated.

ACCH: Association for the Care of Children's Health

ACCP: American College of Chest Physicians

ACDD: Accreditation Council on Services for People with Developmental Disabilities

ACF: Administration for Children and Families

ACHCA: American College of Health Care Administrators

ACIP: Advisory Committee on Immunization Practices

ACOTE: Accreditation Council for Occupational Therapy Education

ACPAC: Annual Conference Program Advisory Committee

ACRE: American Council on Rural Education

ACRM: American Congress of Rehabilitation Medicine

ACSM: American College of Sports Medicine

ACYF: Administration on Children, Youth, and Families

ADA: American Dietetic Association

ADD: Administration on Developmental Disabilities

ADED: Association of Driver Educators for the Disabled

ADHA: American Dental Hygienists Association

ADRDA: Alzheimer's Disease and Related Disorders Association

AERA: American Educational Research Association

AF: Arthritis Foundation

AGA: American Geriatric Association

AGHE: Association for Gerontology in Higher Education

AHA: American Hospital Association

AHCA: American Health Care Association

AHCPR: Agency for Health Care Policy and Research

AHEA: American Home Economics Association

AHPA: Arthritis Health Professional Association

AICPA: American Institute of Certified Public Accountants

AMA: American Medical Association

AMDA: American Medical Directors Association

AMH: Accreditation Manual for Hospitals (JCAHO)

AMSIS: Administrative/Management Special Interest Section (AOTA)

ANA: American Nurses Association

ANSI: American National Standards Institute

AOA: Administration on Aging (DHHS)

AOA: American Optometric Association

AOA: American Osteopathic Association

AOPA: American Orthotic and Prosthetic Association

AOTA: American Occupational Therapy Association

AOTCB: American Occupational Therapy Certification Board (presently called the NBCOT)

AOTF: American Occupational Therapy Foundation

AOTPAC: American Occupational Therapy Political Action Committee (AOTA)

APA: American Psychiatric Association

APA: American Psychological Association

APHA: American Public Health Association

APTA: American Physical Therapy Association

ARC: Association for Retarded Citizens

ARCA: American Rehabilitation Counseling Association

ARF: Association of Rehabilitation Facilities

ASA: American Society on Aging

ASAE: American Society of Association Executives

ASAHP: American Society of Allied Health Professions

ASCOTA: former name for the American Student Committee of the Occupational Therapy Association (AOTA), presently named Assembly of Student Delegates

ASD: Assembly of Student Delegates (AOTA)

ASHA: American Speech-Language-Hearing Association

ASHT: American Society of Hand Therapists

ASI: Assessment Systems, Inc.

ASPA: Association of Specialized and Professional Accreditors

BC/BS: Blue Cross/Blue Shield Association

BCPE: Board for Certification in Professional Ergonomics

BHP: Bureau of Health Professions (DHHS)

BLS: Bureau of Labor Statistics (DOL)

BOC: Board of Commissioners (JCAHO)

BPD: Bureau of Policy Development (HCFA)

BPO: Bureau of Operations (HCFA)

BPPC: Bylaws, Policies, and Procedures Committee (AOTA)

CAAHEP: Commission on Accreditation of Allied Health Education Programs

CAHEA: Committee on Allied Health Education and Accreditation (AMA)

CAPTE: Commission on Accreditation in Physical Therapy Education

CARF: Commission on Accreditation of Rehabilitation Facilities

CBO: Congressional Budget Office

CCB: Child Care Bureau

CCD: Consortium for Citizens with Disabilities

CCR&R: Child Care Resource and Referral Agency

CCY: Coalition for Children and Youth

CDC: Centers for Disease Control and Prevention

CEC: Council for Exceptional Children

CEDC: Certification Exam Development Committee (NBCOT)

CHF: Coalition for Health Funding

CHHA/CHS: Council of Home Health Agencies and Community Health Services (NLN)

CLEAR: Clearinghouse on Licenser, Enforcement, and Regulation

CMD: Conference and Meetings Department (AOTA)

CME: Council on Medical Education (AMA)

CMHS: Center for Mental Health Services (a component of the Substance Abuse and Mental Health Services Administration, U.S. Department of Health and Human Services)

CMS: Centers for Medicare & Medicaid Services

COE: Commission on Education (AOTA)

COP: Commission on Practice (AOTA)

COPA: Council on Postsecondary Accreditation

CORE: Commission on Rehabilitation Education

CRAC: Credentials Review and Accountability Committee (AOTA)

CSAP: Committee of State Association Presidents (AOTA)

CSG: Council of State Governments

CSN: Children's Safety Network

CSS: Children's Specialty Services

CWLA: Child Welfare League of America

DAHEA: Division of Allied Health Education and Accreditation (AMA)

DAHP: Division of Associated Health Professions (DHHS)

DDSIS: Developmental Disabilities Special Interest Section (AOTA)

DHHS: Department of Health and Human Services

DOE: Department of Education

DOL: Department of Labor

DPS: Department of Professional Services (AOTA)

DRC: Documents Review Committee (COE-AOTA)

EB: Executive Board (AOTA)

ECELS: Early Childhood Education Linkage System

EDSIS: Education Special Interest Section (AOTA)

EFA: Epilepsy Foundation of America

EHA: Education of Handicapped Act

ESRC: Educational Standards Review Committee (COE-AOTA)

FAC: Fiscal Advisory Committee (AOTA)

FAHD: Forum on Allied Health Data

FAO: United Nations Food and Agriculture Organization

FAST: Families and Schools Together

FDA: Food and Drug Administration (DHHS)

FEC: Federal Election Commission

FEHBP: Federal Employees Health and Benefits Program

FM: Financial Management Department

F&O: Finance and Operations Division (AOTA)

FRC: Fiscal Review Committee (AOTA)

FTC: Federal Trade Commission

FUSA: Families United for Senior Action

GAO: Government Accounting Office

GMENAC: Graduate Medical Education National Advisory Committee

GSA: Gerontological Society of America

GSIS: Gerontology Special Interest Section (AOTA)

GU: Generations United

GWSAE: Greater Washington Society of Association Executives

HCFA: Health Care Financing Administration (DHHS) renamed Centers for Medicare & Medicaid Services (CMS)

HCHSIS: Home and Community Health Special Interest Section (AOTA)

HCPAC: Health Care Professionals Advisory Committee (AMA)

HCPDG: Health Care Professionals Discussion Group

HFMA: Healthcare Financial Management Association

HIAA: Health Insurance Association of America

HMHB: Healthy Mothers, Healthy Babies Coalition

HMO: health maintenance organization

HRA: Health Resources Administration (DHHS)

HRSA: Health Resources and Services Administration (DHHS)

HSF: Health Services Foundation

HSQB: Health Standards and Quality Bureau (HCFA)

HT CC: Hand Therapy Certification Commission

ICC: Intercommission Council (AOTA)

IDEA: Individuals with Disabilities Education Act

IHS: Indian Health Service

IOM: Institute of Medicine

IRB: Institutional Review Board

IRS: Internal Revenue Service

IRSG: Insurance Rehabilitation Study Group

JCAHO: Joint Commission on Accreditation of Healthcare Organizations

LDA: Learning Disabilities Association

MCH: Maternal and Child Health (DHHS)

MCHB: Maternal and Child Health Bureau (DHHS)

MDAA: Muscular Dystrophy Association of America

MHARC: Mental Health Action Research Connection

MHSIS: Mental Health Special Interest Section (AOTA)

MPI: Meeting Planners International

MRC: Medical Research Council

NAATRP: National Association of Activity Therapy and Rehabilitation Programs

NACCRRA: National Association of Child Care Resource and Referral Agencies

NACOSH: National Advisory Committee on Scouting for the Handicapped

NADT: National Association for Drama Therapy

NAEYC: National Association for Education of Young Children

NAHB/NRC: National Association of Home Builders/National Research Center

NAHC: National Association for Home Care

NAHHA: National Association of Home Health Agencies

NAMI: National Alliance for the Mentally Ill

NAMME: National Association of Medical Minority Educators

NAMT: National Association for Music Therapy

NAPHS: National Association of Psychiatric Health Systems

NAPNAP: National Association of Pediatric Nurse Associates and Practitioners

NAPSO: National Alliance of Pupil Service Organizations

NARA: National Association of Rehabilitation Agencies

NARC: National Association for Retarded Citizens

NARF: National Association of Rehabilitation Facilities

NASA: National Aeronautics and Space Agency

NASDSE: National Association of State Directors of Special Education

NASL: National Association for the Support of Long Term Care

NASMHPR: National Association of State Mental Health Program Directors

NASUA: National Association of State Units on Aging

NASW: National Association of Social Workers

NAVESP: National Association of Vocational Education Special Personnel

NBCOT: National Board for Certification in Occupational Therapy, Inc.

NC: Nominating Committee (COE-AOTA)

NCAHE: National Commission on Allied Health Education

NCBFE: National Center for a Barrier Free Environment

NCCNHR: National Citizens Coalition for Nursing Home Reform

NCD: National Council on Disability

NCDPEH: National Coalition for Disease Prevention and Environmental Health

NCEMCH: National Center for Education in Maternal and Child Health

NCES: National Center for Education Statistics (DHHS)

NCHC: National Council on Health Care Technologists

NCHCA: National Commission for Health Certifying Agencies

NCHHA: National Council of Homemakers and Home Health Aides

NCHP: National Council for Health Planning

NCHS: National Center for Health Statistics (DHHS)

NCIL: National Council on Independent Living

NCMRR: National Center for Medical Rehabilitation Research

NCOA: National Council on Aging

NCSL: National Conference of State Legislatives

NDTA: Neurodevelopmental Treatment Association

NHC: National Health Council

NHLA: National Health Lawyers Association

NHO: National Hospice Organization

NHTSA: National Highway Traffic Safety Administration

NIA: National Institute on Aging

NIAAA: National Institutes on Alcohol Abuse and Alcoholism (Public Health Service)

NICCYD: National Information Center for Children and Youth with Disabilities

NIDA: National Institute of Drug Abuse

NIDRR: National Institute on Disability and Rehabilitation Research

NIH: National Institutes of Health

NIHR: National Institute of Handicapped Research

NIMH: National Institute of Mental Health

NLN: National League for Nursing

NLRB: National Labor Relations Board

NMHA: National Mental Health Association

NMSS: National Multiple Sclerosis Society

NO: National Office (AOTA)

NOS: National Office Staff (AOTA)

NPSRC: National Professional Standards Review Council

NRA: National Rehabilitation Association

NRC: National Research Council

NRCA: National Rehabilitation Counseling Association

NRTI: National Rehabilitation Training Institutes

NSPOT: National Society for the Promotion of Occupational Therapy

NUCEA: National University Continuing Education Association

NVOILA: National Voluntary Organizations for Independent Living for the Aging

OCR: Office of Civil Rights

OE: Office of Education

OH: Office of the Handicapped

OIG: Office of the Inspector General

OMB: Office of Management and Budget (Executive Office of the President)

OPM: Office of Personnel Management

OPRR: Office for Protection from Research Risks (DHHS)

OPRS: Office of Professional Research Services (AOTA)

OSEP: Office of Special Education Programs

OSERS: Office of Special Education and Rehabilitation Services (DOE)

OSG: Office of the Surgeon General

OSHA: Occupational Safety and Health Administration

OTPAC: Occupational Therapy Political Action Committee

OVR: Office of Vocational Rehabilitation

OWH: Office of Women's Health (DHHS)

PAC: Program Advisory Committee (AOTA)

PAC-APTA: Political Action Committee—American Physical Therapy Association

PATH: Partners Appropriate Technology for the Handicapped

PCMA: Professional Convention Management Association

PCPD: President's Committee on People with Disabilities

PDSIS: Physical Disabilities Special Interest Section (AOTA)

PEP: Professional Enhancement Project (AOTA)

PILOT: Project for Independent Living in Occupational Therapy (AOTA)

PIVOT: Planning and Implementing Vocational Readiness in Occupational Therapy (AOTA)

PPO: preferred provider organization

PPS: Prospective Payment System

PROPAC: Prospective Payment Assessment Commission

PRRB: Provider Reimbursement Review Board

PRSA: Public Relations Society of America

PSRO: Professional Standards Review Organization

PTAC: Professional and Technical Advisory Committee (JCAHO)

PVA: Paralyzed Veterans of America

RA: Representative Assembly (AOTA)

RAC: Research Advisory Committee (AOTA)

RAE: Roster of Accreditation Evaluators (AC-AOTA)

RRC: Regional Review Consultants (AOTA)

RSA: Rehabilitation Services Administration (DOE)

SAMHSA: Substance Abuse and Mental Health Services Administration (DHHS)

SAP: State Association President (AOTA)

SEC: Standards and Ethics Commission (AOTA)

SISIS: Sensory Integration Special Interest Section (AOTA)

SISSC: Special Interest Section Steering Committee

SNAP: Society of National Association Publications

SOTA: Student Occupational Therapy Association (AOTA)

SRC: Standards Review Committee (AOTA)

SSA: Social Security Administration (DHHS)

SSSIS: School System Special Interest Section (AOTA)

TASH: The Association for Persons with Severe Handicaps

TRB: Transportation Research Board

TSIS: Technology Special Interest Section (AOTA)

UCPA: United Cerebral Palsy Association
USDA: United States Department of Agriculture

VA: Department of Veterans Affairs
VA DM&S: Veterans Administration Department of Medicine and Surgery
VEWAA: Vocational Evaluation and Work Adjustment Association (NRA)

WCPT: World Confederation of Physical Therapists
WFOT: World Federation of Occupational Therapists
WHCOA: White House Conference on Aging
WHIF: Washington Health Issues Forum
WHO: World Health Organization
WIC: Women in Communication
WPSIS: Work Programs Special Interest Section (AOTA)

Adaptive Nutrition

Claudette L. Peck, LCMHC, RD, LD

Vitamin (Fat-Soluble)	RDA for Most Adults	Function	Food Sources	Drug Interactions*
Vitamin A	Males 900 µg/day Females 700 µg/day	Normal vision, reproduction, gene expression, and immunity	Liver, dairy foods, fish, dark-colored fruits, and leafy vegetables	Aluminum hydroxide, cholestyramine, mineral oil, warfarin (Coumadin)
Vitamin D	200 to 400 IU/day	Maintains serum calcium and phosphorus levels	Fish liver oils, flesh from fatty fish, fortified dairy foods, and cereal	Digoxin, mineral oil, aluminum hydroxide, cholestyramine
Vitamin E	15 mg/day	Antioxidant	Vegetable oils, whole grains, and nuts	Warfarin (Coumadin), mineral oil, aluminum hydroxide, cholestyramine

Jacobs, K., & Simon, L. (Eds.). *Quick Reference Dictionary for Occupational Therapy, Sixth Edition* (pp. 378-388). © 2015 SLACK Incorporated.

Vitamin (Fat-Soluble)	RDA for Most Adults	Function	Food Sources	Drug Interactions*
Vitamin K	Males 120 µg/day Females 90 µg/day	Blood clotting, bone metabolism	Dark leafy green vegetables, broccoli, brussels sprouts, cabbage	Warfarin (Coumadin), mineral oil, aluminum hydroxide, cholestyramine
Thiamin (B$_1$)	Males 1.2 mg/day Females 1.1 mg/day	Coenzyme in metabolism of carbohydrates and branched chain amino acids	Enriched, fortified whole-grain products, breads, cereals, grains	Aluminum hydroxide
Riboflavin (B$_2$)	Males 1.3 mg/day Females 1.1 mg/day	Coenzyme in numerous cellular reactions	Organ meats, milk, fortified cereals and breads	
Niacin (B$_3$)	Males 16 mg/day Females 14 mg/day	Essential for energy metabolism, coenzyme for oxidation reactions	Meat, fish, poultry, enriched and fortified bread and grain products	

Vitamin (Fat-Soluble)	RDA for Most Adults	Function	Food Sources	Drug Interactions*
Vitamin B_6	1.3 to 1.7 mg/day	Coenzyme in metabolism of amino acids and glycogen	Fortified cereals, organ meats, fortified soy-based meat substitutes	Levodopa, phenytoin, hydralazine, isoniazid, penicillamine
Vitamin B_{12}	2.4 µg/day	Coenzyme in nucleic acid metabolism; prevents megaloblastic anemia	Fortified cereals, meats, fish, poultry	Cimetidine, neomycin
Vitamin C	Males 90 mg/day Females 75 mg/day	Cofactor for reactions involving copper and iron; antioxidant	Citrus fruits, tomatoes and tomato products, cauliflower, spinach, strawberries, bell peppers, broccoli	
Folate	400 µg/day	Coenzyme in metabolism of nucleic and amino acids; prevents megaloblastic anemia	Dark leafy green vegetables, enriched cereals and bread products, whole grains	
Pantothenic acid	5 mg/day	Coenzyme in fatty acid metabolism	Chicken, beef, organ meats, potatoes, oats, egg yolk, cereals, whole grains	

Vitamin (Fat-Soluble)	RDA for Most Adults	Function	Food Sources	Drug Interactions*
Biotin	30 µg/day	Coenzyme in synthesis of fats, glycogen, and amino acids	Liver, smaller amounts in fruits and meats	
Choline	Males 550 mg/day Females 425 mg/day	Precursor for acetylcholine and phospholipids	Milk, liver, eggs, peanuts	
Calcium	1000 to 1200 mg/day	Blood clotting, muscle contraction, nerve transmission, and bone and tooth formation	Dairy foods, kale, broccoli, Chinese cabbage, calcium-set tofu	Digitalis, HCTZ, laxative (abuse), phenytoin, verapamil
Copper	900 µg/day	Component of enzymes in iron metabolism	Organ meat, seafood, nuts, seeds, wheat bran, whole grains, cocoa	Penicillamine
Fluoride	Males 4 mg/day Females 3 mg/day	Prevents dental caries, stimulates new bone growth	Fluoridated water, marine fish, dental products	
Iodine	150 µg/day	Component of thyroid hormones, prevents goiter and cretinism	Marine originated foods, iodized salt	

Vitamin (Fat-Soluble)	RDA for Most Adults	Function	Food Sources	Drug Interactions*
Iron	Males 8 mg/day Females 18 mg/day	Component of hemoglobin and numerous enzymes; prevents microcytic hypochromic anemia	Red meats, poultry (heme sources); fortified cereals, vegetables, fruits (non-heme sources)	Penicillamine, aspirin, calcium carbonate
Magnesium	Males 420 mg/day Females 320 mg/day	Cofactor for enzyme systems	Green leafy vegetables, whole kernel grains, nuts, meat, milk	Ethanol
Molybdenum	45 μg/day	Cofactor for enzymes involved in catabolism of sulfur amino acids, purines, pyridines	Legumes, grains, nuts	
Phosphorus	700 mg/day	Maintenance of pH, storage and transfer of energy	Dairy products, meat, eggs, peas, some cereals and breads	Antacids
Potassium	2000 to 3000 mg/day**	Regulates fluid, electrolyte balance, maintains normal blood pressure, transmits nerve and muscle impulses	Potatoes, legumes, dairy products, fish, fruits, fruit juices, and various vegetables	Furosemide, HCTZ, spironolactone, ethanol

Health-Related Condition	Nutrition Intervention
Limited range of motion*	Curved-handled utensils; built-up utensils; cup holder; long, bendable straws; plate guard; nosey cut-out cups/mugs
Chewing/swallowing disorders (dysphagia)*	Mechanical alteration in diet; should be assessed by speech-language pathologist to determine food/liquid consistency; may consider mechanical soft diet, ground diet, puréed diet, full liquid diet, and/or thickened liquids such as syrup-consistency, honey-consistency, or pudding-consistency for better swallowing ability; may need to limit/avoid mixed-consistency foods (i.e., stews, noodle soups, casseroles) to avoid aspiration; ensure proper positioning of posture for optimal swallow during mealtimes; keep upright at 30 to 45 degrees for at least 45 minutes post meals
Dry mouth*	Thicken liquids or thin purées; use gravies, sauces, or creamed soups to moisten foods; if liquids are not restricted, encourage frequent liquids; avoid hot, spicy, or acidic foods

*Adapted from Robinson, G. E., & Leif, B. J. (2001). *Nutrition management and restorative dining for older adults: Practical interventions for caregivers.* Chicago, IL: American Dietetic Association.

Recommended Websites

Diabetes
http://ndep.nih.gov
www.diabetes.org

Heart Disease, Hypertension, Hypercholesterolemia
www.americanheart.org
www.nhlbi.nih.gov

Irritable Bowel Syndrome/Disease, Crohn's Disease
http://digestive.niddk.nih.gov/ddiseases/pubs/crohns
http://digestive.niddk.nih.gov/ddiseases/pubs/ibs

Lactose Intolerance, Celiac Disease/Gluten Intolerance
http://digestive.niddk.nih.gov/ddiseases/pubs/lactoseintolerance
www.csaceliacs.org/recipes.php
www.nlm.nih.gov/medlineplus/celiacdisease.html

Osteoporosis
www.niams.nih.gov/Health_Info/Bone/Osteoporosis/default.asp

Weight Control/Weight Loss/Weight Management
www.healthyweightnetwork.com
www.niddk.nih.gov/health/nutrit/nutrit.htm

American Occupational Therapy Association *Core Values and Attitudes of Occupational Therapy Practice*

INTRODUCTION

In 1985, the American Occupational Therapy Association (AOTA) funded the Professional and Technical Role Analysis study (PATRA). This study had two purposes: to delineate the entry-level practice of OTs and OTAs through a role analysis and to conduct a task inventory of what practitioners actually do. Knowledge, skills, and attitude statements were developed to provide a basis for the role analysis. The PATRA study completed the knowledge and skills statements. The Executive Board subsequently charged the Standards and Ethics Commission (SEC) to develop a statement that would describe the attitudes and values that undergrid the profession of occupational therapy. The SEC wrote this document for use by AOTA members.

The list of terms used in this statement was originally constructed by the American Association of Colleges of Nursing (AACN) (1986). The PATRA committee analyzed the knowledge statements that the committee had written and selected those terms for the AACN list that best identified the values and attitudes of our profession. This list of terms was then forwarded to the SEC by the PATRA committee to use as the basis for the *Core Values and Attitudes* paper.

Jacobs, K., & Simon, L. (Eds.). *Quick Reference Dictionary for Occupational Therapy, Sixth Edition* (pp. 389-394).
© 2015 SLACK Incorporated.

The development of this document is predicated on the assumption that the values of occupational therapy are evident in the official documents of the American Occupational Therapy Association. The official documents that were examined are: (a) "Dictionary Definition of Occupational Therapy" (AOTA, 1986), (b) *The Philosophical Base of Occupational Therapy* (AOTA, 1979), (c) *Essentials and Guidelines for an Accredited Educational Program for the Occupational Therapist* (AOTA, 1991a), (d) *Essentials and Guidelines for an Accredited Educational Program for the Occupational Therapy Assistant* (AOTA, 1991b), and (e) *Occupational Therapy Code of Ethics* (AOTA, 1988). It is further assumed that these documents are representative of the values and beliefs reflected in other occupational therapy literature.

A *value* is defined as a belief or an ideal to which an individual is committed. Values are an important part of the base or foundation of a profession. Ideally, these values are embraced by all members of the profession and are reflected in the members' interactions with those persons receiving services, colleagues, and the society at large. Values have a central role in a profession and are developed and reinforced throughout an individual's life as a student and as a professional.

Actions and *attitudes* reflect the values of the individual. An attitude is the disposition to respond positively or negatively toward an object, person, concept, or situation. Thus, there is an assumption that all professional actions and interactions are rooted in certain core values and beliefs.

SEVEN CORE CONCEPTS

In this document, the *core values and attitudes* of occupational therapy are organized around seven basic concepts: altruism, equality, freedom, justice, dignity, truth, and prudence. How these core values and attitudes are expressed and implemented by occupational therapy practitioners may vary depending on the environments and situations in which professional activity occurs.

Altruism is the unselfish concern for the welfare of others. This concept is reflected in actions and attitudes of commitment, caring, dedication, responsiveness, and understanding.

Equality requires that all individuals be perceived as having the same fundamental human rights and opportunities. This value is demonstrated by an attitude of fairness and impartiality. We believe that we should respect all individuals, keeping in mind that they may have values, beliefs, or lifestyles that are different form our own. Equality is practiced in the broad professional arena but is particularly important in day-to-day interactions with those individuals receiving occupational therapy services.

Freedom allows the individual to exercise choice and to demonstrate independence, initiative, and self-direction. There is a need for all individuals to find a balance between autonomy and societal membership that is reflected in the choice of various patterns of interdependence with the human and nonhuman environment. We believe that individuals are internally and externally motivated toward action in a continuous process of adaptation throughout the life span. Purposeful activity plays a major role in developing and exercising self-direction, initiative, interdependence, and relatedness to the world. Activities verify the individual's ability to adapt, and they establish a satisfying balance between autonomy and societal membership. As professionals, we affirm the freedom of choice for each individual to pursue goals that have personal and social meaning.

Justice places value on the upholding of such moral and legal principles as fairness, equality, truthfulness, and objectivity. This means that we aspire to provide occupational therapy services for all individuals who are in need of these services and that we will maintain a goal-directed and objective relationship with all of those served. Practitioners must be knowledgeable about and have respect for the legal rights of individuals receiving occupational therapy services. In addition, the occupational therapy practitioner must understand and abide by the local, state, and federal laws governing professional practice.

Dignity emphasizes the importance of valuing the inherent worth and uniqueness of each person. This value is demonstrated by an attitude of empathy and respect for the self and others. We believe that each individual is a unique combination of biologic endowment, sociocultural heritage, and life experiences. We view human beings holistically, respecting the unique interaction of the mind, body, and physical and social environment. We believe that dignity is nurtured and grows from the sense of competence and self-worth that is integrally linked to the person's ability to perform valued and relevant activities. In occupational therapy, we emphasize the importance of dignity by helping the individual build on his or her unique attributes and resources.

Truth requires that we be faithful to facts and reality. Truthfulness, or veracity, is demonstrated by being accountable, honest, forthright, accurate, and authentic in our attitudes and actions. There is an obligation to be truthful with ourselves, those who receive services, colleagues, and society. One way that this is exhibited is through maintaining and upgrading professional competence. This happens, in part, through an unfaltering commitment to inquiry and learning, to self-understanding, and to the development of an interpersonal competence.

Prudence is the ability to govern and discipline one's self through the use of reason. To be prudent is to value judiciousness, discretion, vigilance, moderation, care, and circumspection in the management of one's affairs; to temper extremes; to make judgments, and to respond on the basis of intelligent reflection and rational thought.

SUMMARY

Beliefs and values are those intrinsic concepts that underlie the core of the profession and the professional interactions of each practitioner. These values describe the profession's philosophy and provide the basis for defining purpose. The emphasis or priority that is given to each value may change as one's professional career evolves and as the unique characteristics of a situation unfold. The evolution of values is developmental in nature. Although we have basic values that cannot be violated, the degree to which certain values will take priority at a given time is influenced by the specifics of a situation and the environment in which it occurs. In one instance, dignity may be a higher priority than truth; in another, prudence may be chosen over freedom. As we process information and make decisions, the weight of the values that we hold may change. The practitioner faces dilemmas because of conflicting values and is required to engage in thoughtful deliberation to determine where the priority lies in a given situation.

The change for us all is to know our values, be able to make reasoned choices in situations of conflict, and be able to clearly articulate and defend our choices. At the same time, it is important that all members of the profession be committed to a set of common values. This mutual commitment to a set of beliefs and principles that govern our practice can provide a basis for clarifying expectations between the recipient and the provider of services. Shared values empowers the profession and builds trust among ourselves and with others.

REFERENCES

American Association of Colleges of Nursing. (1986). *Essentials of college and university education for professional nursing, Final report.* Washington, DC: Author.

American Occupational Therapy Association. (1979). The philosophical base of occupational therapy. *Am J Occup Ther, 33,* 785.

American Occupational Therapy Association. (1986, April). Dictionary definition of occupational therapy. Adopted and approved by the Representative Assembly to fulfill Resolution #596-83. (Available from AOTA, 4720 Montgomery Lane, Bethesda, MD 20814-3425.)

American Occupational Therapy Association. (1988). Occupational therapy code of ethics. *Am J Occup Ther, 42,* 795-796.

American Occupational Therapy Association. (1991a). Essentials and guidelines for an accredited educational program for the occupational therapist. *Am J Occup Ther, 45,* 1077-1084.

American Occupational Therapy Association. (1991b). Essentials and guidelines for an accredited educational program for the occupational therapy assistant. *Am J Occup Ther, 45,* 1085-1092.

Prepared by Elizabeth Kanny, MA, OTR, for the Standards and Ethics Commission (Ruth Hansen, PhD, OTR, FAOTA, Chairperson).

Approved by the Representative Assembly, July 1993.

SOURCE

AOTA. (1993). Core values and attitudes of occupational therapy practice. *American Journal of Occupational Therapy, 47*, 1085-1086.

American Occupational Therapy Association's Past Presidents

Name	Date
George E. Barton (Architect)	1917
William R. Dunton, MD	1917-1919
Eleanor Clarke Slagle (Social Worker)	1919-1920
Herbert J. Hall, MD	1920-1923
Thomas B. Kidner (Architect)	1923-1928
C. Floyd Havailand, MD	1928-1930
Joseph C. Doane, MD	1930-1939
Everett S. Elwood, MD	1939-1947
Winifred C. Kahmann, OTR	1947-1952
Henrietta W. McNary, OTR	1952-1955
Ruth A. Robinson, OTR	1955-1958
Helen S. Willard, OTR, FAOTA	1958-1961
Wilma L. West, MA, OTR, FAOTA	1961-1964
Ruth Brunyate Wiemer, OTR, FAOTA	1964-1967
Florence S. Cromwell, MA, OTR, FAOTA	1967-1973
Jerry A. Johnson, EdD, MBA, OTR, FAOTA	1973-1978
Mae D. Hightower-Vandamm, OTR, FAOTA	1978-1982
Carolyn M. Baum, MA, OTR, FAOTA	1982-1983
Robert K. Bing, EdD, MA, OTR, FAOTA	1983-1986
Elnora M. Gilfoyle, OTR, FAOTA	1986-1989
Ann P. Grady, MA, OTR, FAOTA	1989-1992

Jacobs, K., & Simon, L. (Eds.). *Quick Reference Dictionary for Occupational Therapy, Sixth Edition* (pp. 395-396). © 2015 SLACK Incorporated.

Name	Date
Mary M. Evert, MBA, OTR, FAOTA	1992-1995
Mary Foto, OT, FAOTA	1995-1998
Karen Jacobs, EdD, OTR/L, CPE, FAOTA	1998-2001
Barbara L. Kornblau, JD, OT/L, FAOTA, DAAPM, ABDA, CCM	2001-2004
Carolyn M. Baum, PhD, OTR/L, FAOTA	2004-2007
Penelope Moyers Cleveland, EdD, OTR/L, BCMH, FAOTA	2007-2010
Florence Clark, PhD, OTR/L, FAOTA	2010-2013
Virginia Stoffel, PhD, OT, BCMH, FAOTA	2013-2016

American Occupational Therapy Association Statements

MISSION STATEMENT

The AOTA advances the quality, availability, use, and support of occupational therapy through standard setting, advocacy, education, and research on behalf of its members and the public.

VISION STATEMENT

The contributions of occupational therapy to health, wellness, productivity and quality of life are widely used, understood, and valued by society.

CENTENNIAL VISION

We envision that occupational therapy is a powerful, widely recognized, science-driven, and evidence-based profession with a globally connected and diverse workforce meeting society's occupational needs (www.aota.org).

Reprinted with permission from the American Occupational Therapy Association.

Jacobs, K., & Simon, L. (Eds.). *Quick Reference Dictionary for Occupational Therapy, Sixth Edition* (p. 397).
© 2015 SLACK Incorporated.

Basic Signs and Tips for Communicating With Individuals With Hearing Impairments

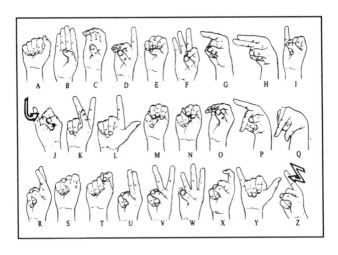

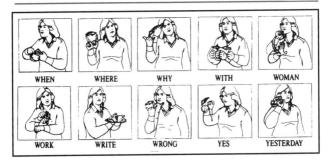

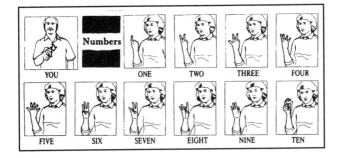

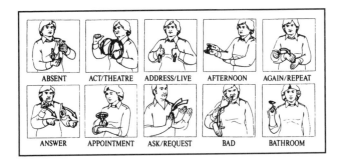

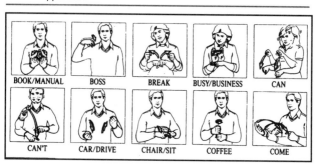

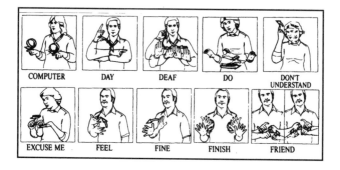

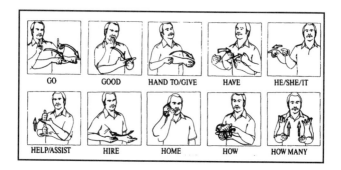

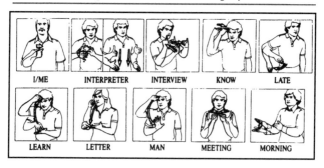

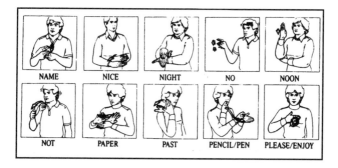

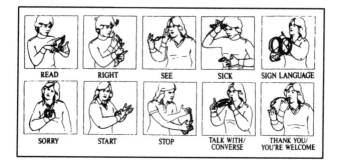

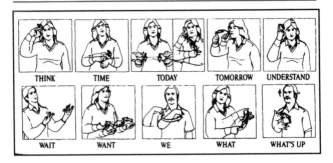

Reprinted with permission from the National Technical Institute for the Deaf, Rochester, NY.

Bones of the Body

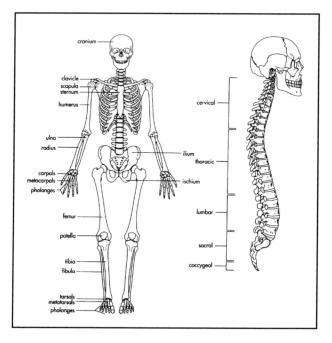

Reprinted with permission from Sladyk, K. (1997). *OT student primer: A guide to college success.* Thorofare, NJ: SLACK Incorporated.

Jacobs, K., & Simon, L. (Eds.). *Quick Reference Dictionary for Occupational Therapy, Sixth Edition* (p. 403).
© 2015 SLACK Incorporated.

Braille Alphabet

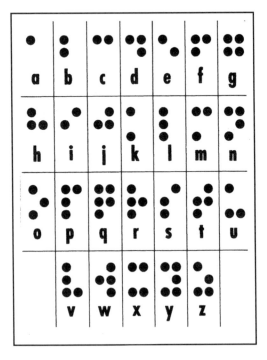

Reprinted with permission from the American Printing House for the Blind, Louisville, KY.

Jacobs, K., & Simon, L. (Eds.). *Quick Reference Dictionary for Occupational Therapy, Sixth Edition* (p. 404).
© 2015 SLACK Incorporated.

Brunnstrom's
Stages of Recovery

1st stage   Predominantly flaccid, no resistance to passive movement.

2nd stage   Spasticity develops and limb synergies or some of their components appear as associated reactions, minimal voluntary movement is present, gross grasp beginning, minimal finger flexion.

3rd stage   Spasticity increases, some voluntary control over limb synergy may occur. Contractures may have a tendency to develop; gross grasp and hook grasp possible.

4th stage   Nonsynergistic muscle movement is possible; spasticity begins to decline, gross grasp present, small amounts of finger extension and lateral prehension develop. Three movements that represent this stage: (1) shoulder flexion to 90 degrees with elbow extended, (2) pronation and supination with elbow flexed at 90 degrees, and (3) internal rotation at the shoulder demonstrating the ability to place affected arm behind back and touch sacral region.

Jacobs, K., & Simon, L. (Eds.). *Quick Reference Dictionary for Occupational Therapy, Sixth Edition* (pp. 405-406).
© 2015 SLACK Incorporated.

5th stage	Limb synergies lose their dominance over motor acts; more movement combinations performed with greater ease. Palmar prehension, cylindrical and spherical grasp may occur. Three movements that represent the 5th stage: (1) shoulder flexion greater than 90 degrees with elbow extended, (2) 90 degrees of shoulder abduction with elbow extended and forearm pronated, and (3) pronation and supination of forearm with extended elbow.
6th stage	Spasticity disappears except with rapid movement; coordination approaches normal, all types of prehension and individual finger motion occur.
Last stage	Motor function is restored.

Burn Chart—Rule of Nines

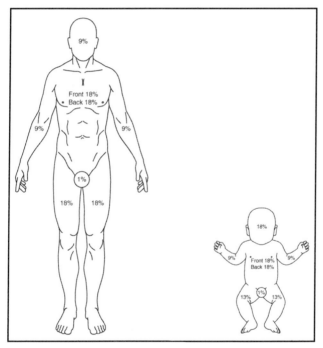

Disclaimer: While all attempts were made to keep this protocol updated, it may or may not represent the most current version of a protocol used in practice. Please use it at your own discretion.

Jacobs, K., & Simon, L. (Eds.). *Quick Reference Dictionary for Occupational Therapy, Sixth Edition* (p. 407). © 2015 SLACK Incorporated.

Classifications of Seizures and Epilepsy

CLASSIFICATIONS OF SEIZURES BY TYPE

Generalized—Excessive electrical discharge over a large portion of the brain; not one localized area.

1. **Absence (Formerly Petit Mal)**

   - Characterized by 5- to 15-second lapses in consciousness without abnormal movements

   - Individual appears to be staring into space or daydreaming, and the eyes may roll upward

   - Absences are not preceded by an aura, and activity can be resumed immediately afterward

   - Attack may go unnoticed

   - Typically occur in children and disappear by adolescence

   - May occur hundreds of times daily and markedly impair school performance

   - May evolve into other seizure types, such as complex-partial or tonic-clonic

   - Occurrence of absences in adulthood are rare

Jacobs, K., & Simon, L. (Eds.). *Quick Reference Dictionary for Occupational Therapy, Sixth Edition* (pp. 408-411).
© 2015 SLACK Incorporated.

2. **Atonic (Drop Attacks)**

   - Characterized by a sudden loss of muscle tone
   - Ranges from only a head drop to complete collapse

3. **Myoclonic**

   - Characterized by brief, involuntary muscle jerks
   - Can be in just the face or over the entire body
   - Individual may have just a simple seizure or several occurring in succession, leading to a tonic-clonic seizure

4. **Tonic-Clonic (Formerly Grand Mal)**

   - A generalized convulsion involving two phases: tonic phase—individual loses consciousness and falls, body becomes rigid; clonic phase—extremities jerk and twitch
   - After the seizure, consciousness is regained slowly
   - If the tonic-clonic seizure begins locally (with a partial seizure), it may be preceded by an aura; these seizures are said to be secondarily generalized

     Status epilepticus: A medical emergency in which an individual experiences continuous/continual tonic-clonic seizures usually lasting 30 minutes or more.

Partial—*Excessive electrical discharge in the brain is limited to one area; however, it may spread over the entire brain and become generalized.*

1. **Simple Partial (Formerly Focal Seizures)**

   - Individual experiences a range of strange or unusual sensations, including sudden, jerky movements or twitching; tingling sensation; hallucination of (or distortions in) smell, vision, hearing, or taste; stomach discomfort; and sudden sense of fear
   - Lasts several minutes
   - Consciousness is not impaired

     If another seizure type follows, these sensations may be referred to as an aura.

2. **Complex Partial (Formerly Psychomotor or Temporal Lobe)**

- Characterized by a complicated motor act involving impaired consciousness

- Individual appears dazed and confused; not responding if addressed

- Involuntary actions called automatisms may be seen, including random walking, mumbling, head turning, pulling at clothing, fumbling with buttons, staring, and lip-smacking

- Individual typically does not remember behaviors

CLASSIFICATIONS OF EPILEPSY BY CAUSE

Ideopathic—Cause is not known.

Symptomatic or Acquired—Cause is known and may be secondary to:

- Traumatic injury—cortico-contusion (a lesion is the focal point of emanating electrical impulses)

- Extremely high fever at birth/infancy

- Tumor

- Stroke

- Infectious process (meningitis, encephalitis)

- Toxic metabolic problems (kidney/liver failure)

- Withdrawal from alcohol, drugs, prescribed medicine (i.e., benzodiazepines, valium antidepressants, lithium, etc.)

- High doses of pharmacological substances (i.e., asthma medications)

OTHER IMPORTANT TERMS

Aura

- Sensations experienced prior to the onset of a seizure

- If the individual is aware of the aura, it may occur far enough in advance to give the person time to avoid possible injury

- These vary from person to person and can include change in body temperature; feeling of tension, anxiety, or fear; musical sound; strange taste; particular curious odor

- If the individual is able to give the physician a good description of this aura, it may provide a clue to the part of the brain where the initial discharges originate

    An aura could occur without being followed by a seizure and in some cases can by itself be called a type of simple partial seizure.

Triggers

- Stimuli that tend to increase seizure evocation, including but not limited to flashing lights (strobe), sleep deprivation, loud noises, certain musical notes, monotonous sounds, alcohol or other mind-altering substances, hypoglycemia, and sexual arousal/orgasm

- Varies from person to person

BIBLIOGRAPHY

Clayman, C. B. (1997). *The American Medical Association home medical encyclopedia.* New York, NY: Random House.

Patrick, A. (1998). *Epilepsy FAQ.* Retrieved from www.faqs.org/faqs/medicine/epilepsy-faq/

Cranial Nerves

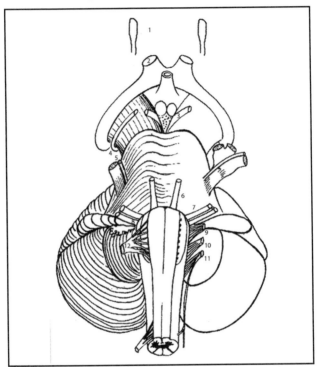

Anterior view of the cerebellum. 1 = olfactory, 2 = optic, 3 = oculomotor, 4 = trochlear, 5 = trigeminal (motor and sensory roots), 6 = abducens, 7 = facial, 8 = vestibulocochlear (acoustic and vestibular), 9 = glossopharyngeal, 10 = vagus, 11 = accessory, 12 = hypoglossal. Figure modified from http://anatmac3.citi2.fr/anatomie/icongraphie/schemas/Dessin/Dessins1/6.GIF. Illustrated by Dr. Dominique Bastian. Reprinted with permission.

Jacobs, K., & Simon, L. (Eds.). *Quick Reference Dictionary for Occupational Therapy, Sixth Edition* (pp. 412-415).
© 2015 SLACK Incorporated.

The positioning of the subject for cranial nerve assessment varies according to the nerve being tested. The examiner's action also will vary according to the cranial nerve being tested. The absence, delay, or asymmetry of a response indicates possible involvement of the particular nerve that is being tested.

CRANIAL NERVE I (OLFACTORY)

The examiner places an object that has a strong, identifiable odor just under the nasal area of the subject in an attempt to assess the ability to perceive the odor. An ammonia capsule is typically used for this test.

CRANIAL NERVE II (OPTIC)

The examiner asks the subject to identify objects within view and to clarify what the subject actually sees (e.g., letters of the alphabet, numbers, pictures of objects, etc.).

CRANIAL NERVE III (OCULOMOTOR)

The examiner asks the subject to elevate the eyelid and elevate, depress, and adduct the eyes. Voluntary motor control of levator palpebrae; superior, medial, and inferior recti; and the inferior oblique eye muscles are the primary function of the oculomotor nerve.

CRANIAL NERVE IV (TROCHLEAR)

The examiner asks the subject to elevate the eyes (look up). The trochlear nerve primarily functions in voluntary motor control of the superior oblique eye muscle.

CRANIAL NERVE V (TRIGEMINAL)

A sensory assessment for integrity of the trigeminal nerve is the ability of the subject to perceive touch along the skin of the face. To test motor function, the examiner asks the subject to perform the motions of elevation, protrusion, retrusion, and lateral deviation of the mandible. The chief function of the trigeminal nerve is the sensation of touch and pain on the skin of the face, mucous membranes of the nose, sinuses, mouth, and anterior tongue. It functions also in voluntary motor control of the muscles of mastication.

CRANIAL NERVE VI (ABDUCENS)

The examiner asks the subject to abduct the eye (keeping head in one place and looking side to side). The chief function of the abducens nerve is voluntary motor control of the lateral rectus muscle of the eye.

CRANIAL NERVE VII (FACIAL)

To test sensation of the facial nerve, the examiner assesses the subject's ability to distinguish identifiable tasting substances with the anterior portion of the tongue. Motor function is tested by having the subject (1) elevate, adduct, or depress the eyebrow; (2) close the eyes; (3) flare and constrict the nose; (4) close the mouth; and (5) close and protrude the lips. The primary function of the facial nerve is taste along the anterior portion of the tongue and voluntary motor control of facial muscles.

CRANIAL NERVE VIII (VESTIBULOCOCHLEAR)

The examiner asks the subject to stand with eyes closed and no support in order to assess the subject's balance. The chief function of the vestibulocochlear nerve is hearing and balance via the ear.

CRANIAL NERVE IX (GLOSSOPHARYNGEAL)

To test sensation of the glossopharyngeal nerve, the examiner assesses the subject's ability to distinguish identifiable objects and/or substances with the posterior portion of the tongue. To establish motor integrity, the examiner asks the subject to swallow. The primary function of the glossopharyngeal nerve is the sensation of touch and pain on the posterior portion of the tongue and pharynx, taste on the posterior portion of the tongue, and voluntary motor control of some muscles of the pharynx.

CRANIAL NERVE X (VAGUS)

The examiner assesses the status of the subject's abdominal and thoracic viscera. The chief function of the vagus nerve is sensation of touch and pain of the pharynx, larynx, and bronchi. Autonomic muscle control of the thoracic and abdominal viscera is also a primary function.

CRANIAL NERVE XI (ACCESSORY)

The examiner asks the subject to elevate (shrug) the shoulders. The primary function of the accessory nerve is voluntary control of the sternocleidomastoid and the trapezius.

CRANIAL NERVE XII (HYPOGLOSSAL)

The examiner asks the subject to protrude the tongue. The primary function of the hypoglossal nerve is voluntary control of the muscles of the tongue.

Text reprinted with permission from Bottomley, J. (2000). *Quick reference dictionary for physical therapy.* Thorofare, NJ: SLACK Incorporated.

Dermatomes

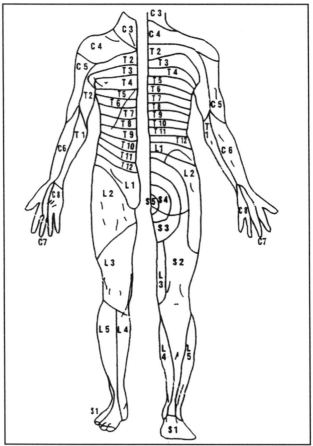

Descriptions of Occupational Therapy

Developed by Scott McNeil, OTD, MS, OTR/L

What is occupational therapy? Every student and practitioner has been asked this very question countless times. The following descriptions of occupational therapy have been collected from professional organizations, leaders in the profession of occupational therapy, and practitioners. These descriptions are designed to provide you with some assistance to help those not familiar with occupational therapy understand what we do.

DESCRIPTIONS OF OCCUPATIONAL THERAPY

- Occupational therapy (noun): Therapy based on engagement in meaningful activities of daily life (such as self-care skills, education, work, or social interaction) especially to enable or encourage participation in such activities despite impairments or limitations in physical or mental functioning (*Merriam Webster Online Dictionary*, 2013).

- Occupational therapy is a skilled rehabilitation service that helps people across the lifespan participate in the things they want and need to do through the therapeutic use of everyday activities (occupations) (American Occupational Therapy Association [AOTA], 2013a).

Jacobs, K., & Simon, L. (Eds.). *Quick Reference Dictionary for Occupational Therapy, Sixth Edition* (pp. 417-429).
© 2015 SLACK Incorporated.

- AOTA's Definition of Occupational Therapy for the Model Practice Act defines occupational therapy as "The therapeutic use of everyday life activities (occupations) with individuals or groups for the purpose of participation in roles and situations in home, school, workplace, community, and other settings. Occupational therapy services are provided for the purpose of promoting health and wellness and to those who have or are at risk for developing an illness, injury, disease, disorder, condition, impairment, disability, activity limitation, or participation restriction. Occupational therapy addresses the physical, cognitive, psychosocial, sensory, and other aspects of performance in a variety of contexts to support engagement in everyday life activities that affect health, well-being, and quality of life" (AOTA, 2010).

- Occupational therapy is a client-centered health profession that assists clients throughout the lifespan who have difficulty engaging in meaningful everyday life activities (occupations). "Occupations include, but are not limited to: self-care, education, social participation, managing household tasks, caring for others, leisure, play, work, and rest/sleep" (AOTA, 2004, 2008, 2010).

- "Occupational therapy is the art and science of enabling engagement in everyday living, through occupation; of enabling people to perform the occupations that foster health and well-being; and of enabling a just and inclusive society so that all people may participate to their potential in the daily occupations of life (Townsend & Polatajko, 2007, p. 372). Occupation refers to everything that people do during the course of everyday life. Each of us have many occupations that are essential to our health and well-being. Occupational therapists believe that occupations describe who you are and how you feel about yourself. A child, for example, might have occupations as a student, a playmate, a dancer and a table-setter" (Canadian Association of Occupational Therapists, 2013).

- "Occupational therapy is a client-centred health profession concerned with promoting health and well-being through occupation. The primary goal of occupational therapy is to enable people to participate in the activities of everyday life. Occupational therapists achieve this outcome by working with people and communities to enhance their ability to engage in the occupations they want to, need to, or are expected to do, or by modifying the occupation or the environment to better support their occupational engagement" (World Federation of Occupational Therapists, 2012).

- Occupational therapy practitioners have specialized training in the physical, social, psychological, neurological, and cognitive aspects of human performance. They also have expertise related to the social, cultural, and physical environment and how its interaction with human performance can maximize self-esteem, independence, and quality of life.

- Occupational therapy is focused on "supporting health and participation in life through engagement in occupation" (AOTA, 2008, p. 3).

- Occupational therapy helps people live life to its fullest!

DESCRIPTIONS OF OCCUPATIONAL THERAPY FROM LEADERS IN THE PROFESSION

"Occupational therapy (I deliberately say this and not just 'OT') is a profession who works with people across their lifespan and enables participation in everyday occupations like living, learning, working, and playing. We know that there is a relationship between active engagement in doing the things you want and need to do and your state of health. You define what it means to be 'living life to its fullest' and an occupational therapy practitioner will help you to accomplish that, thereby helping to achieve health and well-being."

—Virginia Stoffel, PhD, OT, BCMH, FAOTA
President of the American Occupational Therapy Association
June 12, 2013

"Occupational therapy is a health and wellness profession that assists people in developing the skills they need to participate in everyday life where they live, work, and play."

—**Amy Lamb, OTD, OTRL, FAOTA**
Vice President of the American Occupational Therapy Association
March 5, 2013

DEFINITIONS OF OCCUPATIONAL THERAPY FROM MEMBERS OF THE OCCUPATIONAL THERAPY COMMUNITY

- "Occupational therapy is helping a client by having them engage in meaningful activities in order for them to lead what they believe to be an independent life" (E. Wagenhorst, personal communication, July 18, 2008).

- "Occupational therapists use educational, vocational, [and] rehabilitation activities and adaptive approaches to help people of all ages with physical, psychosocial, or environment challenges to learn or regain the skills or adaptive techniques they need to participate fully in valued life roles and activities" (A. Solomon, personal communication, July 19, 2008).

- "The therapeutic use of activities that have meaning to the individual, to maximize their ability to occupy themselves, as they choose, throughout their life" (Y. Hachtel, personal communication, July 19, 2008).

- "Occupational therapy is about enabling people to do whatever they need/want to be able to do, regardless of their issue(s)" (L. Gelnick, personal communication, July 20, 2008).

- "An OT's job is to help you do your job, whether it be mother, student, engineer, etc., to the best of your ability, the way you want to, and with the adaptations and modifications necessary to be successful" (D. Morin, personal communication, July 20, 2008).

- "Occupational therapy is a health profession that empowers people to achieve their goals" (M. Zavala, personal communication, July 20, 2008).

- "Occupational therapists help people help themselves" (J., personal communication, July 20, 2008).

- "Occupational therapy is a helping profession that helps one do the things they do every day, through reengineering those parts of activity one finds difficult or unable to do due to an illness, injury, or genetic difference. More simply put 'OT is the things you do every day'" (J. Harper, personal communication, July 20, 2008).

- "OT helps people with the doing of things" (K. Santos, personal communication, July 20, 2008).

- "I still love the AOTA tag line from a few years back—I suggest 'OT teaches people skills for the job of living'" (T. Jones, personal communication, July 21, 2008).

- "Occupational therapy is used to help a person fulfill his/her life roles and to do it with the most independence possible" (D. Gruber, personal communication, July 21, 2008).

- "Maximum independence in the least restrictive setting" (J. Titus, personal communication, July 21, 2008).

- "Occupational therapy is a unique, creative rehabilitation profession that focuses on helping people of all ages to improve their quality of life in terms of independence, productivity, and/or overall well-being, in spite of whatever physical, mental, situational, or emotional challenges they face" (J. McCabe, personal communication, July 21, 2008).

- "Occupational therapy focuses on a person's ability to engage in the meaningful occupations of day-to-day life such as self-care, education, work, play, and leisure" (C. Clerico, personal communication, July 21, 2008).

- "Occupational therapy helps individuals of all ages with physical, cognitive, emotional, or developmental deficits reach their highest level of functional performance and teaches care providers how to safely help the individuals be as independent as possible" (C. Clerico, personal communication, July 21, 2008).

- "Function...function...function. I help people regain independence and dignity after disease or disability has limited their abilities in daily activities. Occupational therapy not only works on movement, we take it one-step further and bring meaning of a real life activity to rehabilitation" (B. Alwood-Wallace, personal communication, July 21, 2008).

- "Occupational therapy provides treatment and/or new ideas on how to be as independent and self-sufficient as possible in the necessary activities that you do daily" (L. Weber, personal communication, July 21, 2008).

- "Occupational therapy helps people, across the life span, who have physical, cognitive, or visual difficulties be able to engage in all the meaningful daily tasks that 'occupy' their time" (S. Clark, personal communication, July 22, 2008).

- "Occupational therapy: Empowering people since 1917" (J. Neely, personal communication, July 22, 2008).

- "OT is the therapy dedicated to facilitation and promotion of participation of occupations, those tasks and activities most valued by the person, using evidence-based modalities (S. Levandowski, personal communication, July 23, 2008).

- "Occupational therapy: A rehabilitation process to improve performance in life tasks of self-care, work, leisure, education, and social participation by improving skills, abilities, and motivation through preparation for and engagement in purposeful and occupation-based activity" (S. Luster, personal communication, July 23, 2008).

- "Helping people who have sustained a trauma or disability to learn or relearn to do the activities that typically occupy their time" (S. Thanel, personal communication, July 23, 2008).

- "Occupational therapy: The manual and verbal interventions that enable physical, cognitive, and psychosocial recovery of an individual's functional abilities" (J. Perry, personal communication, July 24, 2008).

- "Occupational therapy is therapeutic intervention focused on improving a person's quality of life while addressing deficits impairing [one's] ability to complete any activity [he or she] values during [his or her] daily routine, which can include, but is not limited to, self-care activities, tasks associated with performance of [one's] job, home management, driving, and volitional activities" (R. Reilly, personal communication, July 24, 2008).

- "Occupational therapy is the premier profession that promotes maximum functional independence in the home, workplace, and the community through therapeutic strategies in the rehabilitation or habilitation of individuals with physical, developmental, emotional, and/or behavioral challenges" (D. Tobin, personal communication, July 25, 2008).

- "Occupational therapy is the portion of the rehabilitation team that works with persons of any age or disability to teach them ways to compensate so that they can add life to living" (M. Rinas, personal communication, July 25, 2008).

DESCRIPTIONS OF OCCUPATIONAL THERAPY BY PRACTICE AREA

Children and Youth

- "Occupational therapy practitioners work with infants, toddlers, children, and youth and their families in a variety of settings, including schools, clinics, and homes, to support the occupations that support their health, well-being, and development" (L. Collins, personal communication, February 19, 2013).

- Occupational therapy focuses on various areas of development (physical, cognitive, communication, social-emotional, and adaptive) and the client's ability to participate in daily activities at home, school, day care, and in the community (Clark, Polichino, & Jackson, 2004).

- Occupational therapy is often provided through the school system for children between ages 3 and 21 years. Intervention is focused on identifying student strengths and the barriers that may be interfering with learning and participation in the school setting and is a part of the child's individualized education program.

- "Occupational therapy practitioners facilitate development of sensory, motor, emotional, and social skills to help children be successful in the everyday occupations of play, self-care, education, productivity, and rest and sleep. OT's provide direct service to children, as well as adapt environments, consult, and support teachers, parents, and families in this process" (K. Loukas, personal communication, June 13, 2013).

- "The art and privilege of supporting accessibility, play, function, and participation in the lives of children" (S. Levandowski, personal communication, June 10, 2013).

Mental Health

- "Occupational therapy supports mental health among all client[s], using a shared decision-making process that is person centered and client driven. A primary goal of practitioners is to facilitate resiliency, health, and wellness in the community of the individual's choice, rather than to manage symptoms. Occupational therapy interventions are based on the idea that people with mental illness can and do recover and lead satisfying, meaningful, and productive lives" (L. Collins, personal communication, February 19, 2013).

- Occupational therapy practitioners have specialized training in the psychosocial dimensions of occupation and human performance. They combine this knowledge with the therapeutic use of activity to help people understand and control their feelings to attain the ability to cope and manage daily living roles and occupations (Ramsey, 2004).

- Occupational therapy has its roots in mental health and focuses on the mind-body interrelationship that can lead to a disruption in a client's ability to complete necessary and valued occupations (Ramsey, 2004).

- "Occupational therapists help people identify and achieve their goals related to daily occupations—work or school, play, self-care, and socializing" (J. Froehlich, personal communication, June 10, 2013).

Rehabilitation, Disability, and Participation

- "Occupational therapy practitioners help clients who are recovering from illness or injury, or who have a disability, to become as independent as possible and to participate in all of their valued occupations and roles" (L. Collins, personal communication, February 19, 2013).

- Occupational therapy helps clients manage the physical, psychosocial, and contextual challenges of an acute illness or injury. They work with each client to maximize participation in meaningful, everyday activities, and create a safe plan for discharge from the hospital.

- Occupational therapy emphasizes the strengths and abilities of the client while many other disciplines may focus on impairment and disability.

- Occupational therapy is often the first therapy discipline a client will see on the first morning of his or her rehabilitation program.

- Occupational therapy practitioners assist clients navigate and actively participate at home and in every aspect of the community.

Productive Aging

- "Occupational therapy focuses on ways to help people maintain their independence and valued roles as they age (which often includes a desire to age in place) by addressing community mobility (either driving or other options), home modifications, falls prevention, cognitive disorders, disease or disability management, safety concerns, and any other potential barriers to participation" (L. Collins, personal communication, February 19, 2013).

- Occupational therapists "promote and support occupational engagement and performance to enable adults to remain where they want to live, doing what they want to do" (Dorne & Kurfuerst, 2008).

- "Occupational therapy helps older clients look at the everyday activities that are important to them. Together, we try to come up with ways to make it safer and easier for our clients to get back to their daily routine, while staying safe at home" (J. Romeo, personal communication, June 8, 2013).

Health and Wellness

- Occupational therapy promotes health and well-being through active involvement in meaningful occupations. By helping clients eliminate barriers, enhance their self-management skills, improve their performance of daily activities, and adopt healthy habits and routines, occupational therapy unlocks the door to participation across the lifespan (AOTA, n.d.).

- Occupational therapists believe that "engagement in meaningful occupations supports health and leads to a productive and satisfying life" (AOTA, 2007, p. 2).

- "Occupational therapists can promote healthy lifestyles and access to health maintenance services for all clients and their families in the home communities regardless of wellness, illness, or disability status" (Hildenbrand & Froehlich, 2002).

- Occupational therapists' "ability to recognize and eliminate environmental barriers, analyze promotion program strategies for person-task fit, and facilitate adaptation and accommodation allow us to advocate for services that support healthful behaviors in all people" (Hildenbrand & Froehlich, 2002).

- "Occupational therapy practitioners work with individuals and/or populations of people to facilitate adaptation in lifestyle indicated by occupational engagement in work, positioning, stress management, coping, family changes, physical or mental impairments, caretaking, and aging. Engagement in life-enriching, safe, and meaningful occupation is part of a healthy lifestyle and is the right of all human beings" (K. Loukas, personal communication, June 13, 2013).

Work and Industry

- The goal of occupational therapy is to provide the returning worker with tasks that are meaningful and to facilitate the worker's complete and total independence and function at work (AOTA, 2013b).

- Occupational therapists can recommend environmental and behavioral adaptations to decrease the frequency of musculoskeletal disorders and injuries at various worksites (Dale, 2008).

- Occupational therapists have knowledge of anatomy, physiology, task analysis, and biomechanics, which can be applied to injury prevention, return to work programs, and ergonomics consulting (Fontana, 1999).

- Occupational therapy services provided include "an assessment of ability to work, interventions to enhance work performance, the identification of accommodations necessary for return-to-work, and the prevention of work-related injury, illness, and disability" (AOTA, 2007).

REFERENCES

American Occupational Therapy Association. (n.d.). *Occupational therapy's role in health promotion*. Retrieved from www.aota.org

American Occupational Therapy Association. (2004). Scope of practice. *American Journal of Occupational Therapy, 58*, 673-677.

American Occupational Therapy Association. (2007). *Occupational therapy in the promotion of health and the prevention of disease and disability statement*. Retrieved from www.aota.org

American Occupational Therapy Association. (2008). Occupational therapy practice framework: Domain and process (2nd ed.). *American Journal of Occupational Therapy, 62*, 625-683.

American Occupational Therapy Association. (2010). Scope of practice. *American Journal of Occupational Therapy, 64*(Suppl.), S70-S77. doi: 10.5014/ajot.2010.64S70-64S77

American Occupational Therapy Association. (2013a). *About occupational therapy*. Retrieved from www.aota.org

American Occupational Therapy Association. (2013b). *Returning to work*. Retrieved from www.aota.org

Canadian Association of Occupational Therapists. (2013). *What is occupational therapy?* Retrieved from www.caot.ca/default.asp?pageid=3824

Clark, F. G., Polichino, J., & Jackson, L. (2004). Occupational therapy services in early intervention and school-based programs. *American Journal of Occupational Therapy, 58*, 681-685.

Dale, L. (2008). Occupational therapy, communications, and industry. Partners for learning and OT service delivery. *OT Practice, 13*(12), 10-13.

Dorne, R., & Kurfuerst, S. (2008, March). Productive aging and occupational therapy: A look ahead. *Gerontology Special Interest Section Quarterly, 31*(1), 1-4.

Fontana, P. (1999, December). Pushing the envelope: Entering the industrial arena. *OT Practice Online*. Retrieved from http://fontanacenter.com/site39.php

Hildenbrand, W. C., & Froehlich, K. (2002). Promoting health: Historical roots, renewed vision. *OT Practice 7*(5), 10-15. Retrieved from www.familysuccessbydesign.org/pdf/2008-AOTA-HCH-March08.pdf

Merriam Webster Online Dictionary. (2013). *Occupational therapy*. Retrieved from www.merriam-webster.com/dictionary/occupational-therapy

Ramsey, R. (2004). Psychosocial aspects of occupational therapy. *American Journal of Occupational Therapy, 58,* 669-672.

World Federation of Occupational Therapists. (2012). *Definition of occupational therapy.* Retrieved from www.wfot.org/aboutus/aboutoccupationaltherapy/definitionofoccupationaltherapy.aspx

Diseases, Pathologies, and Syndromes Defined

achlorhydria: A condition resulting in the absence of hydrochloric acid in gastric juice.

acquired brain injury: An injury to the brain that has occurred after birth, usually not caused by blunt force trauma. Examples include brain injuries due to stroke, near drowning, hypoxia, anoxia, tumor, neurotoxins, electric shock, or lightning strike.

acquired immunodeficiency syndrome (AIDS): AIDS is characterized by progressive destruction of cell-mediated (T cell) immunity (as well as humoral immunity) resulting in susceptibility to opportunistic diseases. It is a syndrome caused by the human immunodeficiency virus that renders immune cells ineffective, permitting opportunistic infections, malignancies, and neurologic diseases to develop; it is transmitted sexually or through exposure to contaminated blood.

acromegaly: A disease that develops after closure of the epiphyses of the long bones affecting the bones of the face, jaw, hands, and feet. Acromegaly (hyperpituitarism) occurs as a result of excessive secretion of growth hormone after normal completion of body growth. Results in increased bone thickness and hypertrophy of the soft tissues due to growth hormone-secreting adenomas of the anterior pituitary gland.

Adams-Stokes syndrome: A condition characterized by sudden attacks of unconsciousness, with or without convulsions, which frequently accompanies heart block.

Jacobs, K., & Simon, L. (Eds.). *Quick Reference Dictionary for Occupational Therapy, Sixth Edition* (pp. 430-489).
© 2015 SLACK Incorporated.

Addison's disease: A disease characterized by a bronze-like pigmentation of the skin, severe prostration, progressive anemia, low blood pressure, diarrhea, and digestive disturbance. It is due to disease (hypofunction) of the adrenal glands and is usually fatal.

adhesive capsulitis: *Also known as* periarthritis or frozen joints, it is characterized by diffuse joint pain and loss of motion in all directions, often with a positive painful arc test and limited joint accessory motions.

adult respiratory distress syndrome (ARDS): ARDS is a group of symptoms that accompany acute respiratory failure following a systemic or pulmonary insult. *Also known as* shock lung, wet lung, stiff lung, adult hyaline membrane disease, post-traumatic lung, or diffuse alveolar damage (DAD).

allergy: *See* hypersensitivity disorder.

Alzheimer's disease (AD): Alzheimer's disease is a progressive dementia characterized by a slow decline in memory, language, visuospatial skills, personality, cognition, and motor skills. It is a disabling neurological disorder that may be characterized by memory loss; disorientation; paranoia; hallucinations; violent changes of mood; loss of ability to read, write, eat, or walk; and finally dementia. It usually affects people over the age of 65 and has no known cause or cure.

amyotrophic lateral sclerosis (ALS): A progressive neurodegenerative disease of the nerve cells located in the brain and spinal cord that control voluntary movement. As motor neurons degenerate, they can no longer send impulses to the muscle fibers that normally result in muscle movement. Early symptoms of ALS often include increasing muscle weakness, especially involving the arms and legs, speech, swallowing or breathing. Most commonly diagnosed between ages 40 and 70. *Synonym*: Lou Gehrig's disease.

anemia: A reduction in the oxygen-carrying capacity of the blood owing to an abnormality in the quantity or quality of erythrocytes (RBC). Hemoglobin is < 14 g/dL for men and < 12 g/dL for women. Hematocrit is < 41% for men and < 37% for women.

anencephaly: The most severe form of neural tube defects in which there is no development above the brainstem; absence of the brain.

aneurysm: A condition in which there is an abnormal stretching (dilation) in the wall of an artery, a vein, or the heart. The structure can weaken to the point of rupture.

Angelman syndrome (AS): A neurogenetic disorder that occurs in 1 in 15,000 live births. AS is often misdiagnosed as cerebral palsy or autism. Characteristics of the disorder include developmental delay, lack of speech, seizures, and walking and balance disorders. Individuals with Angelman syndrome will require life-long care (Angelman Syndrome Foundation, 2014).

ankylosing spondylitis: Ankylosing spondylitis is an inflammatory arthropathy of the axial skeleton including the sacroiliac joints, apophyseal joints, costovertebral joints, and the intervertebral disc articulations. Results in the dissolution of a vertebrae.

anorexia nervosa: Anorexia nervosa is an eating disorder in which the individual refuses to eat. It is characterized by severe weight loss in the absence of physical cause and attributed to emotions such as anxiety, irritation, anger, and fear. It is characterized by distortion of body image and fear of becoming fat. The individual does not eat enough to maintain appropriate weight (maintenance of weight 15% below normal for age, height, and body type is indicative of anorexia). Most often occurs in adolescent girls and young women.

anterior cerebral artery syndrome: Infarction in the territory of the anterior cerebral artery is uncommon, but when it occurs it results in profound abulia or a delay in verbal and motor response with paraplegia.

anterior cord syndrome: Damage to the anterior and anterolateral aspect of the cord results in bilateral loss of motor function and pain and temperature sensation due to interruption of the anterior and lateral spinothalamic tracts and corticospinal tract. Frequently associated with flexion injuries.

anterior inferior cerebellar artery syndrome: A stroke-related syndrome in which the principle symptoms include ipsilateral deafness, facial weakness, vertigo, nausea and vomiting, nystagmus (or rhythmic oscillations of the eye), and ataxia. Horner's syndrome ptosis, miosis (constriction of the pupil), and loss of sweating over the ipsilateral side of the face may also occur. A paresis of lateral gaze may be seen. Pain and temperature sensation is lost on the contralateral side of the body.

anterograde amnesia: A disorder of recent memory in which there is failure of new learning.

anxiety disorder: A generalized emotional state of fear and apprehension that is usually associated with a heightened state of physiologic arousal, such as elevation in heart rate and sweat gland activity.

aortic stenosis: Progressive valvular calcification of the bicuspid valve.

Apert syndrome: This is a genetic craniofacial/limb anomaly characterized by specific malformations of the skull, midface, hands, and feet. The skull is prematurely fused and cannot grow normally, the midface (i.e., middle of the eye socket to the upper jaw) appears sunken in, and the fingers and toes are fused together (*see* syndactyly). Apert syndrome occurs in approximately 1 per 160,000 to 200,000 live births (Apert International, 2014).

aphasia: Impairment of the comprehension and production of speech caused by brain injury, can also affect reading and writing.

appendicitis: Inflammation of the vermiform appendix that often results in necrosis and perforation with subsequent localized or generalized peritonitis.

apraxia: A collective term used to describe impairment in carrying out purposeful movements.

Arnold-Hilgartner hemophilic arthropathy: A condition in hemophilic individuals beginning with soft tissue swelling of the joints, osteoporosis and overgrowth of epiphysis with no erosion or narrowing of cartilage space. It leads to subchondral bone cysts, squaring of the patella, significant cartilage space narrowing and ending in fibrous joint contracture, loss of joint cartilage space, marked enlargement of the epiphyses, and substantial disorganization of the joints.

arrhythmia(s): Disturbances of heart rate or rhythm caused by an abnormal rate of electrical impulse generation by the sinoatrial (SA) node or the abnormal conduction of impulses. Sinus arrhythmia is an irregularity in rhythm that may be a normal variation or may be caused by an alteration in vagal stimulation. Atrial fibrillation (involuntary, irregular muscular contractions of the atrial myocardium) is the most common chronic arrhythmia; it occurs in rheumatic heart disease, dilated cardiomyopathy, atrial septal defect, hypertension, mitral valve prolapse, and hypertrophic cardiomyopathy. Ventricular fibrillation (involuntary contractions of the ventricular muscle) is a frequent cause of cardiac arrest. Heart block is a disorder of the heartbeat caused by an interruption in the passages of impulses through the heart's electrical system. Causes include CAD, hypertension, myocarditis, overdose of cardiac medications (such as digitalis), and aging.

arteriosclerosis (obliterans): Artherosclerosis in which proliferation of the intima has caused complete obliteration of the lumen of the artery. Arteriosclerosis represents a group of diseases characterized by thickening and loss of elasticity of the arterial walls, often referred to as "hardening of the arteries."

arteritis: A vasculitis primarily involving multiple sites of the temporal and cranial arteries.

arthrogryposis multiplex congenita (AMC): A nonprogressive neuromuscular syndrome in which multiple congenital contractures, either in flexion or extension, are present at birth. There are three types of AMC: (1) contracture syndromes, (2) amyoplasia (lack of muscle formation or development), and (3) distal arthrogryposis, primarily affecting the hands and feet. The child is born with stiff joints and weak muscles.

ascites: An abnormal accumulation of serous (edematous) fluid within the peritoneal cavity, the potential space between the lining of the liver and the lining of the abdominal cavity. Most often caused by cirrhosis, but other diseases associated with ascites include heart failure, constrictive pericarditis, abdominal malignancies, nephrotic syndrome, and malnutrition.

asthma: An inflammatory condition of the lungs with secondary bronchospasm marked by recurrent attacks of dyspnea, with wheezing due to the spasmodic constriction of the bronchi.

atelectasis: The collapse of normally expanded and aerated lung tissue at any structural level (e.g., lung parenchyma, alveoli, pleura, chest wall, bronchi) involving all or part of the lung.

atherosclerosis: This condition represents a group of diseases characterized by thickening and loss of elasticity of the arterial walls, often referred to as "hardening of the arteries."

athetoid cerebral palsy (Vogt's syndrome): A type of cerebral palsy that is a muscular disorder characterized by continuous, slow, twisting motions of the upper and lower extremities and facial and trunk musculature.

attention deficit disorder (ADD): Characterized by inability to focus attention and impulsiveness; often diagnosed in children.

attention deficit hyperactivity disorder (ADHD): Characterized by inability to focus attention, impulsiveness, and hyperactivity; often diagnosed in children.

autism: Autism is a complex developmental disability that typically appears during the first 3 years of life and affects a person's ability to communicate, read facial expressions, and interact with others. Autism is defined by a certain set of behaviors including repetitive actions, self-stimulation (e.g., rocking, hand flapping, spinning), avoidance of eye contact, and echoalia. Autism is a "spectrum disorder" that affects individuals differently and to varying degrees.

autistic spectrum disorders (ASDs): ASDs are a group of developmental disabilities that can cause significant social, communication, and behavioral challenges. ASDs affect individuals differently, and the spectrum includes those who are severely affected and experience great difficulty in communicating and building relationships to those with more mild forms, such as Asperger's, who mainly have difficulty with obsessive interests and social situations.

autoimmune disease: A category of conditions in which the cause involves immune mechanisms directed against self-antigens. The body fails to distinguish self from non-self, causing the immune system to direct immune responses against normal (self) tissue and become self-destructive.

avascular necrosis (AVN): Death of bone and/or cartilaginous tissue as a result of having a poor or absent blood supply. *See also* osteonecrosis.

bacterial infection(s): An infection process in which a bacterial organism establishes a parasitic relationship with its host.

Barlow's syndrome: Mitral valve prolapse. A slight variation in the shape or structure of the mitral valve occurs, which causes prolapse. *Also known as* floppy valve syndrome or click-murmur syndrome.

basal cell carcinoma: A slow-growing surface epithelial skin tumor originating from undifferentiated basal cells contained in the epidermis. This type of carcinoma rarely metastasizes beyond the skin and does not invade blood or lymph vessels but can cause significant local damage.

basilar artery syndrome: Atheromatous lesions along the basilar trunk resulting in ischemia as a result of occlusion affect the brainstem, including the corticospinal tracts, corticobulbar tracts, medial and superior cerebellar peduncles, spinothalamic tracts, and cranial nerve nuclei. If the basilar artery is occluded, then the brainstem symptoms are bilateral. When a branch of the basilar artery is occluded, the symptoms are unilateral, involving sensory and motor aspects of the cranial nerves.

Bell's palsy: Facial paralysis due to a functional disorder of the seventh cranial nerve. A condition in which the facial nerve is unilaterally affected. Etiology is uncertain, although it is suggested that it is an inflammatory response in the auditory canal. Any agent that causes inflammation and swelling creates a compression that initially causes demyelination.

benign prostatic hyperplasia (BPH): An age-related nonmalignant enlargement of the prostate gland.

biliary cirrhosis: Primary biliary cirrhosis is one type of cirrhosis characterized by chronic, progressive, inflammatory liver disease. Secondary biliary cirrhosis can occur with prolonged partial or complete obstruction of the common bile duct or its branches.

boil: A painful nodule formed in the skin by inflammation of the dermis and subcutaneous tissue enclosing a central slough or "core." *Synonym:* furuncle.

botulism: Classified as a bacterial infection, botulism is a rare paralytic disease that has a predilection for the cranial nerves and then progresses caudally and symmetrically to the trunk and extremities. It is often caused by the ingestion of neurotoxins in food, which resist gastric digestion and proteolytic enzymes and are readily absorbed into the blood from the proximal small intestine.

brain abscess: Occurs when microorganisms reach the brain and cause a local infection.

brainstem syndrome: This syndrome reflects lesions of cranial nerves III through XII at the root, nuclear, or bulbar levels. Common symptoms are gaze palsies, a loss of active control of eye movement; nystagmus, involving rhythmic tremor of the eye; and dysarthria, abnormal speech resulting from poor control of the muscles of speech. Commonly associated with multiple sclerosis.

breast cancer: The most common malignancy of females in the United States. Most breast carcinomas are adenocarcinomas, derived from the glandular epithelium of the terminal duct lobular unit.

Broca's aphasia: Known as "nonfluent aphasia," a language impairment due to injury to the speech-related motor areas of the brain. Affects speech production and limits vocabulary.

bronchiectasis: A form of obstructive lung disease that is actually an extreme form of bronchitis. There is chronic dilation of the bronchi and bronchioles that develops when the supporting structures (bronchial walls) are weakened by chronic inflammatory changes associated with secondary infection.

bronchiolitis: Bronchiolitis is a commonly occurring acute, diffuse, and often severe inflammation of the lower airways (bronchioles) caused by a viral infection.

Brown-Séquard's syndrome: A set of symptoms caused by a primary intraspinal tumor in which there is nerve root pain followed by motor weakness and wasting of muscle supplied by the nerve. This syndrome involves motor changes of extramedullary lesions beginning with segmental weakness at the lesion site and progression to damage of half of the spinal cord. There is paralysis of motion on one side of the body and loss of sensation on the other, dependent on the site of the lesion involving one side of the spinal cord.

Buerger's disease: This condition is a vasculitis that causes inflammatory lesions of the peripheral blood vessels accompanied by thrombus formation and vasospasm occluding blood vessels. The pathogenesis of Buerger's disease is unknown; however, it is generally considered an inflammatory process. *Also known as* thromboangiitis obliterans.

bulimarexia: An eating disorder in which anorexia nervosa and bulimia nervosa coexist. This is characterized by a period of starving to lose weight, alternating with periods of binging and purging.

bulimia nervosa: Bulimia nervosa is a compulsive eating disorder characterized by episodic binge eating (consuming large amounts of food at one time) followed by purging behavior such as self-induced vomiting, fasting, laxative and diuretic abuse, and excessive exercising.

burns: Injuries that result from direct contact or exposure to any thermal, chemical, electrical, or radiation source. The depth of injury is a function of temperature or source of energy and duration of exposure.

cachexia: A state of ill health, malnutrition, and wasting. It may occur in many chronic diseases such as Alzheimer's disease, certain malignancies, and advanced pulmonary tuberculosis.

cancer: A term that refers to a large group of diseases characterized by uncontrolled growth and spread of abnormal cells. Other terms used interchangeably for cancer are *malignant neoplasm*, *tumor, malignancy*, and *carcinoma*. Cancer in its various forms is a genetic disease, characterized by deviations of the normal genetic mechanisms that regulate cell growth.

Caplan's syndrome: A condition associated with pneumoconiosis (see definition), which is characterized by the presence of rheumatoid nodules in the periphery of the lung.

carbuncle: A circumscribed inflammation of the skin and deeper tissues that terminates in a slough and suppuration or boil. Results in a painful node, covered by tight reddened skin and containing pus.

carcinoma: A new growth or malignant tumor enclosing epithelial cells in connective tissue and tending to infiltrate and give rise to metastases. It may affect almost any organ or part of the body and spreads by direct extension, through lymphatics, or the blood stream.

cardiomyopathy (CM): A group of conditions affecting the heart muscle so that contraction and relaxation of myocardial muscle fibers is impaired.

carpal tunnel syndrome (CTS): Entrapment and compression of the median nerve within the carpal tunnel of the wrist. Characterized by pain, tingling, numbness, paresthesia, and progressing to muscular weakness in the distribution of the median nerve.

celiac disease: The condition which is a symptom complex including: (1) steatorrhea (fat in feces), (2) general malnutrition, (3) abdominal distention, and (4) secondary vitamin deficiencies. The disease is defined by an inability to digest gluten, one of the proteins found in wheat, barley, rye, and oats.

central cord syndrome: A result of damage to the central aspect of the spinal cord, often caused by hyperextension injuries in the cervical region. There is characteristically more severe neurologic involvement in the upper extremities than in the lower extremities. Function is typically retained in the thoracic, lumbar, and sacral regions, including the bowel, bladder, and genitals, as peripherally located fibers are not affected.

cerebellar syndrome: Cerebellar syndrome deficits are usually symmetrical with all four limbs involved. Manifestations of cerebellar lesions are ataxia hypotonia and truncal weakness causing postural and movement disorders. Dysarthria of cerebellar origin (scanning speech, producing a prolonged, monotone sound) is common.

cerebral palsy (CP): A nonhereditary and nonprogressive lesion of the cerebral cortex resulting in a group of neuromuscular disorders of posture and voluntary movement, including lack of voluntary control, spasticity, impaired speech, vision, hearing, and perceptual functions, seizure disorder, hydrocephalus, microcephalus, or mental retardation. Damage to the motor area of the brain occurs during fetal life, birth, or infancy.

cerebral syndrome: Characterized by optic neuritis, the manifestation of demyelination of the optic nerve seen in multiple sclerosis and associated with visual field defects, decreased color vision, and reduced clarity of vision.

cerebrovascular accident (CVA): *See* stroke.

cerebrovascular disease: Intrinsic damage to the vessels of the brain causes by atherosclerosis, lipohyalinosis, inflammation, amyloid deposition, arterial dissection, developmental malformation, aneurysm, or venous thrombosis resulting in a stroke.

Charcot-Marie-Tooth disease: Peroneal muscular atrophy that is an inherited autosomal dominant disorder affecting motor and sensory nerves. Initially the disorder involves the peroneal nerve and affects muscles in the foot and lower leg. It later progresses to the hands and forearms.

childhood disintegrative disorder: Marked regression in multiple areas of functioning following a period of at least 2 years of apparently normal development. Onset of disorder takes place before age 10. Loss of previously acquired skills in at least two of the following areas: expressive or receptive language, social skills or adaptive behavior, bowel or bladder control, play, or motor skills.

cholangitis: Sclerosing cholangitis is an inflammatory disease of the bile ducts that has been linked to altered immunity, toxins, and infectious agents, and is thought to be of genetic etiology.

cholecystitis: Inflammation of the gallbladder as a result of impaction of gallstones in the cystic duct causing painful distention of the gall bladder.

choledocholithiasis: Calculi in the common bile duct in persons with gallstones.

cholelithiasis (gallstones): The formation or presence of gallstones that remain in the lumen of the gallbladder or are ejected with bile into the cystic duct.

chondrosarcoma: A tumor in which the neoplastic cells produce cartilage rather than the osteoid seen with the osteosarcoma.

chronic fatigue syndrome (CFS): A combination of symptoms hypothesized to be an autoimmune system response to stress. It is associated with severe and prolonged fatigue, low-grade fever, sore throat, painful lymph nodes, muscle weakness, discomfort or myalgia, sleep disturbances, headaches, migratory arthralgias without joint swelling or redness, photophobia, forgetfulness, irritability, confusion, depression, transient visual scotomata, difficulty thinking, and inability to concentrate.

chronic obstructive bronchitis: This condition is clinically defined as a condition of productive cough lasting for at least 3 months per year for 2 consecutive years. The primary distinction between chronic obstructive bronchitis and COPD is the chronic cough.

chronic obstructive pulmonary disease (COPD): This condition refers to a number of disorders that affect movement of air in and out of the lungs, particularly within the small airways. There is blockage of air and abnormalities of the lungs, causing an effect on expiratory flow. The most important of these disorders are obstructive bronchitis, emphysema, and asthma. *Also known as* chronic obstructive lung disease.

chronic pain disorder (syndrome): Chronic pain has been recognized as pain that persists past the normal time of healing. Chronic pain is often associated with depressive disorders, whereas acute pain appears to be associated with anxiety disorders.

chronic renal failure (CRF): The loss of nephrons results in progressive deterioration of glomerular filtration, tubular reabsorption, and endocrine functions of the kidneys. This ultimately leads to failure of the kidneys and affects all other body systems.

cirrhosis: A group of chronic end-stage diseases of the liver resulting from a variety of chronic inflammatory, toxic, metabolic, or congestive damage most commonly associated with alcohol abuse.

click-murmur syndrome: *See* Barlow's syndrome or mitral valve prolapse.

Clostridium difficile: A species of bacteria of the genus *Clostridium* that causes diarrhea and other intestinal disease. Often occurs when competing healthy bacteria are wiped out by antibiotics. In severely affected patients, the inner lining of the colon becomes severely inflamed with the potential to perforate. *Also known as* C-Diff.

cluster headache: A severe unilateral headache of relatively short duration. The episodic cluster headache is defined by a period of susceptibility to headache, called cluster periods, alternating with periods of remission. *Chronic cluster headache* is a term used when remissions have not occurred for at least 12 months.

coal workers' pneumoconiosis: Lung disease resulting from inhalation of coal dust.

colitis: An irritable bowel syndrome in which there is a suppression of normal gastrointestinal flora, the bacteria normally residing in the lumen of the intestines allowing yeasts and molds to flourish.

collagen vascular disease: This condition is associated with pulmonary manifestations, including exudative pleural effusion, pulmonary nodules, rheumatoid nodules, interstitial fibrosis, and pulmonary vasculitis. *Also known as* connective tissue disease.

congenital heart disease: An anatomic defect in the heart that develops in utero during the first trimester and is present at birth. There are two categories: cyanotic defects resulting from obstruction of blood flow to the lungs or mixing of desaturated blue venous blood with fully saturated red arterial blood within the chambers of the heart and acyanotic defects primarily involving left-to-right shunting of blood through an abnormal opening.

congenital hip dysplasia: Developmental dysplasia of the hip that is unilateral or bilateral and occurs in three forms: (1) unstable hip dysplasia in which the hip is positioned normally but can be dislocated by manipulation, (2) subluxation or complete dislocation in which the femoral head remains intact with the acetabulum, but the head of the femur is partially displaced or uncovered, and (3) complete dislocation in which the femoral head is totally outside the acetabulum.

congestive heart failure (CHF): A heart condition in which the heart is unable to pump sufficient blood to supply the body's needs. Congestive heart disease represents a group of clinical manifestations caused by inadequate pump performance from either the cardiac valves or the myocardium. There is excessive or abnormal accumulation of blood (congestion) in the heart. Causes mechanical or functional inadequacy to fully empty the blood from the heart, due to hypertrophic cardiac muscle changes.

connective tissue disease: A rheumatoid disease such as systemic lupus erythematosus, scleroderma, or polymyositis (see respective definitions).

Conn's syndrome: Conn's syndrome, or primary aldosteronism, is a metabolic disorder that occurs when an adrenal lesion results in hyper-secretion of aldosterone, the most powerful of the mineralocorticoids (aldosterone's primary role is to conserve sodium, and it also promotes potassium excretion). There is an excess of sodium in blood (hypernatremia), indicating water loss exceeding sodium loss; fluid volume excess (hypervolemia), leading to an increase in the volume of circulating fluid or plasma in the body; low blood levels of potassium (hypokalemia); and metabolic alkalosis. All of these factors lead to blood pressure increases.

constipation: A condition in which fecal matter is too hard to pass easily or in which bowel movements are so infrequent that discomfort and other symptoms interfere with activities of daily living.

contact dermatitis: An acute or chronic skin inflammation caused by exposure to a chemical, mechanical, physical, or biologic agent.

conversion disorder: A psychodynamic phenomenon rather than a behavioral response to illness or injury defined as a transformation of an emotion into a physical manifestation.

coronary heart (or artery) disease (CAD): Blockage of the coronary arteries of the heart leading to myocardial infarction, arrhythmias, or failure.

cor pulmonale: *Also known as* pulmonary heart disease, in which there is an enlargement of the right ventricle secondary to pulmonary hypertension that occurs in diseases of the thorax, lung, and pulmonary circulation. It is a term that describes the pathologic effects of lung dysfunction as it affects the right side of the heart. There is hypertrophy or failure of the right ventricle. Heart disease is secondary to disease of the lungs or of the lungs' blood vessels.

corticospinal syndrome: This syndrome involves the corticospinal tract and dorsal column and results in stiffness, slowness, and weakness of the limbs.

Creutzfeldt-Jakob disease: Presenile dementia that is chronic in nature. It is a rapidly dementing disease thought to be activated by a slow virus of genetic predisposition. Results in memory deficits and electroencephalographic changes, and myoclonus is prevalent. Involves the frontal lobe with symptoms of apathy, lack of personal care, and the display of psychomotor retardation. Motor symptoms include incontinence and seizures.

Crohn's disease: A chronic lifelong inflammatory disorder of the bowel that can affect any segment of the intestinal tract and even tissues in other organs. It is characterized by exacerbations and periods of remission.

Cushing's syndrome: A metabolic disorder, *also known as* hypercortisolism (hyperfunction of the adrenal gland), it is a condition in which there is increased secretion of cortisol by the adrenal cortex resulting in liberation of amino acids from muscle tissue with resultant weakening of protein structures. The end result includes a protuberant abdomen with striae ("stretch marks"), poor wound healing, generalized muscle weakness, and marked osteoporosis.

cystic fibrosis (CF): An inherited disease of the exocrine glands affecting the hepatic, digestive, male reproductive (the vas deferens is functionally disrupted in nearly all cases), and respiratory systems. The majority of morbidity and mortality is caused by lung disease, and almost all persons develop obstructive lung disease associated with chronic infection that leads to progressive loss of pulmonary function. Cystic fibrosis is a chronic, progressive disorder characterized by abnormal mucus secretion in the glands of the pancreas and lungs. It is usually diagnosed early in life due to frequent respiratory infections or failure to thrive.

cystitis: Lower urinary tract infection.

cystocele: A herniation of the urinary bladder into the vagina.

cytomegalovirus (CMV): A commonly occurring DNA herpes virus infection occurring congenitally, peri- or postnatally, or disseminated in immunocompromised persons. This infection increases in frequency with age.

dactylitis: Painful swelling of the hands or feet that occurs as a result of clot formation. Occurs most often in those individuals affected by sickle cell disease.

degenerative intervertebral disc disease: A degenerative joint process that applies to any synovial joint, including the facet joints or any intervertebral disc articulation of the spinal column. Events leading to disc degeneration include impaired cellular nutrition, reduced cellular viability, cellular senescence, accumulation of degraded matrix macromolecules, or fatigue failure of the matrix.

dehydration: Removal or loss of water from the body or a tissue; water deficit; severe dehydration may lead to acidosis, accumulation of waste products in the body (uremia), and fatal shock.

dementia: Irrecoverable deteriorative mental state, the common end result of many entities.

depression: A morbid sadness, dejection, or a sense of melancholy, distinguished from grief, which is a normal response to a personal loss.

dermatitis: Infection of the skin. *Eczema* and *dermatitis* are terms that are used interchangeably. A superficial inflammation of the skin due to irritant exposure, allergic sensitization (delayed hypersensitivity), or genetically determined idiopathic factors (e.g., eczema, atopic dermatitis, seborrheic dermatitis, etc.).

dermatomyositis: Diffuse, inflammatory myopathies that produce symmetrical weakness of striated muscle, primarily the proximal muscles of the shoulder and pelvic girdles, neck, and pharynx. This inflammatory disorder is related to the family of rheumatic diseases and has periods of exacerbations and remissions.

dermatophytosis: Fungal infections such as ringworm that are caused by a group of fungi that invade the stratum corneum, hair, and nails. These are superficial infections that live on, not in, the skin and are confined to the dead keratin layers, unable to survive in the deeper layers.

diabetes insipidus: Diabetes insipidus, a rare disorder, involves a physiologic imbalance of water secondary to antidiuretic hormone (ADH) deficiency. Injury or loss of function of the hypothalamus, the neurohypophyseal tract, or the posterior pituitary gland can result in diabetes insipidus.

diabetes mellitus (DM): A metabolic disorder in which the pancreas is unable to produce insulin, a substance the body needs to metabolize glucose as an energy source. A chronic, systemic disorder characterized by hyperglycemia (excess glucose in the blood) and disruption of the metabolism of carbohydrates, fats, and proteins. Insufficient insulin is produced in the pancreas resulting in high blood glucose levels. Over time, DM results in small- and large-vessel vascular complications and neuropathies.

diarrhea: Frequent, watery stools; results in poor absorption of water and nutritive elements and electrolytes, fluid volume deficit, and acidosis as a result of potassium depletion. Other systemic effects of prolonged diarrhea are dehydration, electrolyte imbalance, and weight loss.

diplopia: Damage to the third cranial nerve causing double vision.

discitis: A spinal infection affecting the disc, discitis can range from a self-limiting inflammatory process to a pyogenic infection. It may involve the intervertebral disc, vertebral end plates, or both.

discoid lupus erythematosus: A condition marked by chronic skin eruptions that if left untreated can lead to scarring and permanent disfigurement. Evidence suggests this is an autoimmune defect.

disseminated intravascular coagulation (DIC): Sometimes referred to as consumption coagulopathy, DIC is a thrombotic disease caused by overactivation of the coagulation cascade. It is an acquired disorder of platelet function, with diffuse or widespread coagulation occurring within arterioles and capillaries all over the body.

diverticular disease: The term used to describe diverticulosis (uncomplicated disease) and diverticulitis (disease complicated by inflammation). Diverticulosis refers to the presence of outpouchings (diverticula) in the wall of the colon or small intestine, a condition in which the mucosa and submucosa herniate through the muscular layers of the colon to form outpouching.

Down syndrome: A genetic disorder attributed to a chromosomal aberration referred to as trisomy 21. Down syndrome is characterized by muscle hypotonia, cognitive delay, abnormal facial features, and other distinctive physical abnormalities. Distinct physical characteristics include a large tongue, poor muscle tone, a flat face, and heart problems.

Duchenne's muscular dystrophy: Progressive fatal disorder of the skeletal muscles beginning in early childhood caused by a hereditary sex-linked gene on the X chromosome.

Dupuytren's contracture: A finger deformity characterized by the formation of a flexion contracture and thickening band of palmar fascia, usually involving the third and fourth digits accompanied by pain and decreased extension. Characterized by progressive fibrosis (increase in fibrous tissue) of the palmar aponeurosis, resulting in the shortening and thickening of the fibrous bands that extend from the aponeurosis to the bases of the phalanges. These fibrous bands pull the digits into such marked flexion at the metacarpophalangeal joints that they cannot be straightened.

dysarthria: Refers to a group of speech disorders resulting from weakness, slowness, or lack of coordination of the speech mechanism due to damage to any of a variety of points in the nervous system.

dysphagia: Difficulty swallowing, which may be caused by neurologic conditions, local trauma and muscle damage, or mechanical obstruction.

dysplasia: A general diagnostic category that indicates a disorganization of cells in which an adult cell varies from its normal size, shape, or organization.

dyspraxia: A disorder that affects motor skill development and manifests as difficulty with planning and completing fine motor tasks.

dystonia: A neurologic syndrome dominated by sustained muscle contractions frequently causing twisting and repetitive movements or abnormal postures often exacerbated by active voluntary movements. Dystonia is both a symptom and the name for a collection of neurologic disorders characterized by these movements and postures.

ectopic pregnancy: A pregnancy marked by the implantation of a fertilized ovum outside the uterine cavity.

eczema: *See* dermatitis.

edema: Excessive accumulation of interstitial fluid (fluid that bathes the cells), which may be localized or generalized.

emphysema: Emphysema is defined as a pathologic accumulation of air in tissues, particularly in the lungs. Distention of tissues is caused by gas or air in the interstices. In chronic pulmonary disease there is characteristic increase beyond the normal in the size of air spaces distal to the terminal bronchiole with destructive changes in the alveolar sac walls.

encephalitis: An acute inflammatory disease of the brain caused by direct viral invasion or hypersensitivity initiated by a virus.

encephalocele: Hernia protrusion of brain substance and meninges through a congenital or traumatic opening in the skull.

encephalocystocele: Hernia protrusion of the brain distended by fluid.

enchondroma: A common, benign tumor that arises from residual cartilage in the metaphysis of bone. The hand, femur, and humerus are common sites.

endocarditis: Infective, or bacterial, endocarditis is an infection of the endocardium, the lining inside the heart, including the heart valves.

endometriosis: A condition marked by functioning endometrial tissue found outside the uterus resulting in ectopic pregnancy.

entrapment syndromes: Entrapment or compression of peripheral nerves resulting from their proximity to bony, muscular, and vascular structures (*see* specific disorders: carpal tunnel syndrome, sciatica, Bell's palsy, tardy ulnar palsy, thoracic outlet syndrome, Saturday night palsy).

ependymoma: A neoplasm derived from the ependymal cell lining of the ventricular system and the central canal of the spinal cord. It is usually reddish, lobulated, and well circumscribed, resembling a cauliflower in shape.

epilepsy: A chronic disorder of various causes characterized by recurrent seizures due to excessive discharge of cerebral neurons.

Epstein-Barr virus (EBV): An acute infectious disease caused by EBV, a member of the herpes virus group. *Also known as* infectious mononucleosis.

Erb-Duchenne palsy: A paralysis of the upper limb resulting from a traction injury to the brachial plexus at birth. Erb-Duchenne palsy affects the C5-C6 nerve roots, whole-arm palsy affects C5-T1, and Klumpke's palsy affects the C8 and T1 (lower plexus) nerve roots.

Ewing's sarcoma: A malignant primary bone tumor. The pelvis and lower extremity are the most common sites. This malignant bone tumor often attacks the shaft of the long bones.

facioscapulohumeral muscular dystrophy: A mild form of muscular dystrophy beginning with weakness and atrophy of the facial muscles and shoulder girdle. Inability to close the eyes may be the earliest sign; the face is expressionless when laughing or crying, forward shoulders and scapular winging develop, and the person has difficulty raising the arms overhead.

factitious disorder: A psychophysiologic disorder characterized by somatic symptom production that is intentional or self-induced for the purpose of gaining attention by deceiving health care personnel or for personal gain.

fecal incontinence: Inability to control bowel movements. Psychological factors include anxiety, confusion, disorientation, and depression. Physiologic causes include neurologic sensory and motor impairment; anal distortion secondary to traumatic childbirth, sexual assault, hemorrhoids and hemorrhoidal surgery; altered levels of consciousness; and severe diarrhea.

fibromyalgia: Fibromyalgia or fibromyalgia syndrome, often mislabeled or misdiagnosed as fibrocytis, fibromyositis, nonarticular arthritis, myofascial pain, chronic fatigue syndrome, or systemic lupus erythematosus, is a chronic muscle pain syndrome with no known cause and no known cure. Fibromyalgia has been defined as pain that is widespread with multiple tender points.

fibrositis: A term that means inflammation of the fibrous connective tissue, although muscle biopsy studies have failed to demonstrate an inflammatory process.

floppy valve syndrome: *See* mitral valve prolapse.

fragile X syndrome: Sex-linked disorder, which occurs more frequently in males, that results when the bottom tip of the long arm of the X chromosome is pinched off. Affected individuals can have delayed development of speech and language, intellectual disability, anxiety, hyperactive behavior, and fidgeting or impulsive actions. Some may show features of autism spectrum disorders that manifest in problems with communication and social interaction. Most males and some females with fragile X have characteristic physical features that include a long and narrow face, large ears, prominent jaw and forehead, unusually flexible fingers, and flat feet.

Friedreich's ataxia: A disease involving neurologic degeneration due to cell loss in the dorsal root ganglia and secondary degeneration in the ascending and descending posterior columns and spinocerebellar tracts. It is primarily a disorder of movement with ataxic gait the most common presenting symptom.

frontal lobe syndrome: Lesions affecting the frontal lobe result in change from the premorbid personality in terms of a person's character and temperament, slowness in processing information, lack of judgment based on known consequences, withdrawal, and irritability. Disinhibition and apathy are common clinical dysfunctions of the frontal lobe. The person may lack insight into the deficits and therefore behavior can be difficult to control.

fulminant hepatitis: A rare form of hepatitis (occurs in less than 1% of persons with acute viral hepatitis) defined as hepatic failure with stage III or IV encephalopathy (confusion, stupor, and coma) as a result of massive hepatic necrosis.

furuncle: *See* boil.

furunculosis: Persistent sequential occurrence of boils (furuncles) over a period of weeks or months.

gallstone(s): Gallstones, *also known as* cholelithiasis, is the formation or presence of gallstones that remain in the lumen of the gallbladder or are ejected with bile into the cystic duct. Gallstones are stone-like masses called calculi (singular: calculus) that form in the gallbladder as a result of changes in the normal components of bile.

gangrene: Death of body tissue usually associated with loss of vascular (nutritive, arterial circulation) supply and followed by bacterial invasion and putrefaction. The three major types of gangrene are dry, moist, and gas gangrene. Dry and moist gangrene result from loss of blood circulation due to various causes; gas gangrene occurs in wounds infected by anaerobic bacteria, leading to gas production and tissue breakdown.

gastric adenocarcinoma: A malignant neoplasm arising from the gastric mucosa; constitutes more than 90% of the malignant tumors of the stomach.

gastritis: Inflammation of the lining of the stomach (gastric mucosa). It is not a single disease but represents a group of the most common stomach disorders.

gastroesophageal reflux disease (GERD): *Also known as* esophagitis, may be defined as an inflammation of the esophagus, which may be the result of reflux (backward flow) of gastric juices, infections, chemical irritants, involvement by systemic diseases, or physical agents such as radiation and nasogastric intubation.

gigantism: An overgrowth of the long bones resulting from growth hormone-secreting adenomas of the anterior pituitary gland. Gigantism develops in children before the age when epiphyses of the bones close and results in generalized "largeness," with heights often reaching 8 to 9 feet.

gliomas: Primary tumors of the brain, gliomas are the most prevalent and are tumors of the glial cells, the group of cells that support, insulate, and metabolically assist the neurons.

global aphasia: Severe impairment of both production and comprehension of speech.

goiter: An enlargement of the thyroid gland, which may be the result of lack of iodine, inflammation, or tumors (benign or malignant). Enlargement may also appear in hyperthyroidism, especially Graves' disease.

gout: Gout represents a heterogeneous group of metabolic disorders marked by an elevated level of serum uric acid and the deposition of urate crystals in the joints, soft tissues, and kidneys. Primary gout refers to hyperuricemia in the absence of other disease. Secondary gout refers to hyperuricemia resulting from an antecedent disease.

grand mal seizure: Grand mal or tonic-clonic seizure is the archetypal seizure, which means total loss of control. The seizure begins with a sudden loss of consciousness, generalized rigidity (tonic), followed by jerking movements (clonic), incontinence of bowel and bladder, and in the tonic phase, respiration can cease briefly.

Graves' disease: Hyperthyroidism, the excess secretion of thyroid hormone, creates a generalized elevation of body metabolism that is manifested in almost every system. Graves' disease, which increases T4 production, accounts for 85% of hyperthyroidism. The classic symptoms of Graves' disease are mild symmetrical enlargement of the thyroid (goiter), nervousness, heat intolerance, weight loss despite increased appetite, sweating, diarrhea, tremor, and palpitations.

Guillain-Barré syndrome (GBS): Guillain-Barré syndrome, *also known as* acute inflammatory demyelinating polyradiculoneuropathy (AIDP), which describes the syndrome, is an immune-mediated disorder. Viral and bacterial infections, surgery, and vaccinations have been associated with AIDP. Increased sensitivity response in the peripheral nervous system. Inflammation of the spinal nerve roots, peripheral nerves, and occasionally the cranial nerves. It also results in rapid paralysis of the limbs, accompanied by sensory loss and muscle atrophy.

Gulf War syndrome: Occurring in individuals who served in the Persian Gulf War, symptoms include fatigue, skin rash, headache, muscle and joint pain, memory loss, shortness of breath, sleep disturbances, diarrhea and other gastrointestinal symptoms, and depression. There is no known cause but possible causes include chemical or biologic weapons, insecticides, Kuwaiti oil well fires, parasites, pills protecting against nerve gas, and inoculations against petrochemical exposure.

heart block: *See* arrhythmias.

heartburn: A burning sensation in the esophagus usually felt in the midline below the sternum in the region of the heart, is often a symptom of indigestion and occurs when acidic contents of the stomach move backward or regurgitate into the esophagus. *Also known as* dyspepsia, pyrosis, or indigestion.

hemophilia: A bleeding disorder inherited as a sex-linked autosomal recessive trait in two-thirds of all cases. It is a coagulation (blood-clotting) disorder and caused by an abnormality of plasma-clotting proteins necessary for blood coagulation

hemorrhoids: Hemorrhoids, or piles, are varicose veins in the perineal region and may be internal or external.

hemostasis: The arrest of bleeding after blood vessel injury and involves the interaction between the blood vessel wall, the platelets, and the plasma coagulation proteins. Disorders of hemostasis are caused by defects in platelet number or function or problems in the formation of a blood clot resulting in a bleeding or clotting disorder.

hemothorax: Blood in the pleural cavity following chest trauma.

hepatic encephalopathy: *Also known as* hepatic coma, it refers to a variety of neurologic signs and symptoms in persons with chronic liver failure or in whom portal circulation is impaired.

hepatitis: An acute or chronic inflammation of the liver caused by a virus, a chemical, a drug reaction, or alcohol abuse.

hernia: An acquired or congenital abnormal protrusion of part of an organ or tissue through the structure normally containing it.

herpes simplex: An acute virus disease marked by groups of watery blisters on the skin and mucous membranes, such as the borders of the lips or the nose, or the mucous surface of the genitals. It often accompanies fever. *Also known as* cold sores.

herpes zoster: A local disease brought about by the reactivation of the same virus that causes the systemic disease called varicella (chickenpox). The disease is brought on by an immunocompromised state. *Also known as* shingles.

hiatal hernia: A hiatal or diaphragmatic hernia occurs when the cardiac (lower esophagus) sphincter becomes enlarged, allowing the stomach to pass through the diaphragm into the thoracic cavity.

hip dysplasia: *See* congenital hip dysplasia.

Hodgkin's disease: A neoplastic disease of lymphoid tissue with the primary histologic finding of giant Reed-Sternberg cells in the lymph nodes. These cells are part of the tissue macrophage system and have twin nuclei and nucleoli that give it the appearance of "owl eyes."

Horner's syndrome: Horner's syndrome includes ptosis (drooping of the upper eyelid), miosis (constriction of the pupil), and loss of sweating over the ipsilateral side of the face following an anterior inferior cerebellar artery stroke.

human immunodeficiency virus (HIV): A retrovirus that predominantly infects human T4 (helper) lymphocytes, the major regulators of the immune response, and destroys or activates them. *See also* acquired immunodeficiency syndrome (AIDS).

Huntington's disease (HD): A progressive hereditary disease of the basal ganglia characterized by abnormalities of movement, abnormal posture, postural reactions, trunk rotation, distribution of tone, extraneous movements, personality disturbances, and progressive dementia. Often associated with choreic movement, which is brief, purposeless, involuntary, and random. The disease slowly progresses and death is usually due to an intercurrent infection. *Also known as* Huntington's chorea.

hyaline membrane disease: A respiratory disease of unknown cause in newborn infants, especially if premature, characterized by an abnormal membrane of protein lining the alveoli of the lungs.

hydrocephalus: The increased accumulation of cerebrospinal fluid within the ventricles of the brain. Results from interference with normal circulation and with absorption of fluid, and especially from destruction of the foramina of Magendie and Lushka.

hyperparathyroidism: A metabolic disorder caused by overactivity of one or more of the four parathyroid glands that disrupts calcium, phosphate, and bone metabolism.

hyperpituitarism: An oversecretion of one or more of the hormones secreted by the pituitary gland, especially growth hormone, resulting in gigantism or acromegaly. It is primarily caused by a hormone-secreting pituitary tumor, typically a benign adenoma. Other syndromes associated with hyperpituitarism include Cushing's disease, amenorrhea (absence of the menstrual cycle), and hyperthyroidism.

hypersensitivity disorder: An exaggerated or inappropriate immune response, overreaction to a substance, or hypersensitivity; is often referred to as an allergic response and although the term *allergy* is widely used, the term *hypersensitivity* is more appropriate. Hypersensitivity designates an increased immune response to the presence of an antigen that results in tissue destruction.

hypertension (HTN): Hypertension, or high blood pressure, is defined by the World Health Organization as a persistent elevation of systolic blood pressure above 140 mm Hg and of diastolic pressure above 90 mm Hg measured on at least two separate occasions at least 2 weeks apart.

hyperthyroidism: An excessive secretion of thyroid hormone, sometimes referred to as thyrotoxicosis, a term used to describe the clinical manifestations that occur when the body tissues are stimulated by increased thyroid hormone. Excessive thyroid hormone creates a generalized elevation of body metabolism, the effects of which are manifested in almost every system.

hypochondriasis: A marked preoccupation with one's health and exaggeration of normal sensations and minor complaints into a serious illness.

hypoparathyroidism: Hyposecretion, hypofunction, or insufficient secretion of the parathyroid hormone (PTH) results in hypocalcemia, as the parathyroid's primary role is to regulate calcium balance. The most significant clinical consequence is neuromuscular irritability producing tetany.

hypopituitarism: *Also known as* panhypopituitarism and dwarfism, it results from decreased or absent hormonal secretion by the anterior pituitary gland. It is a generalized condition in which all six of the pituitary's vital hormones (ACTH, TSH, LH, FSH, human growth factor, and prolactin) are inadequately produced or absent.

hypotension: Decrease of systolic and diastolic blood pressure below normal due to a deficiency in tonus or tension. *See also* orthostatic hypotension.

hypothyroidism: Refers to a deficiency of thyroid hormone that results in a generalized slowed body metabolism. In primary hypothyroidism, the loss of thyroid tissue leads to a decreased production of thyroid hormone and the thyroid gland responds by enlarging to compensate for the deficiency (*see* goiter). Secondary hypothyroidism is most commonly the result of failure of the pituitary to synthesize adequate amounts of thyroid-stimulating hormone.

iatrogenic immunodeficiency: A condition induced by immunosuppressive drugs, radiation therapy, or splenectomy in which the immune system is weakened by the intervention.

ichthyosis: A group of skin disorders characterized by dryness, roughness, and scaliness of the skin; results in thickening of the skin, sometimes referred to as "alligator skin," "fish skin," "crocodile skin," or "porcupine skin."

immune complex disease: Normally, excessive circulating antigen-antibody complexes called immune complexes are effectively cleared by the reticuloendothelial system. When circulating immune complexes successfully deposit in tissue around small blood vessels, they activate the complement cascade and cause acute inflammation and local tissue injury. This results in vasculitis, which can affect skin (causing an allergic reaction), synovial joints (such in rheumatoid arthritis), kidneys (causing nephritis), the pleura (causing pleuritis), and the pericardium (causing pericarditis).

impotence: A general term that expresses a problem with libido, penile erection, ejaculation, or orgasm. The contemporary diagnostic term is *erectile dysfunction.*

incontinence: Inability to retain urine, semen, or feces through loss of sphincter control. *See also* fecal incontinence and urinary incontinence.

infection: A process in which an organism establishes a parasitic relationship with its host. This invasion and multiplication of microorganisms produce signs and symptoms as well as an immune response.

infectious diseases: Clinical manifestations of infectious disease are many and varied depending upon the etiologic agent (e.g., viruses, bacteria, etc.) and the system affected (e.g., respiratory, central nervous system, gastrointestinal, genitourinary, etc.). Systemic symptoms can include fever and chills, sweating, malaise, and nausea and vomiting. There may be changes in blood composition, such as an increased number of white blood cells (leukocytes).

inflammatory bowel disease (IBD): Refers to two inflammatory conditions: Crohn's disease and ulcerative colitis (see respective definitions).

insulin resistance syndrome: A syndrome of insulin resistance that is associated with hypertension, carbohydrate intolerance, abdominal obesity, dyslipidemia, and accelerated atherosclerosis associated with non-insulin-dependent diabetes mellitus.

intellectual disability: A disability characterized by significant limitations both in intellectual functioning and in adaptive behavior, which covers many everyday social and practical skills. People with intellectual disabilities may have limitations in skills such as communicating, taking care of oneself, and social skills. Children with intellectual disabilities (sometimes called cognitive disabilities or mental retardation) may take longer to learn to speak, walk, and take care of their personal needs such as dressing or eating.

internal carotid artery syndrome: The clinical picture of internal carotid occlusion varies, depending on whether the cause of ischemia is thrombus, embolus, or low flow. The cortex supplied by the middle cerebral territory is most often affected (*see* middle cerebral artery syndrome). Occasionally, the origins of both the anterior (*see* anterior cerebral artery syndrome) and middle cerebral arteries are occluded at the top of the carotid artery. Symptoms consistent with both syndromes result.

intestinal ischemia: Results from embolic occlusions of the visceral branches of the abdominal aorta, generally in people with valvular heart disease, atrial fibrillation, or left ventricular thrombus. Symptoms include acute abdominal cramps or steady epigastric or periumbilical abdominal pain combined with high leukocyte count. It is sometimes called "intestinal angina," as it is the result of atherosclerotic plaque-induced ischemia. Intermittent back pain at the thoracolumbar junction, particularly with exertion, is also a common complaint.

intracerebral hemorrhage: Bleeding from an arterial source into brain parenchyma (therefore is often referred to as an interparenchymal hemorrhage) and is widely regarded as the most deadly of stroke subtypes. It is characterized by spontaneous bleeding in the absence of an identifiable precipitant and usually associated with hypertension and/or aging.

irritable bowel syndrome (IBS): A group of symptoms that represent the most common disorder of the gastrointestinal system. IBS is referred to as "nervous indigestion," functional dyspepsia, spastic colon, nervous colon, and irritable colon, but because of the absence of inflammation, it should not be confused with colitis or other inflammatory diseases of the intestinal tract. IBS is a functional disorder of motility as a response to diet or stress.

ischemic heart disease: Narrowing or blockage of the coronary arteries causing ischemia in the heart muscle supplied by that artery. Infarction may result. *See also* coronary heart (artery) disease.

Kaposi's sarcoma (KS): A malignancy of angiopoietic tissue that presents as a skin lesion. Growth of this tumor is promoted with a suppressed immune system and is an opportunistic infection associated with AIDS. It is characterized by raised, nontender, purplish lesions.

Kawasaki disease: A cardiovascular pathology, *also known as* mucocutaneous lymph node syndrome, it is an acute systemic vasculitis that can occur in any ethnic group but seems most prevalent in Asian populations. There is extensive inflammation of the arterioles, venules, and capillaries initially, then progressing to the main coronary arteries and larger veins. Vessels develop scarring, intimal thickening, calcification, and formation of thrombi. This syndrome is characterized by high fever, swollen lymph nodes in the neck, rashes, irritated eyes and mucus membranes, with damage to the cardiovascular system. *Synonym*: Kawasaki's syndrome.

keratitis: Inflammation of the cornea.

Klebsiella pneumonia: An organism closely similar to *Aerobacter aerogenes* but occurring in patients/clients with lobar pneumonia and other infections of the respiratory tract.

Klinefelter's syndrome: Characterized by the presence of an extra X chromosome in males, causing failure to develop secondary sex characteristics, enlarged breasts, poor musculature development, and infertility.

Klippel-Feil syndrome: Condition in which one or more vertebrae are fused together in the neck area, causing shortening of the cervical spine.

Korsakoff's psychosis: A chronic subcortical disorder caused by prolonged vitamin B_1 deficiency, which is usually caused by alcoholism.

kyphoscoliosis: *Also known as* Scheuermann's disease, juvenile kyphosis, and vertebral epephysitis, it is a condition of anteroposterior curvature of the spine affecting adolescents between the ages of 12 and 16. Growth retardation and vascular disturbance in the vertebral epiphyses are the two most common theories of pathogenesis of this structural deformity. This condition can also develop with advancing age and is associated with osteoporosis, endocrine disorders, Paget's disease, tuberculosis, poor posture, osteochondritis, and disk degeneration.

lacunar syndrome: Appears when a stroke (CVA) occurs in these deep areas of the brain and is representative of the area of infarct in which the lacunae are predominant. If the posterior limb of the internal capsule is affected, a pure motor deficit may result; in the anterior limb of the internal capsule, weakness of the face and dysarthria may occur. If the posterior thalamus is affected, there is a pure sensory stroke. When the lacunae occur predominantly in the pons, ataxia, clumsiness, and weakness may be seen.

Laënnec's cirrhosis: Alcoholic cirrhosis (*see* cirrhosis).

Landau-Kleffner syndrome: Acquired epileptic aphasia characterized by an acquired aphasia secondary to epileptic seizures in the absence of other neurological abnormalities.

lateral sclerosis: A rare form of involvement in amyotrophic lateral sclerosis that results in neuronal loss in the cortex. Signs of corticospinal tract involvement include hyperactivity of tendon reflexes with spasticity causing difficulty in active movement. Weakness and spasticity of specific muscles represent the level and progression of the disease along the corticospinal tracts. There is no muscle atrophy, and fasciculations are not present.

Legg-Calvé-Perthes disease: *Also known as* coxa plana and osteochondritis deformans juvenilis, Legg-Calvé-Perthes disease is avascular necrosis of the proximal femoral epiphysis with flattening of the head of the femur caused by vascular interruption and ischemic necrosis (affects boys aged 3 to 12).

Legionnaires' disease: An acute respiratory infection, often with pneumonia, caused by bacteria (*Legionella pneumophila*) that may contaminate water or soil (named after an outbreak of the illness at an American Legion convention in July 1976).

Lennox-Gastaut syndrome: A syndrome that occurs with epilepsies of infancy and childhood usually between ages 1 and

6 years. The most common seizures are atonic-akinetic, resulting in loss of postural tone. Violent falls occur suddenly with immediate recovery and resumption of activity, the attack lasting less than 1 second. Tonic attacks consist of sudden flexion of the head and trunk and consciousness is clouded.

leukemia: A malignant neoplasm of the blood-forming cells, specifically replacement of the bone marrow by a malignant clone (genetically identical cell) of lymphocytic or granulocytic cells. Acute leukemia is an accumulation of neoplastic, immature lymphoid or myeloid cells in the bone marrow and peripheral blood, tissue invasion by these cells, and associated bone marrow failure. Chronic leukemia is a neoplastic accumulation of mature lymphoid or myeloid elements of the blood that usually progresses more slowly than an acute leukemic process.

leukocytosis: A condition in which there is an increase in number of leukocytes (greater than 10,000 per cubic mm) in the blood, generally caused by presence of infection. Leukocytosis may occur in response to bacterial infections, inflammation or tissue necrosis, metabolic intoxications, neoplasms, acute hemorrhage, splenectomy, acute appendicitis, pneumonia, intoxication by chemicals, or acute rheumatic fever. It may also occur as a normal protective response to physiologic stressors, such as strenuous exercise, emotional changes, temperature changes, anesthesia, surgery, pregnancy, and some drugs, toxins, and hormones.

leukopenia: A reduction of the number of leukocytes in the blood (less than $5000/\mu L$) that is caused by a variety of factors such as anaphylactic shock and systemic lupus erythematosus, bone marrow failure associated with radiation therapy, dietary deficiencies, and in autoimmune diseases.

limb apraxia: A disorder of skilled and purposeful movement of the arms and legs that occurs with neurological damage or disorders affecting the praxis system. People with limb apraxia often have functional deficits that impede everyday task performance and increase dependence on caregivers.

limbic lobe syndrome: Central nervous system disorder involving primary emotions—those associated with pain, pleasure, anger, and fear.

lupus erythematosus: A chronic inflammatory disorder of connective tissues. It can result in several forms including discoid lupus erythematosus, which affects only the skin, and systemic lupus erythematosus, which affects multiple organ systems, including the skin, and can be fatal (see respective definitions).

Lyme disease: An infectious multisystemic disorder caused by a spiral-shaped form of bacteria. It is carried by a deer tick. Initially, flu-like symptoms accompanied by a rash appear, followed by the appearance of skin lesions that resemble a raised, red circle with a clear center called erythema migrans or bullseye rash, often at the site of the tick bite. Within a few days the infection spreads, more lesions erupt, and a migratory, ring-like rash, conjunctivitis, or diffuse urticaria (hives) occurs. Malaise and fatigue are constant and symptoms include headache, fever, chills, achiness, and regional lymphadenopathy. Lyme disease can progress to include neurologic abnormalities (meningoencephalitis with peripheral and cranial neuropathy, abnormal skin sensations, insomnia and sleep disorders, memory loss, difficulty concentrating, and hearing loss) and cardiac involvement (fluctuating atrioventricular heart block; irregular, rapid, or slowed heartbeat; chest pain; fainting; dizziness; and shortness of breath). Ultimately, the end stage leads to joint changes characteristic of rheumatoid arthritis.

lymphedema: This is not a disease but a symptom of lymphatic transport malfunction that results in an accumulation of lymphatic and edema fluid. Primary lymphedema is defined as impaired lymphatic flow owing to congenital malformation of the lymphatic vessels. Secondary lymphedema is acquired and most common resulting from surgical removal of the lymph nodes, fibrosis secondary to radiation, and traumatic injury to the lymphatic system.

malabsorption syndrome: This is a group of disorders (celiac disease, cystic fibrosis, Crohn's disease, chronic pancreatitis, pancreatic carcinoma, pernicious anemia) characterized by reduced intestinal absorption of dietary components and excessive loss of nutrients in the stool.

malignant melanoma: A neoplasm of the skin originating from melanocytes or cells that synthesize the pigment melanin. The melanomas occur most frequently in the skin but can also be found in the oral cavity, esophagus, anal canal, vagina, meninges, or within the eye.

Mallory-Weiss syndrome: A laceration of the lower end of the esophagus associated with bleeding. The most common cause is severe retching and vomiting as a result of alcohol abuse, eating disorders such as bulimia, or in the case of a viral syndrome.

manic-depressive disorder: Characterized by cyclical mood swings that often include intense outbursts of high energy and activity, elevated mood, a decreased need for sleep, and a flight of ideas (mania) followed by extreme depression. The cause is a biochemical dysfunction. *Also known as* bipolar disorder.

Marfan syndrome: A hereditary disorder characterized by abnormalities of the blood circulation and the eyes, abnormally long bones of the limbs, and very mobile joints.

Meniere's disease: A disorder of the labyrinth of the inner ear function that can cause devastating hearing and vestibular symptoms. It is a disorder of the membranous inner ear. Deficits are related to volume and pressure changes within closed fluid systems. It leads to progressive loss of hearing, characterized by ringing in the ear, dizziness, nausea, and vomiting.

meningitis: Infection of the cerebrospinal fluid within the cranium and spinal cord; meninges of the brain and spinal cord become inflamed. Early features include fever and headache. The cardinal signs are a stiff and painful neck with pain in the lumbar areas and posterior aspects of the thigh. Meningitis may produce damage to the cerebral cortex, which may affect motor function, sensation, and perception, as well as other areas of the central nervous system. Meningitis is almost always a complication of another infection and can be caused by a wide variety of organisms.

meningocele: Hernial protrusion of the meninges through a defect in the vertebral column; a form of spina bifida consisting of a sac-like cyst of meninges filled with spinal fluid. External protrusion of the meninges due to failure of neural tube closure of the spine.

meningomyelocele: Hernial protrusion of a sac-like cyst of meninges, spinal fluid, and a portion of the spinal cord with its nerves through a defect in the vertebral column.

middle cerebral artery syndrome (MCA): A syndrome related to occlusion of the middle cerebral artery that results in contralateral hemiplegia and hemianesthesia, or loss of movement and sensation on one half of the body. If the dominant hemisphere is affected, global aphasia (the loss of fluency, ability to name objects, comprehend auditory information, and repeat language) is the result.

migraine: A headache that is usually confined to one side of the head, is throbbing, and is episodic. The pain associated with migraine is associated with a change in the vasculature in the brain. The pain appears to come from a complex inflammatory process of the trigeminal and cervical dorsal nerve roots that innervate the cephalic arteries and venous sinuses.

mitral regurgitation (MR): There are many possible causes of MR, but mitral valve prolapse accounts for approximately half of all cases. Regurgitation occurs when the valve does not close properly and causes blood to flow back into the heart chamber.

mitral stenosis (MS): A narrowing or constriction of the mitral valve of the heart that prevents the valve from opening fully and may be caused by scars or abnormal deposits on the leaflets. It causes obstruction to blood flow and the left atrium must produce extra work to sustain cardiac output. Because the mitral valve is thickened, it opens early during diastole with a "snap" that is audible on auscultation, and then closes slowly with a resultant murmur.

mitral valve prolapse (MVP): Prolapse of the mitral valve occurs when enlarged leaflets bulge backward into the left atrium. MVP appears to be the result of connective tissue abnormalities in the valve leaflets. *Also known as* floppy valve syndrome, Barlow's syndrome, and click-murmur syndrome.

mononeuropathy: Injury to a single nerve, which is commonly a result of trauma.

motor neuron diseases (MNDs): A group of progressive neurologic disorders that destroy motor neurons, the cells that control essential voluntary muscle activity (e.g., speaking, walking, breathing, and swallowing). Disruptions in the signals between motor neurons and muscle cause muscle weakness, atrophy, spasticity, and in some cases overactive tendon reflexes. Over time, the ability to control voluntary movement can be lost. The most common MND in adults is amyotrophic lateral sclerosis, which affects both upper and lower motor neurons; the most common MND in children is spinal muscular atrophy. Other types of MND may affect only upper or lower motor neurons (National Institutes of Health, 2012).

multiple myeloma: *Also known as* plasma cell myeloma, it is a primary malignant neoplasm of plasma cells arising most often in bone marrow. Malignant plasma cells arise from B cells that produce abnormally large amounts of one class of immunoglobulin (usually IgG, occasionally IgA). The abnormal immunoglobulin produced by the malignant transformed plasma cell is called the M-protein. Bone pain is the most prominent symptom.

multiple organ dysfunction syndrome: Often the final complication of critical illness. It is the progressive failure of two or more organ systems after a serious illness or injury.

multiple sclerosis (MS): A virus-induced autoimmune disease mediated by lymphocytes and macrophages, the cells of the immune system that trigger the demyelination of the central nervous system. It is primarily the white matter that is damaged, but lesions of the gray matter have also been found. Characterized by local inflammation, edema, and demyelination, the disease causes a significant decrease in the conduction rate of the axon.

muscle tension headache: Tension headache associated with muscle contraction occurring in response to stress.

muscular dystrophy (MD): A group of inherited, progressive neuromuscular disorders with a genetic origin characterized by ongoing symmetrical muscle wasting without neural or sensory deficits but with increasing weakness, atrophy, deformity, and disability. Paradoxically, the wasted muscles tend to hypertrophy because of connective tissue and fat deposits. There are four types: (1) Duchenne's (pseudohypertrophic), (2) Becker's (benign pseudohypertrophic), (3) fascioscapulo-humeral (Landouzy-Dejerine), and (4) limb-girdle dystrophy.

myalgia: Tenderness or pain in the muscles, often called muscular rheumatism.

myasthenia gravis (MG): Chronic progressive autoimmune disorder of striated muscles that leads to weakness in the voluntary muscles, particularly those innervated by the bulbar nucleus. A disorder of neuromuscular transmission characterized by fluctuating weakness and fatigability of skeletal muscle. It is a fundamental defect of the neuromuscular junction in which the number of acteylcholine receptors is decreased and those that remain are flattened, which results in decreased efficiency of neuromuscular transmission.

myelodysplasia: A general term used to describe defective development of any part of the spinal cord but especially of the lower spinal cord levels.

myelomeningocele: Protrusion of the meninges and spinal cord due to failure of neural tube closure.

myocardial infarction (MI): The development of ischemia with resultant necrosis of myocardial tissue. Any prolonged obstruction depriving the heart muscle of oxygen can cause an MI. *Also known as* a heart attack or coronary.

myocarditis: A relatively uncommon inflammatory condition of the muscular walls of the heart most often the result of bacterial or viral infection.

myofascial pain dysfunction: A condition marked by the presence of tender myofascial trigger points. The trigger point is viewed as more of a clinical entity than a pathologic entity.

myopathy: Involvement of muscle typically reflected by proximal weakness, wasting, and hypotonia without sensory impairment.

myositis: A rare but potentially life-threatening entity characterized by severe pain and inflammation in the affected muscle. Inflammation is the result of a streptococcal infection and is often referred to as streptococcal myositis.

neuropathy: Any disease of the nerves. *See* peripheral neuropathies.

neuropraxia: Involves segmental demyelination, which slows or blocks conduction of the action potential at the point of demyelination on a myelinated nerve. Often occurs following nerve compression, which induces mild ischemia in nerve fibers.

neurotmesis: The complete severance of nerve fiber and its supporting endoneurium, also producing axonal loss in which the connective tissue coverings are disrupted at the site of injury (e.g., gunshot or stab wounds, or avulsion injuries that disrupt a section of the nerve).

neutropenia: A condition associated with a reduction in circulating neutrophils (less than 2,000/mL). This may occur in severe, prolonged infections when production of granulocytes cannot keep up with demand. Neutropenia may also occur in the presence of decreased bone marrow production, such as happens with radiation, chemotherapy, leukemia, and aplastic anemia.

non–insulin-dependent diabetes mellitus (NIDDM): Associated with obesity through a negative feedback mechanism in which excessive insulin levels decrease the number of insulin receptor sites on adipose cells. The decrease in insulin receptor sites decreases the amount of glucose that can enter cells. This promotes high blood glucose levels.

obesity: A medically defined weight greater than 20% of desirable weight for adults of a given sex, body structure, and height.

orchitis: Inflammation of the testis and can be acute or chronic associated with epididymitis.

orthostatic hypotension: The term *orthostatic (postural) hypotension* signifies a decrease of 20 mm Hg or greater in systolic blood pressure or a decrease of 10 mm Hg or more of both systolic and diastolic arterial blood pressure with a concomitant pulse increase of 15 bpm or more on standing from a supine or sitting position.

Osgood-Schlatter disease: Results from fibers of the patellar tendon pulling small bits of immature bone from the tibial tuberosity. Osgood-Schlatter disease is considered a form of tendinitis of the patellar tendon rather than a degenerative disease. *Also known as* osteochondrosis.

osteoarthritis (OA): A degenerative joint disease that is a slow, progressive degeneration of joint structures due to mechanical stresses, which results in loss of mobility, chronic pain, deformity, and loss of function. Joint degeneration results from periods of inflammation of the joints in response to wear and tear stresses.

osteoblastoma: A benign tumor of the bone similar to osteoid osteoma, only larger, with a tendency to expand.

osteochondroma: The most common primary benign neoplasm of bone.

osteogenesis imperfecta: Autosomal dominant disorder that occurs once in 30,000 births. It is characterized by increased susceptibility to fractures. Normal intelligence and possible hearing loss are associated. Sometimes referred to as "brittle bones," it is a rare congenital disorder of collagen synthesis affecting bones and connective tissue. Clinically, occasional fractures result from brittle bone with growth retardation and long bone deformities.

osteoid osteoma: A benign vascular osteoblastic lesion that is often found in the cortex of long bones, such as the femur, near the end of disphysis. Pathologic study shows areas of immature bone surrounded by prominent osteoblasts and osteoclasts. The lesion is vascular, but no cartilage is present. The tumor can lead to joint pain and dysfunction.

osteomalacia: Softening of bone without loss of bone matrix. It is a generalized bone condition in which insufficient mineralization (deficient bone calcification) of bone matrix results from calcium and/or phosphate deficiency. Sometimes referred to as the adult form of rickets.

osteomyelitis: An inflammation of bone caused by an infectious organism. Acute osteomyelitis is a rapidly destructive pyogenic infection. Chronic osteomyelitis is a recognized complication of treatment of open fractures.

osteonecrosis: The death of bone and bone marrow cellular components in the absence of infection. Avascular necrosis and aseptic necrosis are synonyms for this condition. The femoral head is most commonly affected.

osteopenia: A condition that results in the loss of bone mass, usually in isolated areas. When this condition of demineralization progresses to include the entire skeletal system, it is termed *osteoporosis*.

osteoporosis: A reduction of bone mass per unit of bone volume. Reduction in bone mass associated with loss of bone mineral and matrix occurring when bone resorption is greater than formation; found in sedentary, post-menopausal women or following steroidal therapy.

osteosarcoma: Tumors with malignant properties that are usually destructive lesions with abundant sclerosis both from the tumor itself and from reactive bone formation. A characteristic of osteosarcoma is the production of osteoid by malignant, neoplastic cells.

Paget's disease: Paget's disease, or osteitis deformans, is a progressive disorder of abnormal bone remodeling. Initially, excessive bone resorption occurs followed by disorganized and excessive bone formation. Disease characterized by a greatly accelerated remodeling process in which osteoclastic resorption is massive and osteoblastic bone formation is extensive. As a result, there is an irregular thickening and softening of the bones of the skull, pelvis, and extremities. It rarely occurs in individuals younger than 50.

pancreatitis: A potentially serious inflammation of the pancreas that may result in autodigestion of the pancreas by its own enzymes. Acute pancreatitis is thought to result from "escape" of activated pancreatic enzymes from acinar cells into surrounding tissues. The pathogenesis is unknown, but it may include edema or obstruction of the ampulla of Vater with resultant reflux of bile into pancreatic ducts or direct injury to the acinar cells, which allows leakage of pancreatic enzymes into pancreatic tissue.

paraneoplastic syndromes: Neurologic complications in cancer caused by three phenomena: (1) tumor metastases to the brain,

(2) endocrine, fluid, and electrolyte abnormalities, and (3) para-neoplastic syndromes. When tumors produce signs and symptoms at a site distant from the tumor or its metastasized sites, these "remote effects" of malignancy are collectively referred to as paraneoplastic syndromes. Symptoms include anorexia, malaise, diarrhea, weight loss, and fever (nonspecific symptoms), necrotizing vasculitis, Raynaud's disease, arthralgia, neurologic symptoms, nephrotic syndrome, palmar fasciitis and polyarthritis, scleroderma-like changes, enteric bacteria cultured from joints, bone pain, stress fractures, digital necrosis, and subcutaneous nodules.

Parkinson's disease: A chronic progressive disease of the motor component of the central nervous system characterized by rigidity, tremor, and bradykinesia. It is a degenerative disease of the substantia nigra in the basal ganglia. Abnormal functioning in the area of the basal ganglia in the brain is referred to as parkinsonism. Parkinson's disease usually affects the elderly population.

pediculosis: An infestation by pediculus humanus, a common parasite infecting the head, body, and genital area. More commonly referred to as lice.

peptic ulcer disease (PUD): A break in the protective mucosal lining exposing submucosal areas to gastric secretions. The word *peptic* refers to pepsin, a proteolytic enzyme, the principal digestive component of gastric juice, which acts as a catalyst in the chemical breakdown of protein.

pericarditis: Inflammation of the pericardium.

peripheral neuropathies: Trauma, inherited disorders, environmental toxins, and nutritional disorders may affect the myelin (myelinopathy), axon (axonopathy), or cell body of a peripheral nerve, leading to loss of sensation and subsequent loss of muscle function. Symptoms occur related to the affected nerves, or in many conditions, such as diabetic neuropathy, the pattern of loss is distal and in a sock-like or glove-like pattern.

peripheral vascular disease: Diseases affecting the peripheral blood vessels, including inflammatory diseases (polyarteritis, arteritis, allergies, Kawasaki's disease, Buerger's disease), occlusive disorders (arteriosclerosis, thromboangitis obliterans, arterial thrombosis or embolism), venous disorders (thrombophlebitis, varicose veins, chronic venous insufficiency), and vasomotor dysfunction (Raynard's disease, reflex sympathetic dystrophy).

peritonitis: Inflammation of the serous membrane lining the walls of the abdominal cavity caused by a number of situations that introduce microorganisms into the peritoneal cavity.

pervasive developmental disorder (PDD): The diagnostic category of PDD refers to a group of disorders characterized by delays in the development of socialization and communication skills. Parents may note symptoms as early as infancy, although the typical age of onset is before age 3 years. Symptoms may include problems with using and understanding language; difficulty relating to people, objects, and events; unusual play with toys and other objects; difficulty with changes in routine or familiar surroundings; and repetitive body movements or behavior patterns. Autism (a developmental brain disorder characterized by impaired social interaction and communication skills and a limited range of activities and interests) is the most characteristic and best studied PDD. Other types of PDD include Asperger's syndrome, childhood disintegrative disorder, and Rett's syndrome. Children with PDD vary widely in abilities, intelligence, and behaviors. Some children do not speak at all, others speak in limited phrases or conversations, and some have relatively normal language development. Repetitive play skills and limited social skills are generally evident. Unusual responses to sensory information, such as loud noises and lights, are also common (Office of Communications and Public Liaison, 2013).

phenylketonuria (PKU): Disorder in which a metabolic error occurs when an enzyme fails to convert phenylalanine to tyrosine, resulting in the accumulation of phenylalanine in the blood, causing mental retardation.

Pick's disease: A rare form of dementia involving the frontal and temporal regions of the cortex. Symptoms include prominent apathy as well as memory disturbances, increased carelessness, poor personal hygiene, and decreased attention span. Often severe emotional displays of anxiety and agitation accompany this disease of the brain.

pickwickian syndrome: The complex of exogenous obesity, somnolence, hypoventilation, and erythrocytosis. Named after an obese character in a Dickens novel.

pleural effusion: The collection of fluid in the pleural space (between the membrane encasing the lung and the membrane lining the thoracic cavity) where there is normally only a small amount of fluid to prevent friction as the lung expands and deflates.

pleurisy: An inflammation of the pleura caused by infection, injury (e.g., rib fracture), or tumor. It is often a complication of pneumonia but can also be secondary to tuberculosis, lung abscesses, influenza, systemic lupus erythematosus, rheumatoid arthritis, or pulmonary infarction.

pneumoconiosis: A group of lung diseases resulting from inhalation of particles of industrial substances, particularly inorganic dusts such as that of iron ore or coal with permanent deposition of substantial amount of such particles in the lung ("dusty lungs"). Common pneumoconiosis include coal worker's pneumoconiosis, silicosis, and asbestosis. Other types include talc, beryllium lung disease, aluminum pneumoconiosis, cadmium worker's disease, and siderosis (inhalation of iron or other metallic particles).

***Pneumocystis carinii* pneumonia:** A progressive, often fatal pneumonia that represents the most frequently occurring opportunistic infection in persons with AIDS.

pneumonia: An inflammation affecting the parenchyma of the lungs and can be caused by (1) bacterial, viral, or mycoplasmal infection; (2) inhalation of toxic or caustic chemicals, smoke, dusts, or gases; or (3) aspiration of food, fluids, or vomitus. It often occurs after influenza.

pneumothorax (Ptx): An accumulation of air or gas in the pleural cavity caused by a defect in the visceral pleura or chest wall. The result is collapse of the lung on the affected side.

poliomyelitis: Inflammation of the gray matter of the spinal cord resulting in paralysis, atrophy of muscles, and deformities.

polyarteritis nodosa: Refers to a condition consisting of multiple sites of inflammatory and destructive lesions in the arterial system; the lesions are small masses of tissue in the form of nodes or projections (nodosum). The cause is unknown, although hepatitis B is present in 50% of cases, and polyarteritis occurs more commonly among intravenous drug abusers and other groups who have a high prevalence of hepatitis B.

polycythemia vera: *Also known as* erythrocytosis, it is a neoplastic disease of the bone marrow stem cell primarily affecting the erythoid cells, which produce eryhrocytes, but causing overproduction of all three hematopoietic cell lines. It is characterized by an excessive number of erythrocytes leading to an increased concentration of hemoglobin, increased hematocrit (measure of the volume of packed red blood cells), and an increased hemoglobin level.

polymyalgia rheumatica: A disorder marked by diffuse pain and stiffness that primarily affects the shoulder and pelvic girdle musculature.

polymyositis: A diffuse, inflammatory myopathy that produces symmetrical weakness of striated muscle, primarily the proximal muscles of the shoulder and pelvic girdle, neck, and pharynx.

polyneuropathy: *See* peripheral neuropathies. Indicates involvement of several peripheral nerves.

polyps: A growth or mass protruding into the intestinal lumen from any area of mucous membrane.

polyradiculitis: Injury that affects several nerve roots and occurs when infections create an inflammatory response.

polyradiculoneuropathy: Inflammatory breakdown of myelin usually associated with motor and sensory deficits (*see* Guillain-Barré syndrome).

polyuria: A cardinal sign of diabetes, polyuria is excessive urination. The pathophysiologic basis is that water is not reabsorbed from renal tubules because of osmotic activity of glucose in the tubules.

portal hypertension: An abnormally high blood pressure in the portal venous system of the liver, occurring commonly in conditions such as cirrhosis as a result of obstruction of portal blood flow.

posterior cerebral artery syndrome (PCA): When the proximal posterior cerebral artery is occluded, including penetrating branches, the area of the brain that is affected is the subthalamus, medial thalamus, and ipsilateral (same side) cerebral peduncle and midbrain. Signs include thalamic syndrome, including loss of pain and temperature (superficial sensation), and proprioception and touch (deep sensation). This may develop into intractable, searing pain, which can be incapacitating.

posterior cord syndrome: This is an extremely rare syndrome secondary to injury of the spinal cord. Motor function, pain, and light touch sensation are preserved. There is loss of proprioception below the level of the lesion leading to a wide-based steppage gait.

posterior inferior cerebellar artery (PICA) syndrome: Blood supply to the brainstem, medulla, and cerebellum is provided by the vertebral and posterior cerebellar arteries. When infarction occurs in the posterior inferior cerebellar artery, the lateral medulla and the posteroinferior cerebellum are affected, resulting in Wallenberg's syndrome, which is characterized by vertigo, nausea, hoarseness, and dysphagia (difficulty swallowing). Other symptoms include ipsilateral ataxia (uncoordinated movement), ptosis (eyelid droop), and impairment of sensation in the ipsilateral portion of the face and contralateral portion of the torso and limbs.

post-polio syndrome (PPS): Refers to new neuromuscular symptoms that occur decades (average post-polio interval is 25 years) after recovery from the acute paralytic episode.

post-traumatic stress disorder (PTSD): Development of characteristic symptoms following exposure to an extreme traumatic stressor involving direct personal experience of an event that involves actual or threatened death or serious injury, other threat to one's physical integrity, or witnessing an event that involves death, injury, or threat to someone else. Symptoms include intense fear, helplessness, or horror.

Pott's disease: Vertebral tuberculosis.

Prader-Willi syndrome: Characterized by severe obesity, mental retardation, small hands and feet, and small genitalia. In infancy, problems with poor tone, feeding, and body temperature control are common. More than 50% of children with Prader-Willi syndrome have a deletion of chromosome 15.

pressure ulcer: A lesion caused by unrelieved pressure resulting in damage to the underlying tissue. Pressure ulcers usually occur over bony prominences and are graded or staged to classify the degree of tissue damage observed.

primary lateral sclerosis (PLS): A disease of the upper motor neurons in the arms, legs, and face. Caused by nerve cell degeneration in the motor regions of the cerebral cortex and results in slow and effortful movements. The legs are often affected first, followed by the trunk, arms, and hands, and finally the muscles that control speech, swallowing, and chewing. Symptoms include weakness, muscle stiffness and spasticity, clumsiness, slowing of movement, and problems with balance and speech.

progressive bulbar palsy: A motor neuron disease in which the lowest motor neurons of the brainstem are most affected, causing slurred speech and difficulty chewing and swallowing. There are almost always mildly abnormal signs in the arms and legs.

progressive muscular atrophy: A motor neuron disease that affects only lower motor neurons in the spinal cord. Characterized by muscle weakness, fasciculation, and atrophy.

prostatitis: Inflammation of the prostate gland, which can be acute or chronic and bacterial or nonbacterial.

pseudobulbar palsy: *See* amyotrophic lateral sclerosis.

psoriasis: A chronic, inherited recurrent inflammatory dermatosis characterized by well-defined erythematous plaques covered with a silvery scale.

psoriatic arthritis: A form of arthritis that differs from rheumatoid arthritis in that it more frequently involves the distal interphalangeal joints, asymmetrical distribution, and the presence of spondyloarthropathy. Joints are less tender though pain and stiffness are increased by periods of immobility.

pulmonary edema: An excessive fluid build-up in the lungs that may accumulate in the interstitial tissue, in the air spaces (alveoli), or in both. Pulmonary edema is a complication of many disease processes. *Also known as* pulmonary congestion.

pulmonary embolism: The lodging of a blood clot in a pulmonary artery with subsequent obstruction of blood supply to the lung parenchyma.

pulmonary fibrosis: An excessive amount of fibrous or connective tissue in the lung, predominantly fibroblasts and small blood vessels, that progressively remove and replace normal tissue. Categorized as a restrictive lung disease.

pulmonary hypertension: High blood pressure in the pulmonary arteries defined as a rise in pulmonary artery pressure of 5 to 10 mm Hg above normal (normal is 15 to 18 mm Hg).

pyelonephritis: An infectious, inflammatory disease involving the kidney parenchyma and renal pelvis typically related to a bacterial infection.

pyloric stenosis: An obstruction at the pyloric sphincter (the sphincter at the distal opening of the stomach into the duodenum).

pyoderma: Any purulent (containing or forming pus) skin disease.

rachischisis: Congenital fissure of the vertebral column; seen in spina bifida.

radiculoneuropathy: Indicates involvement of the nerve root as it emerges from the spinal cord.

Raynaud's disease/phenomenon: Intermittent episodes of small artery or arteriole constriction of the extremities causing temporary pallor and cyanosis of the digits and changes in skin temperature is called Raynaud's phenomenon. These episodes occur in response to cold temperature or strong emotion such as anxiety or excitement. When this condition is a primary vasospastic disorder it is called Raynaud's disease. If the disorder is secondary to another disease or underlying cause, the term *Raynaud's phenomenon* is used.

rectocele: Herniation of the rectum into the vagina.

reflex sympathetic dystrophy (RSD): Differentiation syndrome with autonomic nerve changes. Sympathetic dysfunction of the extremity following trauma, nerve injury, or central nervous system disorder; usually occurs secondary to a preexisting condition. For instance, adhesive capsulitis in the shoulder is often accompanied by vasomotor instability of the hand known as reflex sympathetic dystrophy (formerly known as shoulder-hand syndrome). This condition is characterized by severe pain, swelling, and trophic skin changes of the hand (e.g., thinning and shininess of the skin with loss of wrinkling, sometimes with increased hair growth). Skin and subcutaneous tissue atrophy and tendon flexion contractures develop.

Reiter's syndrome: One of the most common reactive arthritic conditions. Reactive arthritis is defined as a sterile inflammatory arthropathy distant in time and place from the initial inciting infectious process. Reiter's syndrome usually follows venereal disease or an episode of bacillary dysentery and is associated with typical extra-articular manifestations of arthritis.

renal calculi: Urinary stone disease is a common urinary tract disorder and can result from sex, age, geography, climate, diet, genetics, and environmental factors. Pathologically there is an increased risk of stone formation due to the urine being super-saturated with calcium, salts, uric acid, magnesium ammonium phosphate, or cystine.

renal cystic disease: A renal cyst is a cavity filled with fluid or renal tubular elements making up a semisolid material. The presence of these cysts can lead to degeneration of renal tissue and obstruction of tubular flow.

renal failure: *See* chronic renal failure.

restrictive lung disease: A major category of pulmonary problems including any condition that limits lung expansion. Pulmonary function tests are characterized by a decrease in lung volume or total lung capacity.

Rett syndrome: Disorder characterized by the development of multiple specific deficits following a period of normal functioning at birth. There is a loss of previously acquired purposeful hand skills between ages 5 and 30 months, with the subsequent development of characteristic stereotyped hand movements resembling hand wringing or hand washing. Problems develop in the coordination of gait or trunk movements. There is also severe impairment in expressive and receptive language development, with severe psychomotor retardation.

Reye's syndrome: Illness that occurs following a viral infection. It is characterized by vomiting and brain dysfunction, such as disorientation, lethargy, and personality disorder, and may progress into coma. Usually affects children and teenagers.

rheumatic fever: One form of endocarditis (infection of the heart), caused by streptococcal group A bacteria. It can be fatal or may lead to rheumatic heart disease, a chronic condition caused by scarring and deformity of the heart valves. It is called rheumatic fever because the two most common symptoms are fever and joint pain.

rheumatoid arthritis (RA): A chronic, systemic inflammatory disease of the joints. Chronic polyarthritis perpetuates a gradual destruction of joint tissues and can result in severe deformity and disability. Pathologically, the indicator of rheumatoid arthritis is a positive rheumatoid factor (antibodies that react with immunoglobulin antibodies found in the blood and in the synovium). Interaction between rheumatoid factor and the immunoglobulin triggers events that initiate an inflammatory reaction. It typically involves the joints of the fingers, hands, wrists, and ankles. Often the hips, knees, and shoulders are severely affected. As a systemic disease, it can affect the juncture at any articulation (e.g., ribs to vertebrae, scapula to clavicle, etc.). The joints are affected symmetrically and there is a considerable range of severity.

rickets: Condition affecting children characterized by soft and deformed bones resulting from inadequate calcium metabolism due to vitamin D deficiency.

right hemisphere syndrome: This syndrome following a stroke represents the inability to orient the body within external space and generate the appropriate motor responses. Hemineglect is a common feature of right hemisphere involvement. The individual does not respond to sensory stimuli on the left side.

sarcoidosis: A systemic disease of unknown origin involving any organ. Sarcoidosis is characterized by granulomatous inflammation present diffusely throughout the body. The lungs and lymph nodes are most commonly affected. Secondary sites include skin, eyes, liver, spleen, heart, and small bones in the hands and feet. Symptoms in dyspnea, cough, fever, malaise, weight loss, skin lesions, and erythem nodosum (multiple, tender nonulcerating nodules).

sarcoma: Refers to a malignant tumor of mesenchymal origin.

Saturday night palsy: This is a radial nerve compression at the spiral groove of the humerus. Compression of the nerve causes segmental demyelination. Paralysis of upper extremity musculature and sensory loss is associated with the level of compression. *Also known as* a crutch palsy.

scabies: This is a skin eruption caused by a mite, *Sarcoptes scabiei*. The mite burrows into the skin and deposits eggs, which hatch and cause the skin eruption.

scapuloperoneal muscular dystrophy: This is a variation of facioscapulohumeral dystrophy (*see* muscular dystrophy) with involvement of the distal muscles of the lower extremities instead of the face and proximal muscles of the shoulder girdle.

Scheuermann's disease: *See* kyphoscoliosis.

sciatica: Radiculopathy in which the nerve root of the sciatic nerve is affected, most typically caused by compression. It results in low back pain with potential radiation down the back of the lower extremity consistent with the innervation of the sciatic nerve.

scleroderma: Systemic sclerosis or scleroderma is an autoimmune disease of connective tissue characterized by excessive collagen deposition in the skin and internal organs.

scoliosis: An abnormal lateral curvature of the spine. The curvature of the spine may be to the right (more common in thoracic curves) or left (more common in lumbar curves). Rotation of the vertebral column around its axis occurs and may cause rib cage deformity. Scoliosis is often associated with kyphosis and lordosis.

septic arthritis: Osteomyelitis is one type of infection that is capable of extending into a joint and causing infection (sepsis). Bacteria, viruses, and fungi can also affect the joints. Infection in the joint causes erosion of the joint capsule, leading to arthritic changes in the septic joint.

shoulder-hand syndrome: *See* reflex sympathetic dystrophy.

sickle cell anemia: A hereditary, chronic form of hemolytic anemia in which the rupture of erythrocytes (forming sickle cells) releases hemoglobin prematurely into the plasma, thereby reducing the delivery of oxygen to tissues.

sick sinus syndrome: *Also known as* brady-tachy syndrome, it is a complex cardiac arrhythmia associated with coronary artery disease or drug therapy (e.g., digitalis, calcium channel blockers, ß-blockers, anti-arrhythmics). Sick sinus syndrome as a result of degeneration of conductive tissue necessary to maintain normal heart rhythm occurs most often among the elderly.

sleep apnea syndrome: Defined as episodes of cessation of breathing occurring at the transition from non-rapid eye movement (NREM) to rapid eye movement (REM) sleep, with repeated wakening and excessive daytime sleepiness.

somatoform disorder: The presence of physical symptoms that suggest a medical condition causing significant impairment in social, occupational, or other areas of functioning. The physical symptoms associated with somatoform disorders are not intentional or under voluntary control. It is a psychophysiologic disorder in which emotional problems or conflicts may develop physical symptoms as a means of coping.

spina bifida: Congenital malformation of the spine in which the walls of the spinal canal do not develop, typically due to the lack of union between vertebrae; the degree of impairment depends on the location of the malformation. A term used to describe various forms of myelodysplasia. A defective closure of the bony encasement of the spinal cord (i.e., the bony vertebral column is divided into two parts through which the spinal cord and meninges may or may not protrude). If the anomaly is not visible, the condition is called spina bifida occulta. If there is an external protrusion of the sac-like structure, it is called spina bifida cystica, which is further classified according to the extent of involvement (e.g., meningocele, meningomyelocele, or myelo-menigocele).

spinal cord injury (SCI): Injury to the spinal cord that results in temporary or permanent paralysis of the muscles of the limbs and the autonomic nervous system. SCI is categorized into traumatic and nontraumatic injuries. Traumatic injury is the most common and is due to a concussion, contusion, or laceration. The spinal cord is violently displaced or compressed. A concussion is an injury caused by a blow or violent shaking and results in temporary loss of function. Contusions are bruises with hemorrhage beneath the unbroken skin often associated with fractured bone segments striking the spinal cord. Laceration (disruption of tissue) results from complete transection of the cord. Nontraumatic SCI is the result of tumors, infection, or bony changes in the spinal column.

spinal muscular atrophy (SMA): A genetic disease caused by the progressive loss of motor neurons, resulting in muscle weakness and atrophy. There are four types that vary in severity with the most severe type (SMA Type I) being the most common among children. SMA is an autosomal recessive disease that has been linked to a gene called the SMN gene. An individual must receive a defective copy of the gene from both parents in order to be affected. Most children are diagnosed at a young age when they fail to hit developmental milestones such as sitting up, rolling over, and walking. *Also known as* Werdnig-Hoffman disease, SMA is the second most common fatal autosomal recessive disorder, after cystic fibrosis.

splenomegaly: The spleen's involvement in the lymphopoietic and mononuclear phagocyte systems predisposes it to multiple conditions causing splenomegaly. The spleen becomes enlarged by an increase in the number of cellular elements, by the deposition of extracellular material, or in the presence of extracellular hemopoiesis, which accompanies reactive bone marrow disorders and neoplasm.

spondylitis: *See* ankylosing spondylitis.

squamous cell carcinoma: The second most common skin cancer, usually arising in sun-damaged skin such as the rim of the ear, face, lips and mouth, and the dorsa of the hands.

staphylococcal infection: *Staphylococcus aureus* is one of the most common bacterial pathogens normally residing on the skin and easily inoculated into deeper tissues where it causes suppurative (pus formation) infections. "Staph" infections are associated with bacteremia, pneumonia, enterocolitis, osteomyelitis, food poisoning, and skin infections.

Still's disease: A form of juvenile rheumatoid arthritis characterized by systemic manifestations including fever and rash. The rash typically appears on the trunk and extremities, leaving palms and soles unaffected. Inflammatory arthritis typically develops at some point.

streptococcal infection: *Streptococcus pyogenes* is one of the most frequent bacterial pathogens of humans and causes many diseases of diverse organ systems ranging from skin infections, to acute pharyngitis, to major-illnesses such as rheumatic fever, scarlet fever, pneumococcal pneumonia, otitis media, meningitis, and endocarditis.

stroke: Stroke, or cerebrovascular accident (CVA), is the result of thrombosis and/or embolic occlusion of a major artery in the brain, causing ischemia and death of brain tissue. An array of neurologic syndromes can result depending on the artery occluded and the area of the brain affected. *See* middle cerebral artery syndrome, anterior cerebral artery syndrome, internal artery syndrome, posterior cerebral artery syndrome, vertebral and posterior inferior cerebellar artery syndrome, basilar artery syndrome, superior cerebellar artery syndrome, anterior inferior cerebellar artery syndrome, and lacunar syndrome. These syndromes reflect the dysfunction associated with disruption of blood flow in specific areas of the brain. The syndromes are named according to the arteries that feed the specific area.

substance abuse: Defined as the excessive use of mood-affecting chemicals, which are a potential or real threat to either physical or mental health.

sudden infant death syndrome (SIDS): Rare form of death in infants from ages 2 to 6 months in which the child dies mysteriously without cause.

superior cerebellar artery syndrome: Occlusion of the superior cerebellar artery results in severe ipsilateral cerebellar ataxia, nausea and vomiting, and dysarthria, which is a slurring of speech. Loss of pain and temperature in the contralateral extremities, torso, and face occurs. Dysmetria, characterized by the inability to place an extremity at a precise point in space, affects the ipsilateral upper extremity.

systemic lupus erythematosus (SLE): Sometimes referred to as lupus, it is a chronic inflammatory autoimmune disorder. The cause of SLE remains unknown but evidence points to interrelated immunologic, environmental, hormonal, and genetic factors. The central immunologic disturbance is auto-antibody production, which destroys the body's normal cells. Arthralgias and arthritis constitute the most common presenting manifestations.

systemic sclerosis: A diffuse connective tissue disease that causes fibrosis of the skin, joints, blood vessels, and internal organs. It is an autoimmune disorder. *See also* scleroderma.

Tay-Sachs disease: Genetic progressive disorder of the nervous system that causes profound mental retardation, deafness, blindness, paralysis, and seizures; life expectancy is 5 years.

temporal lobe syndrome: Temporal lobe syndrome involves the primary emotions, those associated with pain, pleasure, anger, and fear. In this syndrome these emotions are amplified.

tendinitis: Inflammation of any tendon.

tenosynovitis: A rheumatologic condition found most often in diabetics. This is caused by accumulation of fibrous tissue in the tendon sheath and can cause aching, nodularity along the tendons, and contracture. It is most frequently associated with the flexor tendons.

thalassemia: A group of inherited chronic hemolytic anemias predominantly affecting people of Mediterranean or southern Chinese ancestry (thalassa means "sea," referring to early cases of sickle cell disease reported around the Mediterranean). Thalassemia is a sickle cell trait with clinical manifestations inclusive of (1) defective synthesis of hemoglobin, (2) structurally impaired red blood cells, and (3) shortened life span of erythrocytes.

thoracic outlet syndrome (TOS): A nerve entrapment syndrome caused by pressure from structures in the thoracic outlet on fibers of the brachial plexus; in addition, vascular symptoms can occur because of pressure on the subclavian artery. Chronic compression of nerves and arteries between the clavicle and first rib or impinging musculature results in edema and ischemia in the nerves. Initially creates a neurapraxia and segmental demyelination of the nerve.

thromboangiitis obliterans: *See* Buerger's disease.

thrombocytopenia: A decrease in the platelet count below 150,000/ mm^3 of blood caused by inadequate platelet production from the bone marrow, increased platelet destruction outside the bone marrow, or splenic sequestration. Thrombocytopenia is a common complication of leukemia or metastatic cancer (bone marrow infiltration) and aggressive cancer chemotherapy (cytotoxic agents). Presenting symptoms are aplastic anemia and primary bleeding sites in the bone marrow and spleen; and secondary bleeding occurring from small blood vessels in the skin, mucosa, and brain. Other symptoms include petechiae and/or purpura in the skin and mucosa, easy bruising, epistaxis, melena, hematuria, excessive menstrual bleeding, and gingival bleeding.

thrombocytosis: An increase in the number of circulating platelets greater than 400,000/mm^3. Overproduction of platelets is associated with conditions such as chronic nonlymphoblastic leukemia, polycythemia vera, and myelofibrosis (replacement of hematopoietic bone marrow with fibrous tissue). Blood viscosity is increased, leading to an increased risk of thrombosis or emboli.

thrombophlebitis: A partial or complete occlusion of a vein by a thrombus (clot) with secondary inflammatory reaction in the wall of the vein. May affect the deep superficial veins.

torticollis: Torticollis means "twisted neck" and is a contracted state of the sternocleidomastoid muscle producing a bending of the head to the affected side with rotation of the chin to the opposite side.

traumatic brain injury (TBI): A closed head injury occurring when the soft tissue of the brain is forced into contact with the skull. The long-term effects associated with closed head injury vary, depending on the severity of the injury. A mild head injury occurs when there is no skull fracture or laceration of the brain. There is an altered state of consciousness, although loss of consciousness does not always occur. Usually neurologic examination is normal, though post-concussive syndrome may develop, which severely limits an individual's ability to perform activities of daily living. Severe head injuries result from significant bruising and bleeding within the brain. Permanent disability cognitively and physically is often the consequence.

traumatic spinal cord injury: *See* spinal cord injury.

tricuspid atresia: A congenital heart disease in which there is a failure of the tricuspid valve to develop with a lack of communication from the right atrium to the right ventricle. Blood flows through an atrial septal defect or a patent ductus ovale to the left side of the heart and through a ventricular septal defect to the right ventricle and out to the lungs. There is complete mixing of unoxygenated and oxygenated blood in the left side of the heart, resulting in systemic desaturation and varying amounts of pulmonary obstruction.

tricuspid stenosis: Tricuspid stenosis occurs in people with severe mitral valve disease (usually rheumatic in origin) and is rare. A secondary complication is tricuspid regurgitation, which is associated with carcinoid syndrome, systemic lupus erythematosus, infective endocarditis, and in the presence of mitral valve disease. Surgical repair is more common than valvular replacement.

tuberculosis (TB): Respiratory disease caused by the tubercule bacilli. Formerly known as *consumption,* TB is an infectious, inflammatory systemic disease that affects the lungs and may disseminate to involve lymph nodes and other organs. It is caused by infection with *Mycobacterium tuberculosis* and is characterized by granulomas, caseous (resembling cheese) necrosis, and subsequent cavity formation.

Turner's syndrome: Absence of an X chromosome in females, resulting in lower amounts of estrogen produced and tendencies to be shorter in height, have fertility problems, and mild mental retardation or learning difficulties.

ulcerative colitis: An inflammatory intestinal tract disease with prominent erythema and ulceration affecting the colon and rectum. Inflammation and ulceration affect mucosal and submucosal layers. Associated with mild to severe abdominal pain; chronic, severe diarrhea; bloody stools; mild to moderate anorexia; and mild to moderate joint pain.

urinary incontinence: The involuntary loss of urine that is sufficient to be a social and/or hygiene problem. There are five categories of urinary incontinence: (1) stress incontinence is the loss of urine during activities that increase the intra-abdominal pressure such as coughing, laughing, lifting; (2) urge incontinence is the uncontrolled loss of urine that is preceded by an unexpected, strong urge to void; (3) mixed or total incontinence is a combination of stress and urge incontinence; (4) overflow incontinence is the uncontrolled loss of urine when intravesicular pressure exceeds outlet resistance, usually the result of an obstruction (e.g., tumor) or neurologic symptoms; and (5) functional incontinence, which is the functional inability to get to the bathroom or manage the clothing required to go to the bathroom.

urinary tract infection (UTI): An example of urinary tract infection affecting the lower urinary tract (ureter, bladder, urethra) is cystitis. An example of urinary tract infection involving the upper urinary tract (kidneys) is pyelonephritis (see definition). Elder individuals have a higher risk for this due to inactivity or immobility, which causes impaired bladder emptying; bladder ischemia resulting from urine retention; urinary overflow obstruction from renal calculi and prostatic hyperplasia; senile vaginitis; constipation; and diminished bactericidal activity of prostatic secretions. UTI is a bacterial infection with a count greater than 100,000 organisms per milliliter of urine.

urticaria: An eruption of itching wheals (hives); a vascular reaction of the skin with the appearance of slightly elevated patches that are redder or paler than the surrounding skin.

uterine prolapse: Bulging of the uterus into the vagina.

varicose veins: Abnormal dilation of veins, usually the saphenous veins of the lower extremities, leading to tortuosity (twisting and turning) of the vessel, incompetence of the valves, and propensity to thrombosis.

vertebral cerebellar artery syndrome: Blood supply to the brainstem, medulla, and cerebellum is provided by the vertebral and posterior cerebellar arteries. An occlusion of the vertebral artery leading to a medial medullary infarction of the pyramid can result in contralateral hemiparesis of the arm and leg, sparing the face. If the medial lemnicus and the hypoglossal nerve fibers are involved, loss of joint position sense and ipsilateral tongue weakness can occur. The edema associated with cerebellar infarction can cause sudden respiratory arrest due to raised intracranial pressure in the posterior fossa. Gait unsteadiness, dizziness, nausea, and vomiting may be the only early symptoms (vertebral artery syndrome).

vestibular dysfunction: Lesions of the vestibular system that lead to dizziness, lightheadedness, disequilibrium, nystagmus (rhythmic eye movements), abnormalities of saccadic eye movements (fast eye movements), oscillopsia (illusion of environmental movement), and diminished vestibulospinal reflexes. Lesions of the vestibular system can be broadly categorized into five anatomic sites: (1) the vestibular end organ and vestibular nerve terminals, (2) the vestibular ganglia and nerve within the internal auditory canal, (3) the cerbellopontine angle, (4) the brainstem and cerebellum, and (5) the vestibular projections to the cerebral cortex. The causes are varied and include bacterial infection, viral infection, vascular disease, neoplasia, trauma, metabolic disorders, and toxic drugs.

Vogt's syndrome: *See* athetoid cerebral palsy.

von Recklinghausen's disease: Multiple neurofibromata of nerve sheaths that occur along peripheral nerves and on spinal and cranial nerve roots. The area over the tumor may be hyperpigmented. Symptoms may be completely absent or may be those of pain due to pressure on spinal cord and nerves.

Wallenberg's syndrome: *See* posterior inferior cerebellar artery syndrome.

wallerian degeneration: Anterograde (distal) degeneration of the axon (unlike segmental demyelination, which leaves the axon intact as myelin breaks down).

Weber's syndrome: When a third cranial nerve palsy occurs with contralateral hemiplegia. Paralysis of the oculomotor nerve on one side with contralateral spastic hemiplegia is referred to as Weber 's paralysis.

Wernicke's aphasia: Infarct to a specific area of the brain that severely affects the person's level of comprehension. The person is able to visualize but is frequently nonfunctional. Usually involves a vitamin deficiency of vitamin B_1 and vitamin B_{12}.

Williams syndrome: Syndrome caused by a genetic defect, characterized by cardiovascular problems, high blood calcium levels, mental retardation, developmental delays, and a "little pixie face" with puffy eyes and a turned-up nose.

Wilm's tumor: A nephroblastoma that is the most common malignant neoplasm in children. The tumor appears to be fleshy but may have areas of necrosis that lead to cavity formation. The most common presenting feature is a large abdominal mass and abdominal pain. Hematuria may occur, as well as hypertension, anorexia, nausea, and vomiting.

Wilson's disease: This is a progressive disease inherited as an autosomal recessive train that produces a defect in the metabolism of copper, with accumulation of copper in the liver, brain, kidney, cornea, and other tissues. The disease is characterized by the presence of Kayser-Fleischer rings around the iris of the eye (from copper deposition), cirrhosis of the liver, and degenerative changes in the brain, particularly the basal ganglia. *Also known as* hepatolenticular degeneration.

xeroderma: A mild form of ichthyosis; excessive dryness of the skin.

REFERENCES

Angelman Syndrome Foundation. (2014.) *What is Angelman syndrome?* Retrieved from www.angelman.org/understanding-as/

Apert International. (2014). *What is Apert syndrome?* Retrieved from www.apert.org/apert.htm

National Institutes of Health. (2012, March). *Motor neuron diseases fact sheet.* Retrieved from www.ninds.nih.gov/disorders/motor_neuron_diseases/detail_motor_neuron_diseases.htm

Office of Communications and Public Liaison. (2013, December 30). *NINDS Pervasive Developmental Disorders Information Page.* Retrieved from www.ninds.nih.gov/disorders/pdd/pdd.htm

BIBLIOGRAPHY

American Physical Therapy Association. (1997). Guide to physical therapy practice. *Journal of the American Physical Therapy Association, 77,* 11.

Bottomley, J. M., & Lewis, C. B. *Geriatric rehabilitation: A clinical approach.* (2nd ed.). Upper Saddle River, NJ: Prentice Hall Publishers.

Goodman, C. C., & Boissonnault, W. G. (1998). *Pathology: Implications for the physical therapist.* Philadelphia, PA: W. B. Saunders.

Tan, J. C. (1998). *Physical medicine and rehabilitation: Diagnostics, therapeutics, and basic problems.* St. Louis, MO: Mosby-Year Book.

Thomas, C. L. (1997). *Taber's cyclopedic medical dictionary* (18th ed.). Philadelphia, PA: F. A. Davis.

World Health Organization. (1997). International classification of diseases: Clinical modification (9th rev.). New York, NY: Author.

Energy Conservation Techniques

USE GOOD POSTURE

- Avoid excessive bending, reaching, carrying, and lifting. Avoid extra trips by using a cart or trolley to carry items. A small basket keeps cleaning supplies handy. A carpenter's apron works well for small home repairs.

- Consider your own body proportions to determine comfortable work heights. Elbows should form a 90-degree angle, shoulders should be relaxed, and the spine should be straight for a proper work height.

- When carrying, divide the load (e.g., carry two smaller bags of groceries in each arm instead of one large heavy bag).

- Prevent bending and stooping by using long or adjustable handles on dustpans, brushes, shower mops—even paint rollers.

REDUCE FATIGUE

- Consider how you can do some jobs sitting rather than standing, such as chopping vegetables, ironing, and woodworking. Sitting reduces energy use by 25%.

- Alternate postures and take frequent stretch breaks throughout the day.

Jacobs, K., & Simon, L. (Eds.). *Quick Reference Dictionary for Occupational Therapy, Sixth Edition* (pp. 490-492).
© 2015 SLACK Incorporated.

- Incorporate a system of work and rest into activities. Short 5-minute rest breaks during daily activities can help increase overall endurance.

MODIFY ACTIVITIES

- Air-dry dishes and use freezer-to-microwave dishes.

- Use a lightweight steam iron.

- If your laundry room is located downstairs, then toss dirty linen down in a pillowcase rather than making an extra trip.

- To lift items out of the oven, kneel alongside the oven rather than bending over.

- To reduce the amount of bending when making the bed, use a lightweight duvet rather than several layers of sheets and blankets.

CREATE A COMFORTABLE ENVIRONMENT

- If the surrounding conditions are pleasant, then the job will be less tiring and more enjoyable. Listen to your favorite music when doing chores. Good lighting, comfortable clothing, and pleasing colors set the stage for work with less strain.

PRACTICE TIME MANAGEMENT

- Pace yourself; alternate light and heavy tasks.

- Divide activities throughout the week instead of overdoing it in one day. Keep a schedule on the refrigerator to remind you and your family of everyone's responsibilities.

ORGANIZE YOUR WORK

- Plan your activities first to avoid extra trips. Assemble necessary supplies and equipment prior to doing the job. For example, arranging garden supplies and tools prior to planting.

- Group articles that are used together (e.g., cleaning tools and cloths).

- Store heavy articles in the area easiest to reach, light articles in the high and low areas.

Evidence-Based Practice, Levels of Evidence, and Qualitative Research

Developed by Scott McNeil, OTD, MS, OTR/L

The phrase evidence-based practice (EBP) is becoming increasingly popular in health care as insurance companies provide reimbursement. As an occupational therapist, it is important to understand what EBP is, what it is not, and how it can be used to benefit your clients and the occupational therapy profession.

EBP occurs when a practitioner combines his or her clinical expertise with the best available research evidence and the values of the client (Figure 19-1 [Sackett, Straus, Richardson, Rosenberg, & Haynes, 2000]).

Practitioners are encouraged to follow these steps in the EBP process (Lou & Durando, 2006; Wyrick, 2010):

1. Create a clinical question

   a. Practitioners develop clinical questions on a daily basis. It might be a general question, such as "What treatment technique is most effective for a client with a particular diagnosis?" or a more specific one, such as "Is treatment A or treatment B the best option to reduce a particular symptom in a client?"

Jacobs, K., & Simon, L. (Eds.). *Quick Reference Dictionary for Occupational Therapy, Sixth Edition* (pp. 493-498). © 2015 SLACK Incorporated.

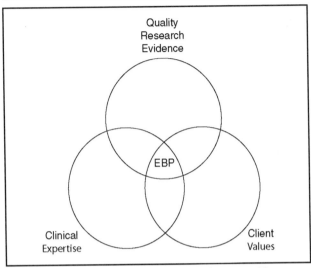

Figure 19-1. Evidence-based practice occurs when a practitioner combines his or her clinical expertise with quality research evidence and client values. (Adapted from Sackett, Straus, Richardson, Rosenberg, & Haynes [2000].)

     i. Develop a PICO question

        1. Population/patient/problem

        2. Intervention

        3. Comparison

        4. Outcome

2. Find research evidence

    a. Take your clinical question and generate keywords to use in online evidence databases, such as Cochrane Library, EBSCOhost, MEDLINE, CINAHL

    b. Scan through the titles and abstracts of available literature to find relevant articles

3. Appraise the research evidence using levels of evidence

   a. To find the best research evidence available, research designs have been organized in a hierarchical order according to design structure, rigor, and sensitivity to eliminate bias or error of results. The higher the level of evidence, the more confident the practitioner can be in using the results to guide practice. It is possible to determine the study research design type by reading the study. This information may be located in the abstract, introduction, or methodology section of the study. It is also possible to filter your search results in an evidence database to produce evidence of a certain level.

   b. Common research designs are placed in a hierarchical order in Figure 19-2 and include meta-analysis, systematic reviews, randomized control trials, cohort design, qualitative studies, case-controlled studies, case report, background information, and expert opinion (Oxford Centre for Evidence-Based Medicine, 2011; Wyrick, 2010).

   c. Read the research article carefully to see whether it is applicable to your clinical question. The evidence may support or contradict your past clinical experience.

4. Apply the findings to clinical practice

   a. Combine the quality research evidence that you located with your clinical experience and a client-centered approach to care

5. Evaluate the outcome and the EBP process itself

   a. Did you make a change in your clinical practice as a result of the evidence? What was the outcome for your client?

EBP is not technically research. Every practitioner can engage in EBP. Research involves the generation of new evidence with the goal of creating new knowledge. A practitioner who engages in EBP uses research and, with practice, can become an expert consumer of the newly created knowledge created by research.

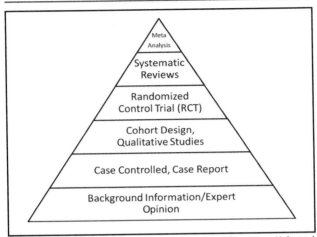

Figure 19-2. Levels of evidence for evidence-based practice. (Adapted from Oxford Centre for Evidence-Based Medicine [2011] and Wyrick [2010].)

The two primary methods of research are qualitative and quantitative. There is value on each method of research, and practitioners are encouraged to include both in their utilization of EBP.

Quantitative research, common in physical sciences, heavily utilizes statistics to test a hypothesis, demonstrate cause and effect, and make predictions. This research method is focused on being objective and often includes standardized procedures with the goal of elaborating on the statistical significance of findings (Kielhofner & Fossey, 2006). Most discussions about EBP emphasize the use of quantitative studies. Statistical procedures common in quantitative research are described in Appendix 55.

Qualitative research methods are common in social sciences and utilize a more descriptive approach to exploring phenomena. These studies are often smaller in size than qualitative studies and typically focus on a person's experiences in his or her unique naturalistic environment. A qualitative researcher is more likely to interview and observe a person to gather as much understanding as possible than to attempt to test a hypothesis. A qualitative study

Characteristic	Quantitative Research	Qualitative Research
Origin	Physical sciences	Study of people
Type of data collected	Numbers and statistics	Words, images, objects
Approach to rigor	Maintain objectivity	Accurately represent those studied
Data presentation/ results	Numbers (statistics), generalizable findings	Descriptions, specific, less generalizable
Data analysis	Describes relationship between variables, tests hypothesis	Identify meaning
Common study designs	Meta-analysis, systematic review, randomized control trials, cohort study, single subject (case controlled), survey research	Case study, survey

provides data that are rich in narrative details but not in statistics, making it more challenging to determine cause-and-effect relationships from data and thus limiting the generalizability of the results.

Fineout-Overholt, Melnyk, and Schultz (2005) described levels of evidence for qualitative studies that focus on meaning/experience questions (Figure 19-3 [Consortium Library, 2007]).

Occupational therapy practitioners use a combination of qualitative and quantitative methods to complete a client's occupational profile and assessment of occupational performance. Without both methods, the practitioner's view of the client would not be complete. The same is true with EBP. To answer your clinical question, qualitative and quantitative research articles should be explored.

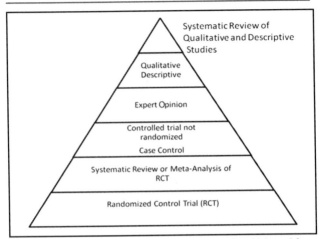

Figure 19-3. Levels of evidence for qualitative studies. (Adapted from Consortium Library [2007].)

REFERENCES

Bennett, S. (n.d.). *Evidence-based practice in occupational therapy: An introduction.* [Powerpoint presentation]. Retrieved from www.otevidence.info/images/Introduction.pdf

Consortium Library. University of Alaska Anchorage. (2007). *Levels of evidence (qualitative).* Retrieved from http://consortiumlibrary.org/aml/researchaids/ebp/ebp_pyramid_qualitative.pdf

Fineout-Overholt, E., Melnyk, B. M., & Schultz, A. (2005). Transforming healthcare from the inside out: Advancing evidence-based practice in the 21st century. *Journal of Professional Nursing, 21*(6), 335-344.

Kielhofner, G., & Fossey, E. (2006). Range of research. In: G. Kielhofner (Ed.), *Research in occupational therapy: Methods of inquiry for enhancing practice* (pp. 20-35). Philadelphia, PA: F. A. Davis.

Lou, J. Q., & Durando, P. (2006). Asking clinical questions and searching for the evidence. In M. Law & J. MacDermid (Eds.), *Evidence-based rehabilitation: A guide to practice* (2nd ed., pp. 95-117). Thorofare, NJ: SLACK Incorporated.

Oxford Centre for Evidence-Based Medicine. (2011). *The Oxford 2011 levels of evidence.* Retrieved from www.cebm.net/mod_product/design/files/CEBM-Levels-of-Evidence-2.1.pdf

Sackett, D. L., Straus, S. E., Richardson, W. S., Rosenberg, W., & Haynes, R. B. (2000). *Evidence-based medicine: How to practice and teach EBM* (2nd ed.). Edinburgh, Scotland: Churchill Livingstone.

Wyrick, A.M. (2010). *Evidence-based practice.* Short course presented at the annual conference of the Virginia Occupational Therapy Association, Richmond, Virginia.

Frames of Reference Used in Occupational Therapy

Originally written by
Emily Firor, MEd; Elizabeth Perras, MS;
Karen Zimmerman, MEd; Kathleen McCarthy, MEd;
and Patricia Kronk, MS, CAS

Updated by Flora Cole, MSOT Student

MODEL OF HUMAN OCCUPATION THEORETICAL CONCEPTS

- Humans are intrinsically motivated to interact with the environment through meaningful activities.

- Positive feedback during purposeful activities and positive interpretation results in positive success cycle. Negative feedback during purposeful activities may result in negative interpretation and a lack of motivation to participate.

DEVELOPMENTAL THEORETICAL CONCEPTS

- View life as an ongoing developmental process.

- Assess and treat to progress the individual toward variable age-appropriate functioning.

- Treatment and evaluation are often done with caregiver involvement.

Jacobs, K., & Simon, L. (Eds.). *Quick Reference Dictionary for Occupational Therapy, Sixth Edition* (pp. 499-506). © 2015 SLACK Incorporated.

Behavioral Theoretical Concepts

- Behavior is shaped by environmental responses.
- Reinforcement can be used to develop and increase desired behaviors.
- Intensity, duration, and frequency of behavior are important to consider.

Psychodynamic Theoretical Concepts

- Unconscious forces affect behaviors as much as conscious ones.
- Treatment is used to develop socially acceptable ways to express drives.
- Treatment makes the unconscious drives conscious and allows them to be expressed appropriately.

Cognitive Disability Theoretical Concepts

- Cognition is the basis for all behavior.
- There are six cognitive levels of processing, which can be determined through assessment.
- Modify the task difficulty to enable success and safety.

Rehabilitation Theoretical Concepts

- Compensate for physical and mental disabilities.
- Use adaptive equipment or techniques to enhance functioning.
- The environment influences the functional level of independence.

Neurodevelopmental Theoretical Concepts

- Neck and trunk control is the foundation for all other body control.

- Brain damage causes abnormal muscle tone and reflexes, which cause impaired functional skills.

- Provide sensory information regarding normal muscle movements to promote normal movement and functioning.

Sensory Integration Theoretical Concepts

- There is difficulty in taking in and combining sensory information and integrating with functional skills.

- Responding adaptively to the environment enhances the intake and combining of sensory information.

- Improved sensory processing provides a foundation for enhanced attention and academic ability.

Biomechanical Theoretical Concept

- Views the body as a machine.

- Improves performance in the component parts of the body (range of motion, strength, endurance), resulting in improved functioning.

Person-Environment Occupational Performance Model

- People are naturally motivated to explore their world and demonstrate mastery.

- Settings in which people experience success help them feel good about themselves.

- Through occupation, people develop their self-identity and derive a sense of fulfillment (Christiansen & Baum, 1997).

OCCUPATIONAL THERAPY INTERVENTION PROCESS MODEL THEORETICAL CONCEPTS

- A professional reasoning model that helps ensure an occupation-centered perspective is used to guide reasoning and plan/implement occupation-based and occupation-focused services.

- The occupational therapy process is depicted as occurring over three global phases: evaluation and goal-setting, intervention, and reevaluation.

- Occupational therapists must document measurable, occupation-focused baselines, goals, and outcomes. Stressing occupational performance in evaluations, interventions, and documentation is an important mechanism for promoting the clients' quality of life (Center for Innovative OT Solutions, 2014).

ECOLOGY OF HUMAN PERFORMANCE THEORETICAL CONCEPTS

- This framework provides a structure for thinking of context as a key variable in assessment and intervention planning, while taking into account the inherent dangers in examining performance out of context.

- Delineates and defines the relevant concepts and describes relationships among variables. Includes a person's experiences and sensorimotor, cognitive, and psychosocial skills and abilities.

- Ecology, or how the interaction between person and the environment affects human behavior and performance, and that performance cannot be understood out of context (Dunn, Brown, & McGuigan, 1994).

INTERNATIONAL CLASSIFICATION OF FUNCTIONING, DISABILITY AND HEALTH THEORETICAL CONCEPTS

- Recognizes disability as a universal human experience, placing all health conditions on an equal footing and allowing the focus to shift from cause to impact.

- Takes into account the social aspects of disability and does not see disability as only a medical or biological dysfunction.

- Includes contextual factors that allow for consideration of the impact of the environment on a person's functioning (World Health Organization, 2001).

HEALTH BELIEF MODEL THEORETICAL CONCEPTS

- This model is based on the concept that a person's health-related behavior depends on the person's perception of four critical areas: the severity of a potential illness or injury, the person's susceptibility to that illness, the benefits of taking preventive action, and the barriers to taking action.

- Emphasizes that a person's perception of the threat caused by a potential illness can be developed by an increased understanding of severity and susceptibility. To promote positive change, the goal is for the perceived severity and susceptibility plus the potential benefits to outweigh the potential barriers.

- Change comes about by the use of cues to action (literature, images, reminders) and development of increased self-efficacy (Boston University, School of Public Health, 2013a).

ADRAGOGICAL EDUCATION (ANDRAGOGY) THEORETICAL CONCEPTS

- Stresses the unique and challenging needs of a mature learner and provides a more engaging and flexible experience of learning.

- This model is appreciative of the existing knowledge base and life experiences of adult learners ("experience rich but theory poor").

- An understanding of why the student is focusing on that particular subject is emphasized, and real-life application is used as much as possible to facilitate mature learning (Donnan, 2008).

TRANSFORMATIVE EDUCATION THEORETICAL CONCEPTS

- Based on the assumption that mature adults go through major transitions in life and adult development is not a linear pathway.

- Adult development is a series of life cycles closely related to life events such as marriage, birth of a child, and career advancement.

- Transformations can be brought about by introduction of transformative learning experiences that can intentionally spur progression and advancement (Pawlak & Bergquist, n.d.).

TRANSTHEORETICAL MODEL CONCEPTS

- The core constructs are the stages of change, which are ordered categories along a continuum of readiness to change behavior. The main focus is on emotions, cognitions, and behavior.

- Transitions between the stages are affected by independent variables known as the processes of change, which include decisional balance (pros and cons), self-efficacy, situational temptations, and psychological, environmental, cultural, socioeconomic, and genetic variables.

- The stages include precontemplation, contemplation, preparation, action, and maintenance. Regression (relapse) can occur when the person moves backward and returns to an earlier stage of change (Boston University, School of Public Health, 2013b).

COMMUNITY OF LEARNERS
THEORETICAL CONCEPTS

- This model views children and adults as active members of a community (classroom, home, neighborhood).

- Adults usually assume the leadership role, but the group defines the direction they will choose. The group dynamic is considered to be a social process in which the adult is the facilitator and the rest of the group are active members.

- The community uses different roles such as supporter, observer, and leader to coordinate and implement activities and endeavors to pursue. Conflicts are expected and resolutions are decided as a group (Charles A. Dana Center at the University of Texas at Austin and Agile Mind, Inc., n.d.).

REFERENCES

Boston University, School of Public Health. (2013a). *The health belief model*. Retrieved from http://sphweb.bumc.bu.edu/otlt/MPH-Modules/SB/SB721-Models/SB721-Models2.html

Boston University, School of Public Health (2013b). *The transtheoretical model (stages of change)*. Retrieved from http://sphweb.bumc.bu.edu/otlt/MPH-Modules/SB/SB721-Models/SB721-Models6.html

Center for Innovative OT Solutions. (2014). *Occupational therapy intervention process model (OTIPM)*. Retrieved from www.innovativeotsolutions.com/content/otipm/

Charles A. Dana Center at the University of Texas at Austin and Agile Mind, Inc. (n.d.). *Learning and the adolescent mind*. Retrieved from http://learningandtheadolescentmind.org/ideas_community.html

Christiansen, C., & Baum, C. (Eds.). (1997). *Occupational therapy: Enabling function and well-being* (2nd ed., p. 48). Thorofare, NJ: SLACK Incorporated.

Donnan, R. *Andragogy*. (2008). Retrieved from www.blog.klpnow.com/2008/01/andragogy.html

Dunn, W., Brown, C., & McGuigan, A. (1994). The ecology of human performance: A framework for considering the effect of context. *American Journal of Occupational Therapy, 48*(7), 595-607.

Pawlak, K., & Bergquist, W. (n.d.). Engaging experience and wisdom in a postmodern age. *Professional School of Psychology*. Retrieved from www.psychology.edu/about/four-models-of-adult-education/

World Health Organization. (2001). *International classification of functioning, disability and health*. Retrieved from www.who.int/classifications/icf/en/

Functional Abilities by Spinal Cord Injury Level

Spinal Cord Levels	Key Muscles Innervated	Movements Possible	Pattern of Weakness	Functional Potential
C1-C3	Sternocleidomastoid Levator scapulae Upper trapezius Diaphragm (C3-C5)	Neck control Chew Swallow Talk Sip Puff Some scapular elevation	Complete paralysis of trunk, upper extremities (UEs), and lower extremities (LEs) Dependence on respirator	Requires full-time attendant care Total dependence with activities of daily living (ADL) and transfers Can propel power wheelchair equipped with portable respirator and chin, head, puff, or sip controls

Spinal Cord Levels	Key Muscles Innervated	Movements Possible	Pattern of Weakness	Functional Potential
				Can operate communication and environmental control systems with head master, head pointer, mouth stick, or pneumatic control
C4	Trapezius (superior, middle, and inferior) Diaphragm Cervical and paraspinal muscles	Respiration Scapula elevation Neck movements	Paralysis of trunk UEs and LEs (except scapula elevation)	Good potential to control breathing without ventilator Requires full-time attendant care Can drink with long straw Total dependence with ADL and transfers Can independently power wheelchair with chin, head, sip, or puff controls

Spinal Cord Levels	Key Muscles Innervated	Movements Possible	Pattern of Weakness	Functional Potential
				Activities can be accomplished through use of mouth stick, head pointer, voice recognition software, or tongue touch key pad
C5	Partial deltoid Biceps brachii Brachialis Brachioradialis Rotator cuff muscles rotation Rhomboids Serratus anterior Teres major	Shoulder abduction, flexion, extension, horizontal abduction, horizontal adduction, internal and external rotation Scapular protraction and retraction Elbow flexion and supination	Total paralysis of trunk and LEs Low endurance because of paralysis of intercostals and low respiratory reserve No active elbow extension, forearm pronation, hand or wrist movement	With adaptive equipment or splints and set-up assistance, can perform eating, handwriting, light hygiene, shaving, telephoning, and typing May be independent in upper body dressing, if muscle strength is good Otherwise may need minimum to moderate assistance

Spinal Cord Levels	Key Muscles Innervated	Movements Possible	Pattern of Weakness	Functional Potential
	All shoulder muscles are at least partially innervated except coracobrachialis and latissimus dorsi			Dependent in lower body with transfers; may be able to assist in rolling in bed, using side rails, or loops; independent with power wheelchair
May drive a van with substantial adaptations
Can write independently with wrist support and writing device
Requires a minimum of at least part-time attendant care

Spinal Cord Levels	Key Muscles Innervated	Movements Possible	Pattern of Weakness	Functional Potential
C6	Extensor carpi radialis longus and brevis Serratus anterior (partial but significant innervation) Pronator teres Coracobrachialis Pectoralis major Latissimus dorsi	Full strength with shoulder movements (flexion, extension, abduction, adduction, external, and internal rotation) Forearm pronation and supination Radial wrist extension Gross grasp and gross prehension via tenodesis action Good stability of scapula on trunk	No elbow extension or ulnar wrist extension Endurance may be low No active wrist flexion Complete paralysis of trunk and LEs	Able to perform many activities independently with tenodesis splint or universal cuff, such as self-feeding with regular utensils, personal hygiene, and grooming Independent in upper body dressing Minimal assistance for lower body dressing Bed mobility, independence in rolling side-to-side Minimal assistance from supine to sitting

Spinal Cord Levels	Key Muscles Innervated	Movements Possible	Pattern of Weakness	Functional Potential
				Assist with transfers by substituting shoulder adduction and external rotation for elbow extension
				May be independent with a sliding board
				Independent with manual wheelchair on level terrain or slight incline
				Requires adaptive equipment and assistance for bathing and bowel care
				Independent at driving car with hand controls
				May participate in wheelchair sports
				May require part-time attendant care

Spinal Cord Levels	Key Muscles Innervated	Movements Possible	Pattern of Weakness	Functional Potential
C7	Triceps brachii	Elbow extension	Limited grasp, release, and dexterity	Independent in ADL
	Pectoralis major	Full strength of all shoulder movements	Complete paralysis of trunk and LEs	Can perform transfers independently
	Latissimus dorsi			Independent bed mobility
	Flexor digitorum superficialis	Finger flexion but weak		Independent for push-up in wheelchair for pressure release
	Extensor digitorum	Finger MP joint extension		
	Flexor carpi radialis	Radial wrist flexion		Independent with driving with hand controls
	Extensor carpi ulnaris	Ulnar wrist extension		Independent with bowel and bladder care
	Extensor pollicis longus and brevis	Thumb extension		Independent with manual wheelchair
	Abductor pollicis longus			

Spinal Cord Levels	Key Muscles Innervated	Movements Possible	Pattern of Weakness	Functional Potential
C8-T1	All the muscles of the UE are now fully innervated Dorsal and palmar interossei Lumbricals Thenar and hypothenar muscles Adductor pollicis Flexor digitorum profundus Flexor pollicis longus and brevis Pronator quadratus	Full control of UEs, including finger flexion, isolated finger and thumb movements, fine coordination, and grasp	Paralysis of LEs Weakness of trunk control Lower respiratory reserves	Independent in ADL, with transfers and bed mobility

Spinal Cord Levels	Key Muscles Innervated	Movements Possible	Pattern of Weakness	Functional Potential
T4-T9	All muscles of UE Partial innervation of intercostal muscles and long muscles of the back	Full arm function Partial trunk stability Increased endurance	Total paralysis of LEs Partial trunk paralysis	Independent in all self-care, independent manual wheelchair use, and transfers Drives car independently with adaptations May use standing frame independently Independent light housekeeping
T10-L2	Intercostal muscles are fully innervated Abdominal muscles are partially to fully innervated	Good trunk stability Increased physical endurance	Paralysis of LEs	Independent in self-care, work, personal hygiene, and housekeeping Drives car with hand controls Often uses wheelchair but can ambulate with difficulty using crutches and braces

Appendix 21

Spinal Cord Levels	Key Muscles Innervated	Movements Possible	Pattern of Weakness	Functional Potential
L3-L4	Lower back muscles Quadriceps Hip flexors Hip adductors	Trunk stability and control Hip flexion Hip adduction Knee extension	Individual cannot perform hip extension, knee flexion, or ankle and foot movements	Can ambulate independently with short leg braces using crutches May still use a wheelchair for energy conservation
L5-S3	Gluteus maximus Hamstrings Knee flexors Ankle and foot muscles	Partial to full control of LEs	May have weakness of ankle and foot Possible decrease in standing and walking tolerance modifications	Independent in all activities Can drive car without modification May require braces for ambulation

Glasgow Coma Scale

The Glasgow Coma Scale (GCS) is a scoring system used to describe the level of consciousness in a person following a traumatic brain injury. It is used to help gauge the severity of an acute brain injury and is a reliable and objective way of recording the initial and subsequent level of consciousness in a person after a brain injury. It is often used by trained staff in the emergency department and intensive care units.

The GCS measures the following functions:
Eye Opening (E)

- 4 = spontaneous
- 3 = to voice
- 2 = to pain
- 1 = none

Verbal Response (V)

- 5 = normal conversation
- 4 = disoriented conversation
- 3 = words, but not coherent
- 2 = no words, only sounds
- 1 = none

Jacobs, K., & Simon, L. (Eds.). *Quick Reference Dictionary for Occupational Therapy, Sixth Edition* (pp. 517-520). © 2015 SLACK Incorporated.

Motor Response (M)

- 6 = normal

- 5 = localized to pain

- 4 = withdraws to pain

- 3 = decorticate posture (an abnormal posture that can include rigidity, clenched fists, legs held straight out, and arms bent inward toward the body with the wrists and fingers bent and held on the chest)

- 2 = decerebrate (an abnormal posture that can include rigidity, arms and legs held straight out, toes pointed downward, and head and neck arched backward)

- 1 = none

Clinicians use this scale to rate the best eye opening response, the best verbal response, and the best motor response an individual makes. The final GCS score or grade is the sum of these numbers.

USING THE GLASGOW COMA SCALE

Every brain injury is different, but generally, brain injury is classified as:

- Severe: GCS 3-8 (you cannot score lower than a 3)

- Moderate: GCS 9-12

- Mild: GCS 13-15

Mild brain injuries can result in temporary or permanent neurological symptoms and neuroimaging tests, such as computed tomography scans or magnetic resonance imaging, may or may not show evidence of any damage.

Moderate and severe brain injuries often result in long-term impairments in cognition (thinking skills), physical skills, and/or emotional/behavioral functioning.

LIMITATIONS OF THE GLASGOW COMA SCALE

Factors such as drug use, alcohol intoxication, shock, or low blood oxygen can alter a patient's level of consciousness. These factors could lead to an inaccurate score on the GCS.

CHILDREN AND THE GLASGOW COMA SCALE

The GCS is usually not used with younger children, especially those too young to have reliable language skills. The Pediatric Glasgow Coma Scale (PGCS), a modification of the scale used on adults, is used instead. The PGCS still uses the three tests—eye, verbal, and motor responses—and the three values are considered separately as well as together.

Here is the slightly altered grading scale for the PGCS:
Eye Opening (E)

- 4 = spontaneous

- 3 = to voice

- 2 = to pain

- 1 = none

Verbal Response (V)

- 5 = smiles, oriented to sounds, follows objects, interacts

- 4 = cries but consolable, inappropriate interactions

- 3 = inconsistently inconsolable, moaning

- 2 = inconsolable, agitated

- 1 = none

Motor Response (M)

- 6 = moves spontaneously or purposefully

- 5 = withdraws from touch

- 4 = withdraws to pain

- 3 = decorticate posture (an abnormal posture that can include rigidity, clenched fists, legs held straight out, and arms bent inward toward the body with the wrists and fingers bent and held on the chest)

- 2 = decerebrate (an abnormal posture that can include rigidity, arms and legs held straight out, toes pointed downward, head and neck arched backward)

- 1 = none

Pediatric brain injuries are classified by severity using the same scoring levels as adults, with 3 to 8 reflecting the most severe, 9 to 12 indicating a moderate injury, and 13 to 15 indicating a mild traumatic brain injury. As in adults, moderate and severe injuries often result in significant long-term impairments.

REFERENCE

Teasdale, G., & Jennett, B. (1974). Assessment of coma and impaired consciousness. A practical scale. *Lancet, 2,* 81-84.

Glossary and Definitions of Terms Used in the Initial Health Assessment/ Refugee Health Assessment

refugee: A person who cannot return to his or her country because of persecution or the well-founded fear of persecution on account of race, religion, nationality, membership in a particular social group, or political opinion. A refugee receives this status before entering the United States. In addition to refugees, the following groups may be eligible for refugee benefits and services: Asylee, Cuban/Haitian Entrant, Certain Amerasians from Vietnam, Certified Victims of a Severe Form of Trafficking, Permanent Residents.

alien: A person who is not a citizen or national of the United States.

Alien Registration Receipt Card: An Immigration and Naturalization Service (INS) document that certifies lawful permanent resident status, commonly called the "green card."

Amerasian: A child fathered by a U.S. citizen in certain Southeast Asian countries (e.g., Vietnam, Laos, Cambodia) during conflicts in that region. Amerasians are granted Lawful/Legal Permanent Resident (LPR) status under special provisions of the Immigration and Nationality Act.

asylee: A foreign-born resident who is not a United States citizen and who cannot return to his or her country because of persecution or a "well-founded fear" of persecution on account of race, religion, nationality, membership in a particular social group, or political opinion, as determined by the Department of State or

Jacobs, K., & Simon, L. (Eds.). *Quick Reference Dictionary for Occupational Therapy, Sixth Edition* (pp. 521-528).
© 2015 SLACK Incorporated.

the INS. An asylee receives asylum (*also called* political asylum) status after entering the United States.

case management agency: An agency under contract with ORI to perform certain functions under MRRP including, but not limited to, (1) working with refugees and employment service agencies to develop a Family Employment Plan designed to employ at least one adult in the shortest possible time and lead to self-sufficiency for the family; (2) tracking the progress of the clients in relation to their Family Employment Plan; (3) linking refugees with appropriate services and programs; (4) determining initial and ongoing eligibility for Refugee Cash Assistance.

Cuban/Haitian entrant: All nationals of Cuba and Haiti who applied for asylum or are in exclusion or deportation proceedings but have not received a final order of deportation, as well as persons who are granted parole status or special status under the United States immigration laws for Cubans and Haitians. Cuban/Haitian entrants are eligible for federal benefits in the same way as refugees.

Department of State: A Federal agency whose Bureau of Refugee programs coordinates with voluntary agencies, state localities the reception and placement of refugees.

deportation: The formal removal of an alien from the United States when the presence of that alien is deemed inconsistent with the public welfare. Deportation is ordered by an immigration judge without any punishment being imposed or contemplated.

diversity transition: A transition towards the permanent diversity program in fiscal year 1995, allocating 40,000 visas annually during the period 1992–1994 to nationals of certain countries identified as having been "adversely affected" by the Immigration and Nationality Act Amendments of 1965 (P.L. 89–236). At least 40% of the visas must be allocated to natives of Ireland.

domestic assistance: Federal programs that provide cash and medical assistance, as well as social services to individual refugees and entrants.

durable self-sufficiency: Family's gross income exceeds 450% of the Federal Poverty Level for the state.

early employment: Job placement within 6 months after the date of arrival in United States.

Employment Services for New Refugee Families (ESNRF): Employment services including pre-employment job skills training and post-placement follow-up for employable TAFDC-eligible refugees. The program encourages (1) early employment by focusing on entry level jobs and (2) self-sufficiency by focusing on successful job retention and upgrades.

Employment Support Services Program (ESSP): Employment services including pre-employment job skills and post-employment job retention and upgrade skills training for refugees and immigrants with time limited TAFDC benefits. The program helps clients enter the work force and retain their employment, advancing them toward economic self-sufficiency.

English for Employment (EE): Language instruction for those refugees determined to be in need of such services in order to be considered employable.

entrant: *See* Cuban/Haitian entrant.

ESL: English as a second language.

extended voluntary departure (EVD): A special temporary provision granted administratively to designated national groups physically present in the United States because the U.S. State Department judged conditions in the countries of origin to be "unstable" or "uncertain" or to have shown a pattern of "denial of rights." Aliens in EVD status are temporarily allowed to remain in the United States until conditions in their home country change. Certain aliens holding EVD status from Afghanistan, Ethiopia, Poland, and Uganda, who have resided in the United States since July 1, 1984, were eligible to adjust to temporary and then to permanent resident status under the legalization program. The term "deferred enforced departure" (DED) has replaced EVD in general use.

federal poverty level: Income level reference used by the federal government in eligibility determinations for certain means-tested benefit programs (e.g., food stamps).

full-time employment: Employment which is at least 35 hours per week.

Governor's Advisory Council on Refugees and Immigrants (GAC): An appointed body established in 1983 by Executive Order 229 to advise the governor and the Office for Refugees and Immigrants on policy and programs for refugees and immigrants.

I-94: The INS control document that records every person's arrival in and departure from the United States. It identifies the period of time for which the person is admitted and the person's immigration status.

Immigration Act of 1990: Public Law 101-649 (Act of November 29, 1990) which increased the total immigration to the United States under an overall flexible cap, revised all grounds for exclusion and deportation, authorized temporary protected status to aliens of designated countries, revised and established new nonimmigrant admission categories, revised and extended the Visa Waiver Pilot Program, and revised naturalization authority and requirements.

Immigration and Naturalization Service (INS): The federal agency under the Department of Justice that administers immigration law.

Immigration Reform and Control Act (IRCA) of 1986: Public Law 99-603 (Act of 11/6/86) which passed in order to control and deter illegal immigration to the United States. Its major provisions stipulate legalization of undocumented aliens, legalization of certain agricultural workers, sanctions for employers who knowingly hire undocumented workers, and increased enforcement at U.S. borders.

job placement: Employment which is at least 20 hours per week.

legal permanent resident: A person who the U.S. Citizenship and Immigration Service has granted permission to permanently reside in the United States as an immigrant.

Massachusetts Office for Refugees and Immigrants (ORI): The state agency which oversees refugee resettlement in Massachusetts. The ORI mission is to (1) support the effective resettlement of refugees and immigrants in the state, (2) promote the full participation of these New Americans in the economic, civic, social, and cultural life of the Commonwealth, and (3) foster a public environment that recognizes the ethnic and cultural diversity of the state.

Massachusetts Refugee Resettlement Program (MRRP): A community-based case management and employment services program which promotes economic self-sufficiency for refugees and their families through (1) early entry into the workforce and (2) post-placement services to help them find, get, and keep better jobs once they are working.

match grant: A public/private partnership agreement between a VOLAG and the Department of State under which refugee resettlement costs are shared between government and a community.

Mutual Assistance Association (MAA): Ethnic-based associations that galvanize ethnic community support for resettlement and provide services to refugees.

naturalization: The act of becoming a citizen, other than by birth.

non-immigrant: A person authorized to be in the United States temporarily and for specific purpose, such as student or tourist.

parolee: An alien who has been given permission to enter the United States under emergency conditions or when that alien's entry is considered to be in public interest.

part-time employment: Employment that is less than 35 and at least 20 hours per week.

Post-Employment English for Self-Sufficiency (PEESS): Additional English instruction to employed refugees and include Vocational English Language Training (VELT) which may be needed for job upgrades. Refugees who achieve early employment are given top priority for post-employment English training.

Post-Employment Vocational Skills Training (PEVST): Services that provide the working refugee with short-term, job-targeted skills (including related VELT) in a specific marketable vocation that will secure a current job and/or lead to an upgraded job. Refugees who achieve early employment are given top priority for PEVST.

PRUCOL: "Persons permanently residing under color of law" (PRUCOL) refers to persons residing in the United States who are known to the immigration authorities and whose extended presence in the United States is tolerated by those authorities although they have not been granted legal status.

reception and placement (R&P): The initial resettlement process and period (generally 30 days) during which a VOLAG or other sponsor under an agreement with the United States Department of State is responsible for assisting a refugee.

refugee: A foreign-born resident who is not a U.S. citizen and who cannot return to his or her country because of persecution or the well-founded fear of persecution on account of race, religion, nationality, membership in a particular social group, or political opinion, as determined by the State Department of the INS. A refugee receives this status before entering the United States.

Refugee Cash Assistance (RCA): A program of temporary financial support for eligible members of the MRRP. Case Management Agencies determine eligibility and grant amount. (*Also called* Transitional Cash Assistance.)

Refugee Employment Services: Services provided to refugees by MRRP Employment Services agencies to help them find a job and achieve self-sufficiency. Refugee Employment Services has four components: (1) Refugee Job Services; (2) English for Employment; (3) Post-Employment English for Self-Sufficiency; and (4) Post-Employment Vocational Skills Training.

Refugee Job Services (RJS): A wide range of services to refugees, including teaching the skills important to get, retain, and upgrade a job; job development; job placement; and post-placement follow-up with the employer and client to ensure long-term success and to promote the attainment of family self-sufficiency.

Refugee Medical Assistance (RMA): A program of temporary medical assistance for eligible members of the MRRP that are not eligible for Medicaid. Case Management Agencies determine eligibility. *Also called* Transitional Medical Assistance.

secondary migrant: Refugee who initially settles elsewhere in the United States and subsequently moves to Massachusetts or moves within Massachusetts yet outside of the jurisdiction of the agency that was responsible for his or her initial resettlement agency.

self-sufficiency: Family's gross income exceeds 150% of the federal poverty level for the state.

sponsor: The person or organization that assists an applicant in their admission to the United States.

TAFDC: Transitional Assistance to Families with Dependent Children, formerly Aid to Families with Dependent Children (AFDC).

Targeted Assistance Discretionary Grant (TAG D): Competitive federal grants that are designated for states or counties that contract out the funds to local and private agencies. The grant is intended to meet the special needs of individual refugees or refugee groups that are unmet through other programs. The purposes for which the funding has been used include employment, mental health, and microenterprise development.

Targeted Assistance Formula Grant (TAG F): Another source of federal funding for eligible counties. The grant is for intensive, individualized employment services for refugees with multiple barriers.

Transitional Cash Assistance: *See* Refugee Cash Assistance.

Transitional Medical Assistance: *See* Refugee Medical Assistance.

Unaccompanied Refugee Minor Program (URMP): A federally funded program that offers foster care and other services to refugee children who arrive in this country without their parents.

undocumented aliens: Foreign-born people who entered the United States unknown to authorities or have no current authorization from immigration authorities to be in the United States.

victim of a severe form of trafficking: A person subject to force, fraud, or coercion for sex trafficking and/or involuntary servitude, peonage, debt bondage, or slavery who is certified as a victim by the U.S. Office of Refugee Resettlement.

visa: A document authorizing a person to enter and remain in the United States for certain periods of time.

VOLAG: National voluntary resettlement agency that has entered into a grant, contract, or cooperative agreement with the Department of State or other appropriate federal agency to provide for the reception, initial placement and resettlement processing of refugees in the United State. The VOLAG assigns continuing responsibility for the refugee to a local affiliated VOLAG or sponsor.

Wilson/Fish Alternative Project: An alternative approach to the state-administered refugee services program that allows grantees to develop their own regulations as well as service and assistance components.

Source: The Official Website of the Executive Office of Health and Human Services. Retrieved from www.mass.gov/eohhs/gov/departments/ori/glossary.html

Grading Edema

Edema is excessive fluid accumulation in the interstitial spaces. Edema may result from the following:

- Increased permeability of the capillary walls
- Lymphatic obstruction
- Increased capillary pressure due to heart failure or venous obstruction
- Decreased renal function
- Decreased plasma protein
- Inflammatory conditions
- Disturbance with fluid and electrolytes, especially those involved in sodium retention
- Malnutrition and/or starvation
- Caustic substances and histamines

Edema is documented according to type (pitting, nonpitting, or brawny).

Jacobs, K., & Simon, L. (Eds.). *Quick Reference Dictionary for Occupational Therapy, Sixth Edition* (pp. 529-530). © 2015 SLACK Incorporated.

To grade edema, palpate area and firmly apply pressure with the thumb for 5 seconds. The degree of edema is based on the depth of indentation in centimeters:

1 cm or less = 1+ edema
2 cm = 2+ edema
3 cm = 3+ edema
4 cm = 4+ edema
5 cm or more = 5+ edema

Grading for Balance: Graded Posture Movement Ability of Individual

GRADING DEFINITIONS FOR BALANCE

- **Static:** Posture without motion
- **Dynamic:** Posture during active motion
- **Grading:** A minus grade in fair and good ranges = inconsistent ability

All grades must be qualified with the assistive device being used by the patient. If no assistive device is used, that must be stated.

Grade	Posture	Movement	Ability of Individual
0	Sitting	Static	Needs maximum assistance to maintain sitting without back support
0	Sitting	Dynamic	N/A
0	Standing	Static	Needs maximum assistance to maintain
0	Standing	Dynamic	N/A
P	Sitting	Static	Needs moderate assistance to maintain
P	Sitting	Dynamic	N/A

Jacobs, K., & Simon, L. (Eds.). *Quick Reference Dictionary for Occupational Therapy, Sixth Edition* (pp. 531-533).
© 2015 SLACK Incorporated.

Grade	Posture	Movement	Ability of Individual
P	Standing	Static	Needs moderate assistance to maintain
P	Standing	Dynamic	Needs moderate assistance during gait
P+	Sitting	Static	Needs minimum assistance to maintain
P+	Sitting	Dynamic	N/A
P+	Standing	Static	Needs minimum assistance to maintain
P+	Standing	Dynamic	Needs minimum assistance during gait
F	Sitting	Static	Maintains without assistance but unable to take any challenges
F	Sitting	Dynamic	N/A, cannot move trunk without losing balance
F	Standing	Static	Maintains without assistance but unable to take any challenges
F	Standing	Dynamic	Needs clinical gait analysis during gait
F+	Sitting	Static	Able to take minimum challenges from all directions
F+	Sitting	Dynamic	Maintains balance through minimal active trunk motion
F+	Standing	Static	Takes minimal challenges from all directions
F+	Standing	Dynamic	Needs close supervision during gait; able to right self with minor loss of balance

Grade	Posture	Movement	Ability of Individual
G	Sitting	Static	Takes moderate challenges in all directions
G	Sitting	Dynamic	Maintains balance through moderate excursion of active trunk motion
G	Standing	Static	Takes moderate challenges in all directions
G	Standing	Dynamic	Needs supervision only during gait; is able to right self with moderate loss of balance
G+	Sitting	Static	Takes maximum challenges in all directions
G+	Sitting	Dynamic	Maintains balance through maximum excursion of active trunk motion
G+	Standing	Static	Takes maximum challenges in all directions
G+	Standing	Dynamic	Independent gait with or without device
N	No deviation seen in posture held statically or dynamically		

Note: This is a basic guideline used at many U.S. facilities. However, there is no evidence-based research to support the values in the scale.

Grasp and Pinch Averages

GRASP DYNAMOMETER NORMS IN POUNDS (APPROXIMATELY)

		Years						
		20	30	40	50	60	70	80
Male	R	125	120	115	100	95	85	80
	L	117	115	100	95	85	80	70
Female	R	64	60	57	55	51	50	48
	L	58	53	52	50	48	45	42

TIP PINCH NORMS IN POUNDS (APPROXIMATELY)

		Years						
		20	30	40	50	60	70	80
Male	R	22.5	22	21	19.5	17.5	16.5	15.5
	L	21	20	18.5	17	16.5	15	14
Female	R	14	13	12.5	12	11	10.5	10
	L	13	12.5	12	11	10	9.5	9

LATERAL PINCH NORMS IN POUNDS
(APPROXIMATELY)

		\multicolumn{7}{c}{Years}
		20	30	40	50	60	70	80
Male	R	23.5	22.5	22	21	20	19.5	18
	L	22	21.4	20.5	20	19	18	17
Female	R	14	13.5	13	12.5	12	11.5	11
	L	13.5	13	12.5	12	11.5	11	10.5

PALMAR PINCH NORMS IN POUNDS
(APPROXIMATELY)

		\multicolumn{7}{c}{Years}
		20	30	40	50	60	70	80
Male	R	23	21.5	19.5	18.5	17	15.5	14.5
	L	21	20	18	17	16	14.5	13.5
Female	R	15	14	13	12	11	9	8.5
	L	14	13	12	11	10	8	7

All tables adapted from Trombly, C. (1983). *Occupational therapy for physical dysfunction.* Baltimore, MD: Williams & Wilkins.

Grip Development and Stages of Writing

supinated grasp/fisted grasp: Palmar/supinated, generally age 1 to 1½ years; 5th digit is closest to the paper and the movement is from the shoulder to get the crayon to move across the paper.

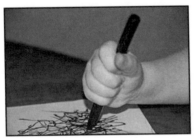

Figure 27-1. Example of fisted grip.

pronate grasp/palmar grasp: Digital/prone, generally age 2 to 3 years; the crayon lies across the palm of the hand and the first and second digits are closest to the paper.

4 or 5 finger grasp: Quadropod, generally age 3½ to 4 years; wrist held off table.

dynamic tripod: Typically age 4 to 6 years; hold the crayon or pencil with the pads of thumb and index and middle digits.

Jacobs, K., & Simon, L. (Eds.). *Quick Reference Dictionary for Occupational Therapy, Sixth Edition* (pp. 536-538).
© 2015 SLACK Incorporated.

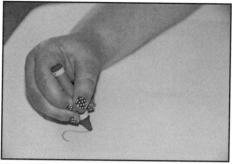

Figure 27-2. Example of dynamic tripod grip.

Children learn in a predictable order how to copy forms, which starts with horizontal and vertical lines, and then moves to circles, crosses, squares, and triangles.

2 to 3 years old:
- Scribble marks
- Horizontal/vertical line

3 to 4 years old:
- Circle
- Cross

4 to 5 years old:
- Square
- Triangle
- Diamond

When teaching children how to write the alphabet, it is important to begin with capital letters because they are symmetrical and distinctive and all take up the same amount of space, whereas lowercase letters are different sizes and easy to confuse.

Begin with letters containing vertical and horizontal strokes:
L, E, F, T, I, H

Next, teach those with circles and curves:
C, O, Q, U, G, J, S, D, P, B

Last, introduce those with diagonals:
K, R, A, V, M, N, W, X, Y, Z

BIBLIOGRAPHY

Gesell, A., Halverson, H. M., Thompson, H., Ilg, F. L., Castner, B. M., Ames, L. B., & Amatruda, C. S. (1940). *The first five years of a life: A guide to the study of the preschool child.* New York, NY: Harper & Brothers.

Growth and Development in Early Childhood

Age	Behavior
1 month	Lifts head, turns head side to side, follows moving object
	Hands fisted
	Exhibits reflexive stepping
	Mass motor response to stimuli
	Reflexive grasp
2 months	Lifts head 45 degrees
	Smiles
	Can maintain head control while supported
	Eyes track pass 90 degrees
	Direct regard
	Head lags on pull to sitting
	Turns from side to back
3 months	Eyes follow 180 degrees
	Can prop self up on forearms
	Head steady
	Regards hands
	Coos, chuckles, and waves arms at toys

Jacobs, K., & Simon, L. (Eds.). *Quick Reference Dictionary for Occupational Therapy, Sixth Edition* (pp. 539-541).
© 2015 SLACK Incorporated.

Age	Behavior
4 to 6 months	Head no longer lags from pull to sitting
	Sits without support
	Rolls over from supine to prone
	Palmar grasp
	Holds and shakes rattle
	Can transfer objects
	Reaches for and picks up toys with one or both hands
7 to 9 months	Sits alone
	Holds toy with one hand
	Creeps or crawls
	Grasps with thumb and forefinger
	Bangs toys
	Waves bye-bye
	Pulls self to stand
	Makes stepping movements
	Equilibrium reactions are present
10 to 12 months	Walks while holding onto furniture
	Stands and begins to walk
13 to 15 months	Can stand and walk without assistance
	Crawls upstairs
	Throws ball while sitting
	Can say some words
	Holds spoon
	Scribbles with crayon
18 months	Sits self in small chair
	Begins to run
	Self-feeds
	Can walk up and down stairs with help
	Builds tower of three blocks
	Improved balance
	Can jump in place
	Can copy a circle
	Grasps with palm

Age	Behavior
2 to 3 years	Runs well
	Can walk on tip toes
	Hand preference emerges
	Can go up and down stairs reciprocally
	Kicks ball
	Can stand on one foot for a moment
4 years	Hops on one foot
	Climbs
	Rides tricycle
	Throws ball overhead
	Can balance on one foot
	Can build a tower of 10 blocks
	Can copy letters
	May be able to tie shoes or button clothes
5 years	Dresses and undresses self
	Can skip and kick a ball
	Can catch a ball
	Can bounce a ball
	Can march to music
	Colors within lines
	Can copy a diamond shape

Guidelines for Blood Pressure Management in Adults and Target Heart Rate

Hypertension is defined as systolic blood pressure greater than 140 mm Hg or a diastolic blood pressure greater than 90 mm Hg:

Category	Systolic, mm Hg	Diastolic, mm Hg
Desired BP	< 120	< 80
Normal BP	< 130	< 85
High Normal BP	130 to 139	85 to 89
Stage 1 HTN	140 to 159	90 to 99
Stage 2 HTN	160 to 179	100 to 109
Stage 3 HTN	> 180	> 110

How to determine target heart rate zone:
1. Subtract patient's age from 220.
2. Multiply the result by 0.65 to find lower end of target zone.
3. Multiply the result by 0.85 to find the upper end of target zone.

Example: 70-year-old patient
$$220 - 70 = 150$$
$$150 * 0.65 = 97.5$$
$$150 * 0.85 = 127.5$$
Target zone is 97 to 127 bpm.

Jacobs, K., & Simon, L. (Eds.). *Quick Reference Dictionary for Occupational Therapy, Sixth Edition* (p. 542). © 2015 SLACK Incorporated.

Appendix 30

Health Literacy

Health literacy is an important issue in service delivery for health care professionals. It is vital for clients to understand the material provided by clinicians and to use that knowledge in their daily lives. Health communication materials should be evidence based and user friendly. Health care professionals can work to create materials that are accessible to a wide range of clients and their families by following several steps:

1. Identify the intended audience and determine what their needs, beliefs/values, and interests are, as well as their level of knowledge of the identified health topic.

2. Determine key concepts and messages based on the knowledge base of the audience.

3. Design a draft of the material that you feel is at the appropriate health literacy level.

4. Pretest materials with the intended audience or other people who are not health care professionals.

5. Adjust or rewrite the draft according to feedback from the audience.

6. Determine the best way to communicate messages to the audience (e.g., print, audio, video).

7. Format the material in an easy-to-read presentation style that feels accessible and not too overwhelming to the reader (seek audience feedback).

Jacobs, K., & Simon, L. (Eds.). *Quick Reference Dictionary for Occupational Therapy, Sixth Edition* (pp. 543-545).
© 2015 SLACK Incorporated.

8. Publish and distribute materials on a small scale to the intended recipients.

9. Evaluate the audience's satisfaction and understanding.

10. Revise materials as needed before distributing on a larger scale.

STYLE AND WORDING TIPS

- Choose your words carefully: use an active voice, short sentences, everyday words, and personal pronouns. Use words with one or two syllables when you can, keep most sentences (if possible) between eight to ten words, and limit paragraphs to three to five sentences.

- Give the most important information first to quickly engage the audience.

- Use presentation elements, such as bulleted lists and graphics that match and reinforce text.

- Limit the number of messages to no more than three or four main ideas per document or section.

- Focus on what your audience needs to know or do and skip details that are not immediately relevant or place them further down in the document.

- Stick to one idea at a time; try not to jump around between subjects.

- Avoid lengthy lists and create short lists (three to seven items) with bullets instead of using commas and long sentences.

- Respect and value your audience; do not talk down to them but do use simple language when possible.

- Use a tone that is encouraging, emphasize practical steps, and give concrete examples.

- Limit the use of jargon, technical, or scientific language. If more complex terms are needed, define them first and then explain them in plain language.

- Use analogies and make comparisons that will be familiar to your audience.

- Avoid unnecessary abbreviations and acronyms, spell the word out at least once in the document, and clearly give the meaning or definition.

- Use visuals to help engage your audience and accommodate different types of learners. Make sure any images you use are culturally relevant and sensitive to your audience.

BIBLIOGRAPHY

Centers for Disease Control and Prevention. *Simply put: A guide for creating easy-to-understand materials.* Retrieved from www.cdc.gov/healthliteracy/pdf/Simply_Put.pdf

U.S. Department of Health and Human Services, Office of Disease Prevention and Health Promotion. *Quick guide to health literacy.* Retrieved from www.health.gov/communication/literacy/quickguide/factsbasic.htm

International Classification of Functioning, Disability and Health

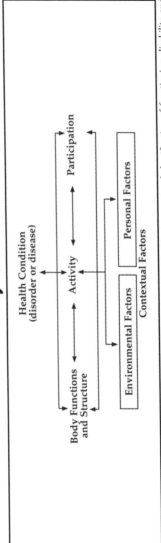

Reprinted with permission from World Health Organization. (2001). *The international classification of functioning, disability and health—Towards a common language for functioning, disability and health.* Geneva, Switzerland: Author. www.who.int/classifications/icf/en/

Jacobs, K., & Simon, L. (Eds.). *Quick Reference Dictionary for Occupational Therapy, Sixth Edition* (p. 546).
© 2015 SLACK Incorporated.

Laboratory Values

Test	Reference Range	Clinical Significance Increased Levels	Clinical Significance Decreased Levels
Glucose	70 to 120 mg/dL	Diabetes mellitus	Hypopituitarism
		Hypothyroidism	Hyperthyroidism
		Pancreatic cancer	Injection too much insulin
		Pancreatitis	Insufficient dietary intake
		Insufficient insulin	Diabetes mellitus
		Excessive food intake	Pancreas
		Acromegaly	Islet cell tumor
		Cushing's syndrome	Malignancy
		Trauma	Sepsis
		Burns	Severe hepatic disease
		Acute myocardial infarction	Reye's syndrome
		Fractures	
		Pituitary adenoma	

Jacobs, K., & Simon, L. (Eds.). *Quick Reference Dictionary for Occupational Therapy, Sixth Edition* (pp. 547-558).
© 2015 SLACK Incorporated.

Test	Reference Range	Clinical Significance Increased Levels	Clinical Significance Decreased Levels
Blood urea nitrogen	10 to 24 mg/dL	Congestive heart failure	Liver failure
		Excessive protein ingestion	Low protein diet
		Gastrointestinal bleed	Malnutrition
		Hypovolemia	Overhydration
		Myocardial infarction	Nephritic syndrome
		Renal disease	Pregnancy
		Renal failure	
		Shock	
		Urinary tract obstruction	
		Addison's disease	
		Fever	
		Prerenal azotemia	
		Post-renal obstruction	
		Stress	

Test	Reference Range	Clinical Significance Increased Levels	Clinical Significance Decreased Levels
Creatinine	0.7 to 1.5 mg/dL	Dehydration Diabetic nephropathy Eclampsia Glomerulonephritis Muscular dystrophy Reduced renal flow Renal failure Rhabdomyolysis Urinary tract obstruction Gigantism Congestive heart failure Hyperthyroidism Rheumatoid arthritis	Muscular dystrophy (late stages) Myasthenia gravis

Test	Reference Range	Clinical Significance Increased Levels	Clinical Significance Decreased Levels
Sodium (Na)	133 to 145 mEq/L	Dehydration	Ascites
		Diabetes insipidus	Congestive heart failure
		Extensive thermal burns	Diarrhea
		Osmotic diuresis	Excessive sweating
		Diabetes mellitus	Intraluminal bowel loss
		Hypothalamic tumor	Ketoacidosis
		Cushing's syndrome	Kidney disease
			Osmotic dilution
			Acute renal failure
			Pleural effusion
			Cirrhosis
			Severe hypoaluminemia
			Vomiting or nasogastric aspiration

Test	Reference Range	Clinical Significance Increased Levels	Clinical Significance Decreased Levels
Potassium (K)	3.3 to 5.1 mEq/L	Crush injury (tissue trauma)	Deficient K intake in diet
		Hemolytic (red blood cell destruction)	Diarrhea
		Metabolic or respiratory acidosis	Vomiting
		Renal failure	Acute myeloid leukemia
		Transfusion	
		Hyperkinetic periodic paralysis	
		Addison's disease	
		Thrombocytosis	
		Dehydration	
		Acidosis	
		Tumor lysis syndrome	
		Adrenal insufficiency	
		Muscle necrosis	

Test	Reference Range	Clinical Significance Increased Levels	Clinical Significance Decreased Levels
Chloride (Cl)	96 to 108 mEq/L	Chronic hyperventilation	Addison's disease
		Cushing's syndrome	Burns
		Dehydration	Chronic respiratory acidosis
		Eclampsia	Congestive heart failure
		Excess infusion of normal saline	Excessive sweating
		Kidney dysfunction	Gastric suction
		Metabolic acidosis	Overhydration
		Renal tubular acidosis	Salt-losing nephritis
		Diarrhea	Vomiting
		Diabetes insipidus	Diabetes mellitus
			Metabolic alkalosis
			Hyponatremia
			Syndrome of inappropriate antidiuretic hormone secretion

Test	Reference Range	Clinical Significance Increased Levels	Clinical Significance Decreased Levels
Carbon dioxide (CO_2)	22 to 33 mEq/L	Excessive vomiting	Ketoacidosis
		Respiratory dysfunction	Lactic acidosis
		Hyper aldosteronism	Kidney disease
		Cushing's syndrome	Diarrhea
		Acidosis	Methanol poisoning
		Emphysema	Ethyl glycol poisoning
			Addison's disease
			Respiratory alkalosis
			Starvation
			Acute renal failure

Test	Reference Range	Clinical Significance Increased Levels	Clinical Significance Decreased Levels
Calcium	8.4 to 10.5 mg/dL	Hyperparathyroidism	Hyperparathyroidism
		Metatastic bone tumor	Malabsorption
		Milk alkali syndrome	Osteomalacia
		Paget's disease	Renal failure
		Tumor producing a parathyroid hormone substance	Rickets
		Vitamin D intoxication	Vitamin D deficiency
		Multiple myeloma	Pancreatitis
		Osteoporosis	Hypoalbuminemia
		Chronic renal failure	Wilson's disease
		Cancer (breast, lungs, renal)	
		Hyperthyroidism	

Test	Reference Range	Clinical Significance Increased Levels	Clinical Significance Decreased Levels
Albumin	3.4 to 4.8 mg/dL	Dehydration Multiple myeloma Chronic infection Sarcoidism Liver disease Collagen Autoimmune disease Lupus Scleroderma Rheumatoid arthritis Hemolysis	Ascites Burns Glomerulonephritis Liver disease Malabsorption syndrome Malnutrition Nephritic syndrome Inflammatory bowel disease Hodgkin's disease Renal disease Leukemia
White blood cell count	4.8 to 10.8 X (1,000) cumm	Infectious disease Inflammatory disease Leukemia Severe emotional or physical stress Tissue damage	Bone marrow failure Presence of catatonic substance Collagen vascular disease Disease of liver or spleen Radiation

Test	Reference Range	Clinical Significance Increased Levels	Clinical Significance Decreased Levels
Red blood cell count	4.2 to 5.7 X (1,000,000) cumm		Anemia Hemorrhage Bone marrow failure Erythroprotein deficiency Hemolytic from transfusion reaction Multiple myeloma Malnutrition
Hematocrit	40% to 50%	Congenital heart disease Polycythemia vera Severe dehydration Erythrocytes Severe diarrhea Eclampsia Burns Dehydration Chronic obstructive pulmonary disease	Anemia hyperthyroidism Cirrhosis Hemolytic reaction Hemorrhage Dietary deficiency Bone marrow failure Normal pregnancy Rheumatoid arthritis Multiple myeloma Leukemia hemoglobinopathy

Test	Reference Range	Clinical Significance Increased Levels	Clinical Significance Decreased Levels
Hemoglobin	13.5 to 17.5 mg/dL	Congenital heart disease	Anemia
		Polycythemia vera/	Severe hemorrhage
		heme concentration of the blood	Hemolytic
		Chronic obstructive pulmonary	Cancer
		disease	Nutritional deficiency
		Congestive heart failure	Lymphoma
		High altitudes	Systemic lupus erythematosus
		Severe burns	Acidosis
		Dehydration	Kidney disease
			Chronic hemorrhage
			Splenomegaly
			Sickle cell anemia
			Neoplasia

Test	Reference Range	Clinical Significance Increased Levels	Clinical Significance Decreased Levels
Platelet count	150 to 440,000 cumm	Malignant disorder	Hypersplenism
		Polycythemia vera	Hemorrhage
		Post-splenectomy syndrome	Immune thrombocytopenia
		Rheumatoid arthritis	Leukemia
		Iron deficiency anemia	Thrombotic thrombocytopenia
			Disseminated intravascular coagulation
			Systemic lupus
			Pernicious anemia
			Cancer
			Chemotherapy
			Infection

Legislation and Policy Decisions Affecting Rehabilitation

Americans with Disabilities Act (1990) (ADA): This U.S. federal act protects persons with disabilities from discrimination in employment, transportation, public accommodations, telecommunications, and activities of state and local government.

ADA Amendments Act (2008) (ADAAA): This federal act amended the Americans with Disabilities Act of 1990. The changes, which apply to both the ADA and the Rehabilitation Act, include an updated definition of the term *disability*, which clarifies and broadens the words used in order to protect more people under the ADA and other federal disability nondiscrimination laws. The definition of major life activities was expanded to include bodily functions, which will allow many people with internal function disorders, such as gastrointestinal disorders, cancer, sleep disorders, insulin-dependent diabetes, and heart disease, to now be covered under the ADA. The act also required the Equal Employment Opportunity Commission to adopt the changes into their regulations in order to protect the rights of a greater number of employees.

Architectural Barriers Act (1969): U.S. federal legislation that requires accessibility to certain facilities.

Balanced Budget Act (BBA): Enacted in 1997 in an attempt to balance the national budget of the United States, which placed an annual $1,500 cap on Medicare recipient benefits for combined physical therapy and speech therapy services under

Jacobs, K., & Simon, L. (Eds.). *Quick Reference Dictionary for Occupational Therapy, Sixth Edition* (pp. 559-566). © 2015 SLACK Incorporated.

Medicare Part B. The Prospective Payment System fixes the amount that hospitals are reimbursed for the primary diagnosis for each hospital stay. A moratorium was placed on this cap in a legislative decision in November 1999 that was in effect for the years 2000 and 2001.

Civilian Industrial Rehabilitation Act (1920): First U.S. federal legislation to help occupational therapy. It commissioned federal aid for vocational rehabilitation for those disabled by accident or illness in industry.

Community Mental Health Act (1963): Under this act, the National Institute of Mental Health was mandated to establish community mental health centers as part of a national movement to take more responsibility for individuals with mental illness.

Consolidated Omnibus Budget Reconciliation Act of 1985 (COBRA): Federal legislation that requires that all employers with 20 or more employees continue health coverage for up to 18 months after a worker loses benefits due to reduced work hours or loss of employment.

Deficit Reduction Legislation Acts (1984, 1985, 1986): Extended U.S. Federal coverage for health and social services through modification of Medicare legislation.

Developmental Disabilities Act Amendments (1984): U.S. federal legislation that ensured that people with developmental disabilities receive necessary services and established a monitoring system.

Developmental Disabilities Services and Facilities Construction Act (1970): U.S. law giving the states broad responsibility for planning and implementing a comprehensive program of services to individuals with developmental delays, epilepsy, cerebral palsy, and other neurological impairments.

Disability Insurance Benefit Program (1956): U.S. federal legislation that provided benefits to qualified workers with disabilities.

Education of All Handicapped Children Act (1975): U.S. federal legislation that is intended to ensure that children with disabilities receive education in the least restrictive environment.

Education of the Handicapped Act Amendments (1986): Increase in U.S. federal funds for special education and other services provided to preschoolers ages 3 to 5 years.

Employment Retirement Income Security Act (ERISA): A federal act passed by Congress in 1974 that defines requirements and exemptions for self-insuring firms.

Fair Housing Amendment Act (1988): U.S. federal law meant to prohibit discriminatory housing for those with disabilities.

Handicapped Children's Early Education Assistance Act: U.S. federal law in which funds were authorized for the development, evaluation, and dissemination of different projects for persons with disabilities aged birth to 8 years and their families.

Health Insurance Portability and Accountability Act of 1996 (HIPAA): Title I of HIPAA protects health insurance coverage for workers and their families when they change or lose their jobs. Title II of HIPAA, known as the Administrative Simplification provisions, requires the establishment of national standards for electronic health care transactions and national identifiers for providers, health insurance plans, and employers. The act gives the right to privacy to individuals from age 12 through 18 years. The provider must have a signed disclosure from the patient before giving out any information on provided health care to anyone, including parents. The Administrative Simplification provisions also address the security and privacy of health data.

Health Maintenance Organization Act of 1973: U.S. federal law that provided for the planning and development of health maintenance organizations and encourage less ambulatory care.

Health Professions Educational Assistance Act: U.S. federal law that provided incentives for medical schools to increase the number of family practice physicians to half of their graduates and also attempted to attract physicians to underserved areas by subsidizing their medical education.

Individuals with Disabilities Education Act (IDEA): U.S. federal legislation that provides resources to school-aged children with disabilities.

Insurance Coverage for Telemedicine (2013): Updates the New Mexico insurance code, health maintenance organization law, and the nonprofit health care plan law to require coverage for telemedicine services. Also provides for utilization review and appeal rights for denials of telemedicine coverage.

Interim Payment System (IPS): Enacted in 1997 in an attempt to balance the national budget of the United States. The IPS fixes the amount that home care agencies are reimbursed for services for the primary diagnosis.

Maryland Medical Assistance Program—Telemedicine (2013): Requires the Maryland Medical Assistance Program to provide certain reimbursement for certain services delivered by telemedicine.

Mississippi Telemedicine Services (2013): Requires health insurance plans to provide coverage to same extent as in-person services.

Montana Telemedicine Services (2013): Requires that each group or individual policy, certificate of disability insurance, subscriber contract, membership contract, or health care services agreement that provides coverage for health care services must provide coverage for health care services provided via telemedicine if the service is otherwise covered by the policy, certificate, contract, or agreement.

National Consumer Health Information and Health Promotion Act of 1976: U.S. federal legislation that attempted to set rational goals for health information and education.

National Health Planning and Resource Development Act of 1974: U.S. federal legislation that established regional health systems agencies to assume responsibility for health care planning for community needs and cost containment.

Nebraska LB 556 (2013): Provides for telehealth services for children, changes the medical assistance program, and provides duties for the Department of Health and Human Services.

North Carolina Require Pulse Oximetry Newborn Screening Act (2013): Allows screenings for congenital heart defects in newborns to take place over telemedicine.

Oklahoma Repealing Informed Consent Provisions Related to Telemedicine (2013): Repeals Section 6804, which relates to informed consent relating to telemedicine and provides an effective date.

Older Americans Act: Enacted in 1965 as the major piece of legislation for provision of social and health-related services to older Americans; established a federal, state, and local government network for advocacy and service delivery.

Omnibus Budget Reconciliation Act of 1987 (OBRA '87): U.S. federal legislation that recognizes quality of life as most important to nursing home residents. Contains a section of the Federal Nursing Home Reform Act, which made sweeping changes in the standards for provision of nursing home care. These mandated changes address areas such as patient care planning, nursing, staffing, nurse's aide training, nurse's aide registry, patient's rights, transfers and discharges, and administrator standards.

Omnibus Reconciliation Act (1981): U.S. federal legislation designed to finance community-based services for people with developmental disabilities when that treatment is less expensive than an institution.

Omnibus Social Security Act (1983): U.S. federal legislation that established a prospective payment system based on a fixed price per diagnosis-related group for inpatient services.

Osteopathic Medicine Act (2013): Allows the Oklahoma State Board of Osteopathic Examiners to issue telemedicine licenses.

Patient Protection and Affordable Care Act (2010) (PPACA): This U.S. federal statute is aimed at decreasing the number of uninsured Americans and reducing the overall costs of health care. It includes mandates, subsidies, and tax credits to employers and individuals with the goal of increasing the coverage rate and streamlining the delivery of health care.

Insurance companies are now required to cover all applicants and offer the same rates regardless of preexisting conditions or gender. Sometimes referred to as ObamaCare, the act also includes telehealth provisions, which create ways to promote evidence-based medicine and patient engagement, report on quality and cost measures, and coordinate care through the use of telehealth, remote patient monitoring, and other such enabling technologies. The PPACA directs the new Center for Medicare and Medicaid Innovation to explore as a care model how to facilitate inpatient care at local hospitals through the use of electronic monitoring by specialists. The legislation also provides states with a "health home" option for chronic conditions that includes the use of health information technology in providing health home services, including the use of wireless patient technology to improve coordination and management of care and increase patient adherence to recommendations made by their provider.

Rehabilitation Act (1973): Services were expanded to the severely disabled; affirmative action provided in employment and non-discrimination in facilities by federal contractors and grantees.

Servicemen's Readjustment Act (GI Bill) of 1944: U.S. federal legislation that provided for the education and training of individuals whose education or career had been interrupted by military service.

Social Security Acts and Amendments (1935): U.S. federal legislation that provided financial support for workers with disabilities and retirement income for the elderly.

Social Security Amendments of 1972: U.S. federal legislation that provided for the establishment of Professional Standard Review Organizations to ensure that federally funded programs were used in an efficient and effective manner.

Sunset Review Occupational Therapy Practice Act (2013): A bill passed in Colorado that recognizes telehealth as an allowable method of delivering consultative services for the practice of occupational therapy.

Tax Equity and Fiscal Responsibility Act (TEFRA) (1982): U.S. federal act that put limits on Medicare and Medicaid reimbursements (including physical and occupational therapy); also limits items such as inpatient hospital costs.

Technology-Related Assistance for Individuals with Disabilities Act of 1988: U.S. federal legislation that requires assistive technology be made available to persons with disabilities to enhance their functional capabilities.

Telehealth and Telemedicine Services Reimbursement Under Medicaid (2013): Requires the Indiana State Office of Medicaid Policy and Planning to reimburse home health agencies, federally qualified health centers, rural health clinics, community mental health centers, and critical access hospitals for telehealth services under the Medicaid program, regardless of the distance between the provider and the patient.

Telemedicine Practice for Osteopathic Physicians (2013): This bill would clarify that an osteopathic physician may engage in telemedicine from within or outside the state or United States if he or she possesses an osteopathic license from Nevada. Also clarifies that a bona fide physician-patient relationship can be established through telemedicine. In addition, it stipulates that an osteopathic physician can supervise a physician assistant electronically or telephonically or by using fiber optics.

Telemedicine Services Outside of Health Care Facility (2013): Focuses on a pilot program in Vermont to study effects of telemedicine when delivered outside of health care facilities.

Telepharmacy and Telemedicine Practice for Physicians (2013): Authorizes certain providers of health care in Nevada to engage in telemedicine under certain circumstances. It also sets forth certain requirements concerning the practice of telemedicine; providing that authorization to engage in telemedicine does not modify, expand, or alter the scope of practice of a provider of health care.

Title VII of the Medicare Prospective Payment Legislation (1983): U.S. federal legislation that provides incentives for cost containment and better management of resources by a reimbursement structure based on client's diagnosis rather than direct cost of care.

Title XVIII and Title XIX of the Social Security Act (1965): U.S. federal legislation that established reimbursement based on reasonable cost for medical services for the elderly and through state grants to the poor.

Vocational Rehabilitation Act and Amendments (1943): U.S. federal legislation that brought about a change to include payment for medical services, thus allowing occupational therapy services (physical therapy services already covered) to be covered as a legitimate service.

Welsh-Clark Act (World War II Disabled Veterans Rehabilitation Act): U.S. federal legislation that provided vocational rehabilitation for veterans of World War II.

West Virginia Practice of Pharmacist Care Bill (2013): Clarifies that a valid patient-practitioner relationship can be established via telemedicine.

BIBLIOGRAPHY

American Telemedicine Association. (2010). *Telemedicine in the Patient Protection and Affordable Care Act.* Retrieved from www.americantelemed. org/docs/default-source/policy/telehealth-provisions-within-the-patient-protection-and-affordable-care-act.pdf?sfvrsn=14

Levels of Assistance

Total assistance (TOT)	Individual requires 100% assistance to safely complete task. Individual does not assist at all.
Maximum assistance (MAX)	Individual requires 75% of physical/cognitive assistance to safely complete task. Individual assists 25%.
Moderate assistance (MOD)	Individual requires 50% of physical/cognitive assistance to safely complete task. Individual assists 50%.
Minimal assistance (MIN)	Individual needs no more than 25% physical/cognitive assistance. Individual assists 75%.
Standby assistance (SBA)	Supervision or standby assistance for safe, effective task performance.
Set-up assistance	Individual requires set-up of necessary items to perform tasks.
Independent (IND)	No assistance or supervision is required. Able to perform independently. Safety is demonstrated during tasks.

Jacobs, K., & Simon, L. (Eds.). *Quick Reference Dictionary for Occupational Therapy, Sixth Edition* (p. 567).
© 2015 SLACK Incorporated.

Manual Muscle Testing

Number Grade	Word/Letter Grade	Definition
Against Gravity		
5/5	Normal (N)	The part moves through full range of motion against maximum resistance and gravity
4+/5	Good plus (G+)	The part moves through full range of motion against less than maximum resistance but more than moderate resistance
4/5	Good (G)	The part moves through full range of motion against gravity and moderate resistance
4-/5	Good minus (G-)	The part moves through full range of motion against gravity and less than moderate resistance
3+/5	Fair plus (F+)	The part moves through full range of motion against gravity and takes minimal resistance
3/5	Fair (F)	The part moves through full range of motion against gravity with no added resistance

Jacobs, K., & Simon, L. (Eds.). *Quick Reference Dictionary for Occupational Therapy, Sixth Edition* (pp. 568-569). © 2015 SLACK Incorporated.

Number Grade	Word/Letter Grade	Definition
Against Gravity		
3-/5	Fair minus (F-)	The part moves less than full range of motion against gravity (more than 50%)
2+/5	Poor plus (P+)	The part moves through full range of motion on a gravity-eliminated plane with minimal resistance
Gravity Eliminated		
2/5	Poor (P)	The part moves through full range of motion on a gravity-eliminated plane with no added resistance
2-/5	Poor minus (P-)	The part moves less than full range of motion on a gravity-eliminated plane
1/5	Trace	No joint motion but contraction felt when muscle palpated
0/5	Zero (0)	No tension or contraction is palpated in the muscle or tendon

Measures and Weights

LINEAR MEASURE

12 inches = 1 foot
3 feet = 1 yard (0.9144 meter)
5½ yards = 1 rod
40 rods = 1 furlong/220 yards
8 furlongs = 1 statute mile/1,760 yards
5,280 feet = 1 statute or land mile
3 miles = 1 league
6,076.11549 feet = 1 international nautical mile (1,852 meters)

DRY MEASURE

2 pints = 1 quart
8 quarts = 1 peck
4 pecks = 1 bushel/2,150.42 cubic inches

ANGULAR AND CIRCULAR MEASURE

60 seconds = 1 minute
60 minutes = 1 degree
90 degrees = 1 right angle
180 degrees = 1 straight angle
360 degrees = 1 circle

Jacobs, K., & Simon, L. (Eds.). *Quick Reference Dictionary for Occupational Therapy, Sixth Edition* (pp. 570-571). © 2015 SLACK Incorporated.

SQUARE MEASURE

144 square inches = 1 square foot
9 square feet = 1 square yard
30¼ square yards = 1 square rod
160 square rods = 1 acre
640 acres = 1 square mile

TROY WEIGHT

24 grains = 1 pennyweight
20 pennyweights = 1 ounce
12 ounces = 1 pound, Troy

CUBIC MEASURE

1,728 cubic inches = 1 cubic foot
27 cubic feet = 1 cubic yard

LIQUID MEASURE

4 gills = 1 pint
2 pints = 1 quart
4 quarts = 1 gallon/231.0 cubic inches

AVOIRDUPOIS WEIGHT

27 11/32 grains = 1 dram
16 drams = 1 ounce
16 ounces = 1 pound/0.45359237 kilogram
100 pounds = 1 short hundredweight
20 short hundredweights = 1 short ton

Medical Roots Terminology

a-: negative prefix (n is added before words beginning with a vowel) (e.g., ametria)

ab-: away from (e.g., abducent)

abdomin-: abdomen (e.g., abdominis, abdominoscopy)

ac-: *see* ad- (e.g., accretion)

ac-: pertaining to

acet-: acid (e.g., acetum vinegar, acetometer)

acid-: acid (e.g., acidus sour, aciduric)

acou-: hear (e.g., acouesthesia); *also spelled* acu-

acr-: extremity; peak (e.g., acromegaly)

act-: drive; act (e.g., reaction)

actin-: ray, radius (e.g., actinogenesis)

acu-: hear (e.g., osteoacusis)

ad-: toward (d changes to c, f, g, p, s, or t before words beginning with those consonants) (e.g., adrenal)

aden-: gland (e.g., adenoma)

adeno-: gland

adip-: fat (e.g., adipocellular, adipose)

-aemia: blood (e.g., polycythaemia)

aer-: air (e.g., anaerobiosis)

aero-: air

aesthe-: sensation (e.g., aesthesioneurosis)

af-: *see* ad- (e.g., afferent)

ag-: *see* ad- (e.g., agglutinant)

Jacobs, K., & Simon, L. (Eds.). *Quick Reference Dictionary for Occupational Therapy, Sixth Edition* (pp. 572-593). © 2015 SLACK Incorporated.

-agogue: leading, inducing (e.g., galactagogue)

-agra: catching, seizure (e.g., podagra)

al-: pertaining to

alb-: white (e.g., albocinereous)

albo-: white

alg-: pain (e.g., neuralgia, algesia)

all-: other, different (e.g., allergy)

alve-: channel, cavity (e.g., alveolar, alveous trough)

amb-: both, on both sides (e.g., ambulate)

amph-: *see* amphi-, around, on both sides (e.g., ampheclexis)

amphi-: both, doubly (i is dropped before words beginning with a vowel) (e.g., amphicelous)

amyl-: starch (e.g., amylosynthesis)

an-: pertaining to

an-: *see* ana- (e.g., anagogic)

ana-: up, positive (final a is dropped before words beginning with a vowel) (e.g., anaphoresis)

andr-: man (e.g., gynandroid)

angi-: vessel (e.g., angiemphraxis)

angio-: vessel

ankyl-: crooked, looped (e.g., ankylodactylia); *also spelled* ancyl-

ant-: *see* anti- (e.g., antophthalmic)

ante-: before (e.g., anteflexion)

anti-: against, counter (i is dropped before words beginning with a vowel or the word is hyphenated) (e.g., antipyrogenic, anti-inflammatory); *see also* contra-

antr-: cavern (e.g., antrodynia)

ap-: *see* ad- (e.g., append)

-aph-: touch (e.g., dysaphia); *see also* hapt-

apo-: away from, detached, opposed (o is dropped before words beginning with a vowel) (e.g., apophysis)

ar-: pertaining to

arachn-: spider (e.g., arachnodactyly)

arch-: beginning, origin (e.g., archenteron)

arter(i)-: elevator, artery (e.g., arteriosclerosis, periarteritis)

arthr-: joint (e.g., synarthrosis); *see also* articul-

arthro-: joint

articul-: articulus joint (e.g., disarticulation); *see also* arthr-

as-: *see* ad- (e.g., assimilation)

-ase: enzyme

at-: *see* ad- (e.g., attrition)

audio-: hearing

aur-: ear (e.g., aurinasal); *see also* ot-

aut-: self (e.g., autechoscope)

auto-: self (e.g., autoimmune)

aux-: increase (e.g., enterauxe)

ax-: axis (e.g., axofugal)

axon-: axis (e.g., axonometer)

ba-: go, walk, stand (e.g., hypnobatia)

bacill-: small staff, rod (e.g., actinobacillosis); *see also* bacter-

bacter-: small staff, rod (e.g., bacteriophage); *see also* bacill-

ball-: throw (e.g., ballistics); *see also* bol-

bar-: weight (e.g., pedobarometer)

bi-^{1}: life (e.g., aerobic)

bi-^{2}: two, twice, double (e.g., bipedal)

bil-: bile (e.g., biliary)

bio-: life

blast-: bud, child, a growing thing in its early stages (e.g., blastoma, zygotoblast)

blep-: look, see (e.g., hemiablepsia)

blephar-: eyelid (e.g., blepharoncus)

bol-: ball (e.g., embolism)

brachi-: arm (e.g., brachiocephalic)

brachy-: short (e.g., brachycephalic)

brady-: slow (e.g., bradycardia)

brom-: stench (e.g., podobromidrosis)

bronch-: windpipe (e.g., bronchoscopy)

bry-: be full of life (e.g., embryonic)

bucc-: cheek (e.g., distobuccal)

cac-: bad, evil, abnormal (e.g., cacodontia, arthrocace); *see also* mal-, dys-

calc-^{1}: stone, limestone, lime (e.g., calcipexy)

calc-²: heel (e.g., calcaneotibial)

calor-: heat (e.g., calorimeter); *see also* therm-

cancr-: cancer, crab (e.g., cancrology); *see also* carcin-

capit-: head (e.g., decapitate); *see also* cephal-

caps-: container (e.g., encapsulation)

carbo-: coal, charcoal (e.g., carbohydrate, carbonuria)

carcin-: crab, cancer (e.g., carcinoma); *see also* cancr-

cardi-: heart (e.g., lipocardiac)

cardio-: heart

cat-: *see* cata- (e.g., cathode)

cata-: down, negative (final a is dropped before words beginning with a vowel) (e.g., catabatic)

caud-: tail (e.g., caudate)

cav-: hollow (e.g., concave)

cec-: blind (e.g., cecopexy)

-cele: tumor, hernia, cyst (e.g., gastrocele)

cell-: room (e.g., celliferous)

cen-: common (e.g., cenesthesia)

cent-: one hundred (e.g., centimeter, centipede)

cente-: puncture (e.g., enterocentesis, amniocentesis)

centr-: central point, center (e.g., neurocentral)

cephal-: relating to the head (e.g., encephalitis)

cept-: take, receive (e.g., receptor)

cer-: wax (e.g., ceroplasty, ceromel)

cerebr-: relating to the cerebrum (e.g., cerebrospinal)

cervic-: neck (e.g., cervicitis, cervical)

chancr-: crab, cancer (e.g., chancriform)

chir-: hand (e.g., chiromegaly)

chlor-: green (e.g., achloropsia)

chloro-: green

chol-: bile (e.g., hepatocholangeitis)

chondr-: cartilage (e.g., chondromalcia)

chondro-: cartilage

chord-: string, cord (e.g., perichordal)

chori-: protective fetal membrane (e.g., endochorion)

chrom-: color (e.g., polychromatic)

chron-: time (e.g., synchronous)

chy-: pour (e.g., ecchymosis)

-cid(e): causing death, cut, kill (e.g., infanticide, germicidal)

cili-: eyelid (e.g., superciliary); *see also* blephar-

cine-: move (e.g., autocinesis)

-cipient: take, receive (e.g., incipient)

circum-: around (e.g., circumferential); *see also* peri-

-cis-: cut, kill (e.g., excision)

clas-: break (e.g., osteoclast, cranioclast)

clin-: bend, incline, make lie down (e.g., clinometer)

clus-: shut (e.g., malocclusion)

co-: *see* con- (e.g., cohesion)

cocc-: seed, pill (e.g., gonococcus)

coel-: hollow (e.g., coelenteron); *also spelled* cel-

col-[1]: pertaining to the lower intestine (e.g., colic)

col-[2]: *see* con- (e.g., collapse)

colic-: large intestines

colon-: lower intestine (e.g., colonic)

colp-: hollow, vagina (e.g., endocolpitis)

com-: *see* con- (e.g., commasculation)

con-: with, together (becomes co- before vowels or h)

col-: before l; com- before b, m, or p; cor- before r (e.g., contraction)

contra-: against, counter (e.g., contraindication); *see also* anti-

copr-: dung (e.g., coproma); *see also* sterco-

cor-[1]: doll, little image, pupil (e.g., isocoria)

cor-[2]: *see* con- (e.g., corrugator)

corpor-: body (e.g., intracorporal); *see also* somat-

cortic-: bark, rind (e.g., corticosterone)

cost-: rib (e.g., intercostal); *see also* pleur-

crani-: skull, cranium (e.g., pericranium)

cranio-: skull

creat-: meat, flesh (e.g., creatorrhea)

-crescent: grow (e.g., excrescent)

cret-[1]: grow (e.g., accretion)

cret-[2]: distinguish, separate off (e.g., discrete)

crin-: distinguish, separate off (e.g., endocrinology)

crur-: shin, leg (e.g., brachiocrural)

cry-: cold (e.g., cryesthesia)

crypt-: hide, conceal (e.g., cryptorchism)

cult-: tend, cultivate (e.g., culture)

cune-: wedge (e.g., sphencuneiform)

cut-: skin (e.g., subcutaneous); *see also* derm(at)-

cyan-: blue (e.g., anthocyanin)

cycl-: circle, cycle (e.g., cyclophoria)

cyst-: bag, bladder (e.g., nephrocystitis); *see also* vesic-

cyt-: cell (e.g., plasmocytoma); *see also* cell-

cyto: cell

dacry-: tear (e.g., dacryocyst)

dactyl-: finger, toe, digit (e.g., hexadactylism)

de-: down from (e.g., decomposition)

dec-[1]: ten, indicates multiple in metric system (e.g., decagram)

dec-[2]: ten, indicates fraction in metric system (e.g., decimeter)

deci-: tenth (e.g., decibel)

demi-: half (e.g., demipenniform)

dendr-: tree (e.g., neurodendrite)

dent-: tooth (e.g., interdental); *see also* odont-

dento-: teeth

derm-: skin (e.g., endoderm, dermatitis); *see also* cut-

derma-: skin

desm-: band, ligament (e.g., syndesmopexy)

dextr-: handedness (e.g., ambidextrous)

di-[1]: two (e.g., dimorphic); *see also* bi-[2]

di-[2]: *see* dia- (e.g., diuresis)

di-[3]: *see* dis- (e.g., divergent)

dia-: through, apart, between, asunder (a is dropped before words beginning with a vowel) (e.g., diagnosis)

didym-: twin, gemini (e.g., epididymal)

digit-: finger, toe (e.g., digital); *see also* dactyl-

diplo-: double (e.g., diplomyelia)

dips-: thirst

dis-: apart, away from, negative, absence of (s may be dropped before a word beginning with a consonant) (e.g., dislocation)

disc-: disk (e.g., discoplacenta)

dors-: back (e.g., ventrodorsal)
drom-: course (e.g., hemodromometer)
-ducent: lead, conduct (e.g., adducent)
duct-: lead, conduct (e.g., oviduct)
dur-: hard, sclera (e.g., induration)
dynam(i)-: power (e.g., dynamoneure, neurodynamic)
-dynia: pain (e.g., coxodynia)
dys-: bad, improper, malfunction, difficult (e.g., dystrophic)

e-: out from (e.g., emission)
-eal: pertaining to
ec-: out of, on the outside (e.g., eccentric)
-ech-: have, hold, be (e.g., synechotomy)
ect-: outside (e.g., ectoplasm); *see also* extra-
ecto-: out, without, away
-ectomy: a cutting out (e.g., mastectomy)
ede-: swell (e.g., edematous)
ef-: out of (e.g., efflorescent)
-elc-: sore, ulcer (e.g., enterelcosis); *see also* helc-
electr-: amber (e.g., electrotherapy)
em-: in, on (e.g., embolism, empathy, emphlysis); *see also* en-
-em-: blood (e.g., anemia); *see also* hem(at)-
-emesis: vomiting (e.g., nemesis)
-emia: blood (e.g., bacteremia)
en-: in, on, into (n changes to m before b, p, or ph) (e.g., encelitis)
encephal-: brain
end-: inside (e.g., endangium); *see also* intra-
endo-: within (e.g., endocardium)
enter-: intestine (e.g., dysentery)
epi-: upon, after, in addition (i is dropped before words beginning with a vowel) (e.g., epiglottis, epaxial)
erg-: work, deed (e.g., energy)
erythr-: red, rubor (e.g., erythrochromia)
erythro-: red
eso-: inside (e.g., esophylactic); *see also* intra-, endo-
esthe-: perceive, feel, sensation (e.g., anesthesia)
eu-: good, normal, well (e.g., eupepsia, eugeric)

ex-: out of (e.g., excretion)
exo-: outside (e.g., exopathic); *see also* extra-
extra-: outside of, beyond (e.g., extracellular)

faci-: face (e.g., brachiofaciolingual)
-facient: make (e.g., calefacient)
-fact-: make (e.g., artifact)
fasci-: band (e.g., fascia)
febr-: fever (e.g., febrile, febricide)
-fect-: make (e.g., defective)
-ferent: bear, carry (e.g., efferent, afferent)
ferr-: iron (e.g., ferroprotein)
fibr-: fiber (e.g., chondofibroma)
fibro-: fiber
fil-: thread (e.g., filament, filiform)
fiss-: split (e.g., fissure)
flagell-: whip (e.g., flagellation)
flav-: yellow (e.g., riboflavin)
-flect-: bend, divert (e.g., deflection)
-flex-: bend, divert (e.g., reflexometer, flexion)
flu-: flow (e.g., fluid)
flux-: flow (e.g., affluxion)
for-: door, opening (e.g., foramen, perforated)
fore-: before, in front of (e.g., forefront)
-form: shape, form (e.g., ossiform, cuniform)
fract-: break (e.g., fracture, refractive)
front-: forehead, front (e.g., nasofrontal)
-fug(e): to drive away, flee, avoid (e.g., vermifuge, centrifugal)
funct-: perform, serve, function (e.g., functional, malfunction)
fund-: pour (e.g., infundibulum)
fus-: pour (e.g., diffusible)

galact-: milk (e.g., dysgalactia)
gam-: marriage, reproductive union (e.g., agamont)
gangli-: swelling, plexus (e.g., neurogangliitis)
gastro-: stomach, belly (e.g., gastrostomy)
gelat-: freeze, congeal (e.g., gelatin)

gemin-: twin, double (e.g., quadrigeminal)

gen-: become, be produced, originate, formation (e.g., genesis, cytogenic, gene)

-genesis: beginning

germ-: bud, a growing thing in its early stages (e.g., germinal, ovigerm)

gest-: bear, carry (e.g., congestion)

gland-: acorn (e.g., intraglandular)

-glia: glue (e.g., neuroglia)

gloss-: relating to the tongue (e.g., lingutrichoglossia)

glott-: tongue, language (e.g., glottic)

gluc-: sweet (e.g., glucose)

glutin-: glue (e.g., agglutination)

glyco-: sugar

glyc(y)-: sweet (e.g., glycemia, glycyrrhia)

gnath-: jaw (e.g., orthognathous)

gno-: know, discern (e.g., diagnosis)

gon-: produce, formulate (e.g., gonad, amphigony)

grad-: walk, take steps (e.g., retrograde)

-gram: scratch, write, record (e.g., cardiogram)

gran-: grain, particle (e.g., lipogranuloma, granulation)

graph-: scratch, write, record (e.g., histography)

grav-: heavy (e.g., multigravida)

gyn(ec)-: woman, wife (e.g., androgyny, gynecologic)

gyr-: ring, circle (e.g., gyrospasm)

haem(at)-: pertaining to blood (e.g., haemorrhagia, haematoxylon)

hapt-: touch (e.g., haptometer)

hect-: one hundred, indicates multiple in metric system (e.g., hectometer)

helc-: sore, ulcer (e.g., helcosis)

hem(at)-: blood (e.g., hematocyturia, hemangioma)

hemi: half (e.g., hemiageusia); *see also* semi-

hemo-: blood

hen-: one (e.g., henogenesis)

hepat-: liver (e.g., gastrohepatic)

hept(a)-: seven (e.g., heptatomic, heptavalent)

hered-: heir (e.g., heredity)

hetero-: other, indicating dissimilarity (e.g., heterogeneous)

hex-^{1}: six, sex-, hexly- (e.g., hexagram)

hex-^{2}: have, hold, be (e.g., cachexy)

hexa-: six, sex-, hexly- (e.g., hexachromic)

hidr-: sweat (e.g., hyperhidrosis)

hist-: web, tissue (e.g., histodialysis)

hod-: road, path (e.g., hodoneuromere)

holo-: all (e.g., hologenesis)

homo-: common, same (e.g., homomorphic)

horm-: impetus, impulse (e.g., hormone)

hydat-: water (e.g., hydatism)

hydr-: pertaining to water (e.g., achlorhydria)

hydro-: water

hyp-: under (e.g., hypaxial, hypodermic)

hyper-: over, above, beyond, extreme (e.g., hypertrophy)

hypn-: sleep (e.g., hypnotic)

hypo-: under, below (o is dropped before words beginning with a vowel) (e.g., hypometabolism)

hyster-: womb (e.g., hysterectomy)

-ia: condition of

-iasis: condition, pathological state (e.g., hemiathriasis); *see also* -osis

iatr-: specialty in medicine (e.g., pediatrics)

-ic: pertaining to

idio-: peculiar, separate, distinct (e.g., idiosyncrasy)

il-: negative prefix (e.g., illegible); in, on (e.g., illinition)

ile-: pertaining to the ileum (ile- is commonly used to refer to the portion of the intestines known as the ileum) (e.g., ileostomy)

ili-: lower abdomen, intestines, (ili- is commonly used to refer to the flaring part of the hip bone known as the ilium) (e.g., iliosacral)

im-: in, on (e.g., immersion; negative prefix (e.g., imperfection)

in-^{1}: fiber (e.g., inosteatoma)

in-^{2}: in, on (n changes to l, m, or r before words beginning with those consonants) (e.g., insertion)

in-³: negative prefix (e.g., invalid)

infra-: beneath (e.g., infraorbital)

insul-: island (e.g., insulin)

inter-: among, between (e.g., intercarpal)

intra-: inside (e.g., intravenous)

ir-: in, on (e.g., irradiation; negative prefix (e.g., irreducible)

irid-: rainbow, colored circle (e.g., keratoiridocyclitis)

is-: equal (e.g., isotope)

ischi-: hip, haunch (e.g., ischiopubic)

-ism: condition, theory (e.g., hemiballism, agism)

iso-: equal (e.g., isotonic)

-ist: specialist

-itis: inflammation (e.g., neuritis)

-ive: pertaining to

-ize: to treat by special method (e.g., specialize)

jact-: throw (e.g., jactitation)

ject-: throw (e.g., injection)

jejun-: hungry, not partaking of food (e.g., gastrojejunostomy)

jug-: yoke (e.g., conjugation)

junct-: yoke, join (e.g., conjunctiva)

juxta-: near (e.g., juxtaposed)

kary-: nut, kernel, nucleus (e.g., megakaryocyte)

kerat-: horn (e.g., keratolysis, keratin)

kil-: one thousand, indicates multiple in metric system (e.g., kilogram)

kine-: move (e.g., kinematics)

kinesio-: movement

-kinesis: movement (e.g., orthokinesis)

labi-: lip (e.g., gingivolabial)

lact-: milk (e.g., glucolactone, lactose)

lal-: talk, babble (e.g., glossolalia)

lapar-: flank, loin, abdomen (e.g., laparotomy)

laryng-: windpipe (e.g., laryngendoscope)

lat-: ear, carry (e.g., translation)

later-: side (e.g., bentrolateral)
lent-: lentil (e.g., lenticonus)
lep-: take, seize (e.g., cataleptic, epileptic)
lepto-: small, soft (e.g., leptotene)
leuk-: white (e.g., leukocyte); *also spelled* leuc-
lien-: spleen (e.g., lienocele)
lig-: tie, bind (e.g., ligate)
lingu-: tongue (e.g., sublingual)
lip-: fat (e.g., glycolipid)
lipo-: fat
lith-: stone (e.g., nephrolithotomy)
litho-: stone
loc-: place (e.g., locomotion)
log-: speak, give an account (e.g., logorrhea, embryology)
-logy: study of
lumb-: loin (e.g., dorsolumbar)
lute-: yellow (e.g., xanthluteoma)
ly-: loose, dissolve (e.g., keratolysis)
lymph-: water (e.g., hydrolymphadenosis)
-lysis: setting free, disintegration (e.g., glycolysis)

macro-: long, large (e.g., marcromyoblast)
mal-: bad, abnormal (e.g., malfunction)
malac-: soft (e.g., osteomalacia)
mamm-: breast (e.g., mammogram, mammary)
man-: hand (e.g., maniphalanx, manipulation)
mani-: mental aberration (e.g., kleptomania)
-mania: excessive preoccupation
mast-: breast (e.g., mastectomy, hypermastia)
medi-: middle (e.g., medial, medifrontal)
mega-: great, large, indicates multiple (1 million) in metric system
(e.g., megacolon, megadyne)
megal-: great, large (e.g., cardiomegaly, acromegaly)
mel-: limb, member (e.g., symmelia)
melan-: black (e.g., melanoma, melanin)
melano-: black
men-: month (e.g., menopause, dysmenorrhea)

mening-: membrane (e.g., encephalomeningitis)

ment-: mind (e.g., dementia)

mer-: part (e.g., polymeric)

mes-: middle (e.g., mesoderm)

meso-: middle

met-: after, beyond, accompanying (e.g., metallergy)

meta-: after, beyond, accompanying (a is dropped before words beginning with a vowel) (e.g., metacarpal, metatarsal)

-meter: measure)

metr-[1]**:** measure (e.g., stereometry)

metr-[2]**:** womb (e.g., endometritis)

micr-: small (e.g., photomicrograph)

micro-: small

mill-: one thousand, indicates fraction in metric system (e.g., milligram, millipede)

mio-: smaller, less (e.g., mionectic)

miss-: send (e.g., intromission)

-mittent: send (e.g., intermittent)

mne-: remember (e.g., pseudomnesia)

mon-: only, sole, single (e.g., monoplegia)

mono-: single

morph-: form, shape (e.g., morphonuclear)

mot-: move (e.g., vasomotor, locomotion)

multi-: many (e.g., multiple)

my-: muscle (e.g., myopathy)

-myces: fungus (e.g., myelomyces)

myc(et)-: fungus (e.g., ascomycetes, streptomycin)

myel-: marrow (e.g., poliomyelitis)

myo-: muscle

myx-: mucus (e.g., myxedema)

narc-: numbness (e.g., toponarcosis, narcolepsy)

nas-: nose (e.g., nasal)

necr-: corpse, dead (e.g., necrocytosis, necrosis)

necro-: dead

neo-: new, young (e.g., neocyte, neonate)

nephr-: kidney (e.g., nephron, nephric)

nephro-: kidney
neur-: nerve (e.g., neurology, estesioneure)
neuro-: nerve and brain
nod-: knot (e.g., nodosity)
nom-: deal out, distribute, law, custom (e.g., nominal, taxonomy)
non-: nine, no (e.g., nonacosane)
nos-: disease (e.g., nosology)
nucle-: nut, kernel (e.g., nucleus, nucleide)
nutri-: nourish (e.g., malnutrition)

ob-: against, toward (b changes to c before words beginning with that consonant) (e.g., obtuse)
oc-: *see* ob- (e.g., occlude)
ocul-: eye (e.g., oculomotor)
-od-: road, path (e.g., periodic)
-ode[1]: road, path (e.g., cathode)
-ode[2]: form (e.g., nematode)
odont-: tooth (e.g., orthodontia)
-odyn-: pain, distress (e.g., gastrodynia)
-oid: form (e.g., hyoid; resembling)
-ol: oil (e.g., cholesterol)
-old: form, shape, resemblance (e.g., scaffold)
ole-: oil (e.g., oleorsin)
olig-: few, small (e.g., oligospermia)
-oma: tumor (e.g., blastoma)
omo-: shoulder (e.g., omosternum)
omphal-: navel (e.g., periomphalic)
onc-: bulk, mass (e.g., oncology, hematoncometry)
onych-: claw, nail (e.g., anonychia)
oo-: egg, ovum (e.g., perioothecitis)
oophor-: pertaining to the ovary (e.g., oophorectomy)
ophthalm-: eye (e.g., ophthalmic)
or-: mouth (e.g., intraoral)
orb-: circle (e.g., suborbital)
orchi-: testicle (e.g., orchiopathy)
organ-: implement, instrument (e.g., organoleptic)
-orrhage: excessive bleeding

-**orrhagia:** hemorrhage
-**orrhaphy:** suture
-**orrhea:** flow, discharge
-**orrhexis:** rupture
orth-: straight, right, normal (e.g., orthopedics)
-**osis:** condition, disease (e.g., osteoporosis)
oss-: bone (e.g., osseous, ossiphone)
ost(e)-: bone (e.g., enostosis, osteonecrosis)
-**ostomy:** new opening
ot-: ear (e.g., parotid); *see also* aur-
oto-: ear
-**otomy:** cutting (e.g., osteotomy)
-**ous:** pertaining to
ov-: egg (e.g., synovia)
oxy-: sharp, acid (e.g., oxycephalic)

pachy(n)-: thicken (e.g., pachyderma, myopachynsis)
pag-: fix, make fast (e.g., thoracopagus)
pan-: entire, all (e.g., pancytosis, pandemic)
par-[1]: bear, give birth to (e.g., primiparous)
par-[2]: *see* para- (e.g., parepigastric)
para-: beside, beyond, alongside of (final a is dropped before words beginning with a vowel) (e.g., paramastoid)
part-: bear, give birth to (e.g., parturition)
path-: that which one undergoes, sickness, disease (e.g., pathology, psychopathic)
patho-: disease
pec-: fix, make fast (e.g., sympectothiene); *see also* pex-
ped-: child (e.g., pediatric, orthopedic)
pell-: skin, hide (e.g., pellagra)
-**pellent:** drive (e.g., repellent)
pen-: need, lack (e.g., erythrocytopenia)
pend-: hang down (e.g., appendix)
-**penia:** deficiency
pent(a)-: five (e.g., pentose, pentaploid)
peps-: digest (e.g., bradypepsia)
pept-: digest (e.g., dyspeptic)

per-: through, excessive (e.g., pernasal)
peri-: around (e.g., periphery)
pet-: seek, tend toward (e.g., centripetal)
pex-: fix, make fast (e.g., hepatopexy)
-pexy: fixation
pha-: say, speak (e.g., dysphasia)
phac-: lentil, lens (e.g., phacosclerosis); *also spelled* phak-
phag-: eat (e.g., lipphagic)
phak-: lentil, lens (e.g., phakitis)
phan-: show, be seen (e.g., diaphanoscopy)
pharmac-: drug (e.g., pharmacology)
pharyng-: throat (e.g., glossopharyngeal)
phen-: show, be seen (e.g., phosphene)
pher-: bear, support (e.g., periphery)
phil-: like, have affinity for (e.g., eosinophilia, philosophy)
phleb-: vein (e.g., periphlebitis, phlebotomy)
phleg-: burn, inflame (e.g., adenophlegmon)
phlog-: burn, inflame (e.g., antiphlogistic)
phob-: fear, dread (e.g., claustrophobia)
-phobia: fear
phon-: sound (e.g., echophony)
phono-: voice
phor-: bear, support (e.g., exophoria)
phos-: light (e.g., phosphorus)
phot-: light (e.g., photerythrous)
phrag-: fence, wall off, stop up (e.g., diaphragm)
phrax-: fence, wall off, stop up (e.g., emphraxis)
phren-: mind, midriff (e.g., metaphrenia, metaphrenon)
phthi-: decay, waste away (e.g., opthalmophthisis)
phy-: beget, bring forth, produce, be by nature (e.g., nosophyte, physical)
phyl-: tribe, kind (e.g., phylogeny)
phylac-: guard (e.g., prophylactic)
-phylaxis: protection (e.g., prophylaxis)
-phyll: leaf (e.g., xanthophyll)
phys(a)-: blow, inflate (e.g., physocele, physalis)
physe-: blow, inflate (e.g., emphysema)

pil-: hair (e.g., epilation)
pituit-: phlegm (e.g., pituitous)
placent-: cake (e.g., extraplacental)
plas-: mold, shape (e.g., cineplasty, plastazode)
-plasty: surgical repair
platy-: broad, flat (e.g., platyrrhine)
pleg-: strike (e.g., diplegia, paraplegia)
plet-: fill (e.g., depletion)
pleur-: rib, side (e.g., peripleural)
plex-: strike (e.g., apoplexy)
plic-: fold (e.g., complication)
plur-: more (e.g., plural)
pne-: breathing (e.g., traumatopnea)
-pnea: breathing
pneum(at)-: breath, air (e.g., pneumodynamics, pneumothorax)
pneumo(n)-: lung (e.g., pneumocentesis, pneumontomy)
pod-: foot (e.g., podiatry)
poie-: make, produce (e.g., sarcopoietic)
pol-: axis of a sphere (e.g., peripolar)
poly-: much, many (e.g., polyspermia)
pont-: bridge (e.g., pontocerebellar)
por-[1]: passage (e.g., myelopore)
por-[2]: callus (e.g., porocele)
posit-: put, place (e.g., deposit, repositor)
post-: after, behind in time or place (e.g., postnatal, postural)
pre-: before in time or place (e.g., prenatal, prevesical)
press-: press (e.g., pressure, pressoreceptive)
pro-: before in time or place (e.g., progamous, prolapse)
proct-: anus (e.g., ecteroproctia)
prosop-: face (e.g., prosopus)
proto-: first (e.g., prototype)
pseud-: false (e.g., pseudoparaplegia)
psych-: soul, mind (e.g., psychosomatic)
pto-: fall (e.g., nephroptosis)
-ptosis: prolapse
pub-: adult (e.g., puberty, ischiopubic)
puber-: adult (e.g., puberty)

pulmo(n)-: lung (e.g., cardiopulmonary, pulmolith)
puls-: drive (e.g., propulsion)
punct-: prick, pierce (e.g., puncture, punctiform)
pur-: pus (e.g., puration)
py-: pus (e.g., nephropyosis)
pyel-: trough, basin, pelvis (e.g., nephropyelitis)
pyl-: door, orifice (e.g., pylephlebitis)
pyo-: pus
pyr-: fire (e.g., galactopyra)

quadr-: four (e.g., quadraplegic, quadrigeminal)
quinque-: five (e.g., quinquecuspid)

rachi-: spine (e.g., alorachidian)
radi-: ray (e.g., irradiation)
re-: back, again (e.g., retraction)
ren-: kidneys (e.g., adrenal)
ret-: net (e.g., retothelium)
retro-: backward (e.g., retrodeviation, retrograde)
rhag-: break, burst (e.g., hemorrhagic)
rhaph-: suture, stitching (e.g., gastrorrhaphy)
rhe-: flow, discharge (e.g., disrrheal)
rhex-: break, burst (e.g., metrorrhexis)
rhin-: nose (e.g., basirhinal)
rhino-: nose
rot-: wheel (e.g., rotator)
rub(r)-: red (e.g., bilirubin, rubrospinal)

sacchar-: sugar (e.g., saccharin)
sacro-: pertaining to the sacrum (e.g., sacroiliac)
salping-: tube, trumpet (e.g., salpingitis)
sanguin-: blood (e.g., sanguineous)
sarc-: flesh (e.g., sarcoma)
schis-: split (e.g., schistorachis, rachischisis)
scler-: hard (e.g., sclerosis, scleraderma)
sclero-: hardening
scop-: look at, observe (e.g., endoscope)

sect-: cut (e.g., sectile, resection)

semi-: half (e.g., semiflexion)

sens-: perceive, feel (e.g., sensory)

sep-: rot, decay (e.g., sepsis)

sept-[1]: fence, wall off, stop up (e.g., septal)

sept-[2]: seven (e.g., septan)

ser-: whey, watery substance (e.g., serum, serosynovitis)

sex-: six (e.g., sexdigitate)

sial-: saliva (e.g., polysialia)

sin-: hollow, fold (e.g., sinobronchitis)

sit-: food (e.g., parasitic)

solut-: loose, dissolve, set free (e.g., dissolution)

-solvent: loose, dissolve (e.g., dissolvent)

somat-: body (e.g., somatic, psychosomatic)

-some: body (e.g., dictyosome)

spas-: draw, pull (e.g., spasm, spastic)

spectr-: appearance, what is seen (e.g., spectrum, microspectroscope)

sperm(at)-: seed (e.g., spermacrasia, spermatozoon)

spers-: scatter (e.g., dispersion)

sphen-: wedge (e.g., sphenoid)

spher-: ball (e.g., hemisphere)

sphygm-: pulsation (e.g., sphygmomanometer)

spin-: spine (e.g., cerebrospinal)

spirat-: breathe (e.g., inspiratory)

splanchn-: entrails, vicera (e.g., neurosplanchnic)

splen-: spleen (e.g., splenomegaly)

spor-: seed (e.g., sporophyte, sygospore)

squam-: scale (e.g., squamus, desquamation)

sta-: make stand, stop (e.g., genesistasis)

stal-: send (e.g., peristalsis); *see also* stol-

staphyl-: bunch of grapes, uvula (e.g., staphylococcus, staphylectomy)

-stasis: stopping, controlling

stear-: fat (e.g., stearodermia)

steat-: fat (e.g., steatopygous)

sten-: narrow, compressed (e.g., stenocardia)

ster-: solid (e.g., cholesterol)

sterc-: dung (e.g., stercoporphyrin)

sthen-: strength (e.g., asthenia)

stol-: send (e.g., diastole)

stom(at)-: mouth, orifice (e.g., anastomosis, stomatogastric)

strep(h)-: twist (e.g., strephosymbolia, streptomycin); *see also* stroph-

strict-: draw tight, compress, cause pain (e.g., constriction)

-stringent: draw tight, compress, cause pain (e.g., astringent)

stroph-: twist (e.g., astrophic); *see also* strep(h)-

struct-: pile up (against) (e.g., obstruction)

sub-: under, below (b changes to f or p before words beginning with those consonants) (e.g., sublumbar)

suf-: *see* sub- (e.g., suffusion)

sup-: *see* sub- (e.g., suppository)

super-: above, beyond, extreme (e.g., supermobility)

supra-: above, beyond

sy-: *see* syn- (e.g., systole)

syl-: *see* syn- (e.g., syllepsiology)

sym-: *see* syn- (e.g., symbiosis, symmetry, sympathetic, symphysis)

syn-: with, together (n dropped before s; changes to l before l; and changes to m before b, m, p, and ph) (e.g., myosynizesis)

ta-: stretch, put under pressure (e.g., ectasis)

tac-: order, arrange (e.g., atactic)

tachy-: over

tact-: touch (e.g., contact)

tax-: order, arrange (e.g., ataxia, taxotomy)

tect-: cover (e.g., protective)

teg-: cover (e.g., integument)

tel-: end (e.g., telosynapsis)

tele-: at a distance (e.g., teleceptor, telescope)

tempor-: time, timely or fatal spot, temple (e.g., temporomalar)

ten(ont)-: tight stretched band (e.g., tenodynia, tenonitis, tenontagra)

tens-: stretch (e.g., extensor)

test-: pertaining to the testicle (e.g., testitis)

tetra-: four (e.g., tetragenous)
the-: put, place (e.g., synthesis)
thec-: repository, case (e.g., thecostegnosis)
thel-: teat, nipple (e.g., thelerethism)
thera-: therapy
therap-: treatment (e.g., hydrotherapy)
therm-: heat (e.g., diathermy)
thermo-: heat
thi-: sulfur (e.g., thiogenic)
thorac-: chest (e.g., thoracoplasty)
thromb-: lump, clot (e.g., thrombophlebitits, thrombopenia)
thym-: spirit (e.g., dysthymia)
thyr-: shield, shaped like a door (e.g., thyroid)
tme-: cut (e.g., axonotmesis)
toc-: childbirth (e.g., dystocia)
tom-: cut (e.g., appendenctomy)
ton-: stretch, put under pressure (e.g., tonus, peritoneum)
top-: place (e.g., topesthesia)
tors-: twist (e.g., extorsion)
tox-: arrow poison, poison (e.g., toxemia)
trache-: windpipe (e.g., tracheotomy)
trachel-: neck (e.g., tracheloplexy)
tract-: draw, drag (e.g., protraction)
trans-: across (e.g., transport)
traumat-: wound (e.g., traumatic)
tri-: three (e.g., trigonad)
trich-: hair (e.g., trichoid)
trip-: rub (e.g., entripsis)
trop-: turn, react (e.g., sitotropism)
troph-: nurture, relating to nourishment (e.g., atrophy)
-trophy: nutrition, growth
tuber-: swelling, node (e.g., tubercle, tuberculosis)
typ-: type (e.g., atypical)
typh-: for, stupor (e.g., adenotyphus)
typhl-: blind (e.g., typhlectasis)

uni-: one (e.g., unioval)
ur-: urine (e.g., polyuria)
uro-: urine

vacc-: cow (e.g., vaccine)
vagin-: sheath (e.g., invaginated)
vas-: vessel (e.g., vascular)
ventro-: abdomen, in front of (e.g., ventrolateral, ventrose)
vers-: turn (e.g., inversion)
vert-: turn (e.g., diverticulum)
vesic-: bladder (e.g., vesicovaginal)
vit-: life (e.g., devitalize)
vuls-: pull, twitch (e.g., convulsion)

xanth-: yellow, blond (e.g., xanthophyll)
xantho-: yellow

-yl: substance (e.g., cacodyl)

zo-: life, animal (e.g., microzoaria)
zyg-: yoke, union (e.g., zygote, zygodactyly)
zym-: ferment (e.g., enzyme)

Metabolic Equivalent (MET) Values for Activity and Exercise

Approximate Metabolic Cost of Activities[a,b]

MET Levels	Self-Care Activities	Occupational/Work Activities	Recreational Activities
1.5 to 2.0 METs[c] 4 to 7 mL O_2/min/kg 2 to 2.5 kcal/min (70 kg BW)[d] Very light/minimal	Eating Shaving, grooming Getting in and out of bed Standing Walking (1.6 km or 1 mph)	Desk work Typing, writing Auto driving[e]	Standing Walking (1.6 km or 1 mph) Flying[e] Motorcycling[e] Playing cards[e] Knitting, sewing

Jacobs, K., & Simon, L. (Eds.). *Quick Reference Dictionary for Occupational Therapy, Sixth Edition* (pp. 594-600). © 2015 SLACK Incorporated.

MET Levels	Self-Care Activities	Occupational/Work Activities	Recreational Activities
2 to 3 METs 7 to 11 mL O$_2$/min/kg 2.25 to 4 kcal/min (70 kg BW) Light	Showering in warm water Walking (3.25 km or 2 mph)	Ironing Light woodworking Riding lawn mower Auto repair Radio/TV repair Janitorial work Manual typing Bartending	Walking (3.25 km or 2 mph) Level biking (8 km or 5 mph) Billiards, bowling Skeet Shuffleboard Powerboat driving Power golf cart driving Canoeing (4 km or 2.25 mph) Horseback riding (walk) Playing a musical instrument

MET Levels	Self-Care Activities	Occupational/Work Activities	Recreational Activities
3 to 4 METs 11 to 14 mL O$_2$/min/kg 4 to 5 kcal/min (70 kg BW) Moderate	Dressing, undressing Walking (5 km or 3 mph)	Cleaning windows Making beds Mopping floors, vacuuming Bricklaying, plastering Machine assembly Wheelbarrow (100-kg or 220-lb load) Trailer truck in traffic Welding (moderate load) Pushing light power mower	Walking (5 km or 3 mph) Biking (10 km or 6 mph) Horseshoe pitching Volleyball (noncompetitive) Golf (pulling bag cart) Archery Sailing (handling small boat) Fly fishing (standing in waders) Horseback riding (sitting to trot) Badminton (social doubles) Energetic musician

MET Levels	Self-Care Activities	Occupational/Work Activities	Recreational Activities
4 to 5 METs 14 to 18 mL O$_2$/min/kg 5 to 6 kcal/min (70 kg BW) Heavy	Showering in hot water Walking (5.5 km or 3.5 mph)	Scrubbing floors Hoeing Raking leaves Light carpentry Painting, masonry Hanging wallpaper	Walking (5.5 km or 3.5 mph) Biking (13 km or 8 mph) Table tennis Golf (carrying clubs) Dancing (foxtrot) Badminton (singles) Tennis (doubles) Calisthenics
5 to 6 METs 18 to 21 mL O$_2$/min/kg 6 to 7 kcal/min (70 kg BW) Very heavy	Walking (6.5 km or 4 mph)	Digging in garden Shoveling light earth	Walking (6.5 km or 4 mph) Biking (16 km or 10 mph) Canoeing (6.5 km or 4 mph) Horseback ("posting" or trot) Stream fishing Ice/roller skating (15 km or 9 mph)

MET Levels	Self-Care Activities	Occupational/Work Activities	Recreational Activities
6 to 7 METs 21 to 25 mL O$_2$/min/kg 7 to 8 kcal/min (70 kg BW) Very heavy	Walking (8 km or 5 mph)	Snow shoveling 10/min (10 kg or 22 lbs) Manual lawn mowing	Walking (8 km or 5 mph) Biking (17.5 km or 11 mph) Badminton (competitive) Tennis (singles) Folk/square dancing Light downhill skiing Ski touring (4 km or 2.5 mph) Water skiing
7 to 8 METs 25 to 28 mL O$_2$/min/kg 8 to 10 kcal/min (70 kg BW)		Digging ditches Carrying 80 kg or 175 lbs Sawing hardwood	Jogging (8 km or 5 mph) Biking (19 km or 12 mph) Horseback riding (gallop) Vigorous downhill skiing Basketball Mountain climbing Ice hockey Canoeing (8 km or 5 mph) Touch football Paddleball

MET Levels	Self-Care Activities	Occupational/Work Activities	Recreational Activities
8 to 9 METs 28 to 32 mL O_2/min/kg 10 to 11 kcal/min (70 kg BW)		Shoveling 10 min (14 kg or 31 lbs)	Running (9 km or 5.5 mph) Biking (21 km or 13 mph) Ski touring (6.5 km or 4 mph) Squash/handball (social) Fencing Basketball (vigorous)
10+ METs 32+ mL O_2/min/kg 11+ kcal/min (70 kg BW)		Shoveling 10 min (16 kg or 35 lbs)	Running 6 mph = 10 METs 7 mph = 11.5 METs 8 mph = 13.5 METs 9 mph = 15 METs 10 mph = 17 METs Ski touring (8+ km or 5+ mph) Squash/handball (competitive)

aIncludes resting metabolic needs.

bSource of MET listing: American Heart Association.

c1 MET is the energy expenditure at rest, equivalent to approximately 3.5 mL O_2/min/kg.

dBW = body weight.

eA major increase in metabolic requirements may occur due to excitement, anxiety, or impatience, which are common responses during some activities. The individual's emotional reactivity must be assessed when prescribing or sanctioning certain activities.

Reprinted with permission from Neistadt, M., & Crepeau, E., *Willard & Spackman's occupational therapy*, Lippincott Williams & Wilkins, 1998.

Metric and English Conversion

LINEAR MEASURE

1 centimeter = 0.3937 inch
1 inch = 2.54 centimeters
1 foot = 0.3048 meter
1 meter = 39.37 inches/1.0936 yards
1 yard = 0.9144 meter
1 kilometer = 0.621 mile
1 mile = 1.609 kilometers

SQUARE MEASURE

1 square centimeter = 0.1550 square inch
1 square inch = 6.452 square centimeters
1 square foot = 0.0929 square meter
1 square meter = 1.196 square yards
1 square yard = 0.8361 square meter
1 hectare = 2.47 acres
1 acre = 0.4047 hectare
1 square kilometer = 0.386 square mile
1 square mile = 2.59 square kilometers

Jacobs, K., & Simon, L. (Eds.). *Quick Reference Dictionary for Occupational Therapy, Sixth Edition* (pp. 601-602). © 2015 SLACK Incorporated.

WEIGHT MEASURE

1 gram = 0.03527 ounce
1 ounce = 28.35 grams
1 kilogram = 2.2046 pounds
1 pound = 0.4536 kilogram
1 metric ton = 0.98421 English ton
1 English ton = 1.016 metric tons

VOLUME MEASURE

1 cubic centimeter = 0.061 cubic inch
1 cubic inch = 16.39 cubic centimeters
1 cubic foot = 0.0283 cubic meter
1 cubic meter = 1.308 cubic yards
1 cubic yard = 0.7646 cubic meter
1 liter = 1.0567 quarts
1 quart dry = 1.101 liters
1 quart liquid = 0.9463 liter
1 gallon = 3.78541 liters
1 peck = 8.810 liters
1 hectoliter = 2.8375 bushels

Metric System

LINEAR MEASURE

10 millimeters = 1 centimeter
10 centimeters = 1 decimeter
10 decimeters = 1 meter
10 meters = 1 dekameter
10 dekameters = 1 hectometer
10 hectometers = 1 kilometer

LIQUID MEASURE

10 milliliters = 1 centiliter
10 centiliters = 1 deciliter
10 deciliters = 1 liter
10 liters = 1 dekaliter
10 dekaliters = 1 hectoliter
10 hectoliters = 1 kiloliter

SQUARE MEASURE

100 square millimeters = 1 square centimeter
100 square centimeters = 1 square decimeter
100 square decimeters = 1 square meter
100 square meters = 1 square dekameter
100 square dekameters = 1 square hectometer
100 square hectometers = 1 square kilometer

Jacobs, K., & Simon, L. (Eds.). *Quick Reference Dictionary for Occupational Therapy, Sixth Edition* (pp. 603-604).
© 2015 SLACK Incorporated.

WEIGHTS

10 milligrams = 1 centigram
10 centigrams = 1 decigram
10 decigrams = 1 gram
10 grams = 1 dekagram
10 dekagrams = 1 hectogram
10 hectograms = 1 kilogram
100 kilograms = 1 quintal
10 quintals = 1 ton

CUBIC MEASURE

1,000 cubic millimeters = 1 cubic centimeter
1,000 cubic centimeters = 1 cubic decimeter
1,000 cubic decimeters = 1 cubic meter

Muscles of the Body

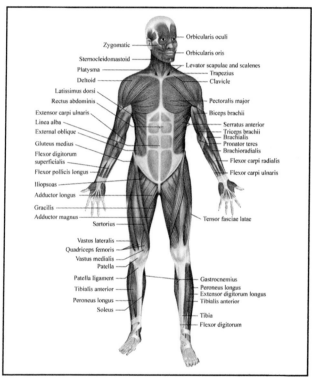

Figure 41-1. Superficial anterior (front) muscles of the body. (Adapted from Leonard, P. [1995]. *Quick and easy terminology* [2nd ed.]. Philadelphia, PA: WB Saunders.)

Jacobs, K., & Simon, L. (Eds.). *Quick Reference Dictionary for Occupational Therapy, Sixth Edition* (pp. 605-608).
© 2015 SLACK Incorporated.

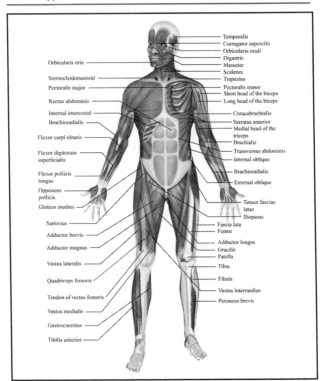

Figure 41-2. Deep anterior (front) muscles of the body. (Adapted from Leonard, P. [1995]. *Quick and easy terminology* [2nd ed.]. Philadelphia, PA: WB Saunders.)

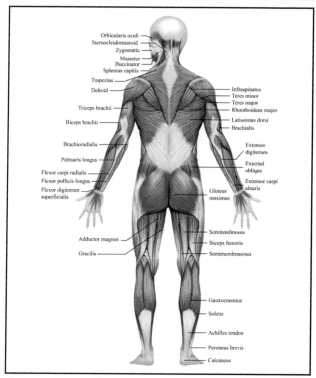

Figure 41-3. Superficial posterior (back) muscles of the body. (Adapted from Leonard, P. [1995]. *Quick and easy terminology* [2nd ed.]. Philadelphia, PA: WB Saunders.)

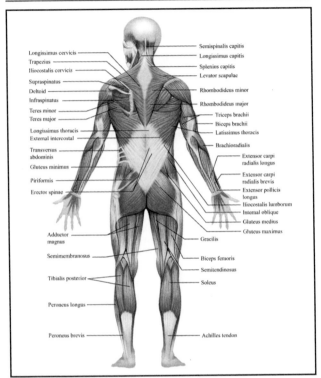

Figure 41-4. Deep posterior (back) muscles of the body. (Adapted from Leonard, P. [1995]. *Quick and easy terminology* [2nd ed.]. Philadelphia, PA: WB Saunders.)

Muscles: Origin/Insertion/Action—Innervation—Blood Supply*

Muscle *Neck*	Origin	Insertion	Action	Nerve	Artery
Sternocleido-mastoid (SCM)	Med or sternal head cranial part of ventral surface of manubrium; lat or clavicular head—sup border & ant surface of med 1/3 clavicle	Lat surface mastoid process & lat 1/2 sup nuchal line of occipital bone	↻ opp side lat √ same √ forward	Spinal accessory n. C2 & C3 ant rami	Subclavian a.
Platysma	Fascia covering sup part of pectoralis major & deltoid	Some fibers into bone below oblique line, others into skin	Draws lip inf & post	Cervical branch of facial n.	Subclavian a. (branch)
Suprahyoid Group					
Digastricus	Post belly: mastoid notch of temporal bone; Ant belly: a depression on inner side of inf border of mandible	Post belly: hyoid bone by fibrous loop; Ant belly: same as post belly	▲ hyoid bone Post draws backward Ant draws forward	Post: facial n. Ant: mylohyoid n.	Lingual a.

*Note: Please refer to key on page 634.

Jacobs, K., & Simon, L. (Eds.). *Quick Reference Dictionary for Occupational Therapy, Sixth Edition* (pp. 609-634). © 2015 SLACK Incorporated.

Muscle	Origin	Insertion	Action	Nerve	Artery
Stylohyoideus	Post & lat surface of styloid process	Body of hyoid bone	Draws hyoid sup & post ▲ hyoid & tongue	Facial n. (branch)	Lingual a.
Mylohyoideus	Whole length of mylohyoid line of mandible	Body of hyoid bone		Mylohyoid n.	Lingual a.
Geniohyoideus	Inf medial spine on inner surface of symphysis menti	Ant surface of hyoid	Draws & tongue	1st cervical n. (through hypo-glossal n.)	Lingual a.
Infrahyoid Group					
Sternohyoideus	Post surface of med end of clavicle, post sterno-clav lig & sup & post part of manubrium sterni	Inf border of hyoid bone	Draws hyoid inferiorly	Branch of ansa cervicalis (1st three cervical nerves)	Lingual a. Subclavian a.
Sternothyroideus	Dorsal surface of manubrium sterni (caudal of origin of sternohyoideus)	Oblique line on lamina of thyroid cartilage	Draws thyroid caudally	Branch of ansa cervicalis (1st three cervical nerves)	Lingual a. Subclavian a.
Thyrohyoideus	Oblique line on lamina of thyroid cartilage	Inf border of greater cornu of hyoid bone	Draws hyoid inferiorly Draws thyroid cartilage sup	1st & 2nd cervical n.	Lingual a. Subclavian a.

Muscle	Origin	Insertion	Action	Nerve	Artery
Omohyoideus	Cranial border of scapula (near or crossing scapular notch)	Caudal border of hyoid bone	Draws hyoid caudally	Branch of ansa cervicalis (1st three cervical nerves)	Subclavian a.
Longus Colli	Vertical: ant surface of C5-C7, T1-T3; Sup: ant tubercles of transverse processes C3-C5; Inf: ant surface of T2 & T3	Vertical: ant surface of C2-C4; sup: narrow tendon into tubercle on ant arch of atlas; Inf: ant tubercles of transverse processes C5 & C6	√ of neck ↻ neck (min)	Branches of 2nd to 7th cervical nerves	Subclavian a. (thyrocervical)
Longus Capitus	Four tendinous slips from ant tubercles of transverse processes C3-C6	Inf surface of the basilar part of occipital bone	Head √	Branches from 1st, 2nd, & 3rd cervical nerves	Subclavian a.
Rectus Capitus Anterior	Ant surface of lat mass of the atlas & from root of its transverse process	Inf surface of basilar part of occipital bone	Head √	Branch of 1st & 2nd cervical nerves	Subclavian a.
Rectus Capitus Lateralis	Sup surface of transverse process of atlas	Inf surface of jugular process of occipital bone	Lat √ head	Branch of 1st & 2nd cervical nerves	Subclavian a.

Muscle	Origin	Insertion	Action	Nerve	Artery
Scalenus Anterior	Ant tubercles of transverse processes of C3-C6 of rib	Scalene tubercle on inner border of 1st rib & ridge on cranial surface	▲ 1st rib √ head ↻ head	Branches of lower cervical nerves	Subclavian a. (thyrocervical)
Scalenus Medius	Post tubercles of transverse processes of C2-C7	Cranial surface of 1st rib between tubercle & subclavian groove	▲ 1st rib √ head ↻ head	Branches from cervical nerves	Subclavian a. (thyrocervical)
Scalenus Posterior	Post tubercles of transverse processes of C5-C7	Outer surface of 2nd rib (deep to serratus anterior)	▲ 2nd rib √ head ↻ head	Ventral primary branches C5-C7	Subclavian a.
Back/Neck					
Serratus Posterior Superior	Caudal part of ligamentum nuchae, spinous processes C7, T1, T2 & T3; supraspinal ligament	Four digitations— cranial borders of ribs 2-5	Respiratory ▲ ribs	Ventral rami T1-T4	Subclavian a.
Inferior	Spinous processes T11, T12, L1-L3; supraspinal ligament	Four digitations into inf borders of last 4 ribs (a little beyond their angles)	Respiratory Draws ribs ◄▶ & ▶	Ventral rami T9-T12	Subclavian a.

Muscle	Origin	Insertion	Action	Nerve	Artery
Splenius Capitis Cervicis	Caudal 1/2 ligamentum nuchae & spinous processes C7, T1-T3 & sometimes T4	Occipital bone just inf to lat 1/3 of sup nuchal line; into mastoid process of temporal bone	/ head & neck lat ✓ same side ↻ same side	Lat branches dorsal primary cervical nerves	Subclavian a. (branches)
Spinalis Capitis	Usually inseparable from semispinalis capitis		/ spine	Branch dorsal primary spinal nerves	Thoracic aorta (branch)
Semispinalis Capitis	Tips of transverse processes C7, T1-T6 & sometimes T7	Between sup & inf nuchal lines of occipital bone	/ head & neck ↻ opp side	Dorsal rami	Subclavian a. (branches)
Longissimus Capitis	Transverse processes T4 & T5 and cervicis & articular processes C4-C7	Post margin of mastoid process (deep to splenius capitus & SCM)	/ head ↻ same side ✓ same side	Dorsal primary mid & lower cervical nerves	Subclavian a. (branches)
Obliquus Capitus Inferior	Arises from apex of spinous process of axis	Inf & dorsal transverse process of atlas	↻ same side	Branch dorsal primary division suboccipital n.	Subclavian a. (branch)
Superior	Tendinous fibers from sup surface transverse process of atlas	Occipital bone between sup & inf nuchal lines (lat to semispinalis capitis)	/ head	Branch dorsal primary division suboccipital n.	Subclavian a. (branch)

Muscle	Origin	Insertion	Action	Nerve	Artery
Rectus Capitis Posterior Major	Spinous process of the axis	Lat part of inf nuchal line of occipital bone and surface immediately inf	/ head ↻ same side	Branch dorsal primary division suboccipital n.	Subclavian a. (branch)
Posterior Minor	Tendon from tubercle on post arch of atlas	Med part of the inf nuchal line of occipital bone & surface between it & foramen magnum	/ head	Branch dorsal primary division suboccipital n.	Subclavian a. (branch)
Longissimus Cervicis	Long, thin tendons from apex transverse processes of upper 4 or 5 thoracic vertebrae	Post tubercles of transverse processes of C2-C6	/ spine lat ✓ ▶ ribs	Dorsal primary branch spinal nerves	Thoracic aorta (branches)
Iliocostalis Cervicis	Angles of the 3rd-6th ribs	Post tubercles of transverse processes of C4-C6	/ spine lat ✓ ▶ ribs	Dorsal primary branch spinal nerves	Thoracic aorta (branches)
Spinalis Cervicis	Caudal part of ligamentum nuchae, spinous process C7; sometimes T1 & T2	Spinous processes of axis; sometimes spinous process C1 & C2	/ spine	Dorsal primary branch spinal nerves	Thoracic aorta (branch)
Semispinalis Cervicis	Transverse processes of 1st five or six thoracic vertebrae	Cervical spinous processes from axis to C5	/ spine ↺ opp side	Dorsal primary branch spinal nerves	Thoracic aorta (branch)

Muscle *Back*	Origin	Insertion	Action	Nerve	Artery
Longissimus Thoracis	Arising from erector spinae & post surfaces transverse & accessory processes of lumbar vertebrae & ant layer lumbocostal aponeurosis	Transverse processes of all thoracic vertebrae and lower 9 or 10 ribs between tubercles and angles	/ spine lat ✓ ▼ ribs	Dorsal primary branch spinal nerves	Thoracic aorta (branch)
Iliocostalis Thoracis	Flattened tendons from upper borders of angles of lower 6 ribs (med to iliocostalis lumborum)	Cranial borders of angles of 1st six ribs and into dorsum of transverse process C7	/ spine lat ✓ ▼ ribs	Dorsal primary branch spinal nerves	Thoracic aorta (branch)
Spinalis Thoracis	Med continuation of sacrospinalis. Arises from spinous processes of T11, T12, L1, & L2	Spinous processes of upper thoracic vertebrae	/ spine	Dorsal primary branch spinal nerves	Thoracic aorta (branch)
Semispinalis Thoracis	Transverse processes of T6–T10	Spinous processes of C6, C7, T1–T4	/ spine ↻ opp side	Dorsal primary branch spinal nerves	Thoracic aorta (branch)
Iliocostalis Lumborum	Flattened tendons from upper portion of erector	Inf borders of angles of last six or seven ribs	/ spine lat ✓ ▼ ribs	Dorsal primary branch spinal nerves	Thoracic aorta (branch)

Muscle	Origin	Insertion	Action	Nerve	Artery
Sacrospinalis (Erector Spinae)	Arises from broad tendon attached to mid crest of sacrum; spinous processes T11-T12 & lumbar vertebrae; supraspinal ligament to lip of iliac crests & lat crest of sacrum	Splits into longissimus, iliocostalis, spinalis, & semispinalis muscles (see respective muscles)	/ spine ↻ spine ▶ ribs lat ✓	Spinal nerves	Thoracic aorta
Multifidus	Spinous processes of each vertebra from sacrum to axis. Arises from back of sacrum from aponeurosis of sacrospinalis, from med surface of post sup iliac spine & post sacroiliac ligaments	Each ascends obliquely crossing over two to four vertebrae and inserted into spinous process of vertebra from last lumbar to axis	/ spine ↻ opp side nerves	Branches of dorsal primary spinal nerves	Thoracic aorta
Rotatores	Transverse process of one vertebra & insert at base of spinous process of vertebra above from the sacrum to the axis	Rotatores longi cross one vertebra in their oblique course. Rotatores breves insert in next succeeding vertebra & run horizontal	/ spine ↻ opp side	Branches of dorsal primary spinal nerves	Thoracic aorta

Muscle	Origin	Insertion	Action	Nerve	Artery
Quadratus Lumborum	Sup borders of the transverse processes L2-L5	Inf border of last rib & transverse process L1-L4	▼ last rib lat ✓	12th thoracic n. 1st lumbar n.	Iliac circumflex
Shoulder Girdle					
Trapezius	Ext occipital protuberance; med 1/3 sup nuchal line; spinous process C7, T1-T12	Post border of lat 3rd clavicle; med margin acromion; spine of the scapula	▲ & /shoulder Abd same side ↺ opp side Retraction ▲↺ glen fossa ▲ glenoid fossa	Spinal accessory n. C3 & C4 spinal nerves	Suprascapular
Levator Scapulae	Transverse processes C1-C4	Med border scapula between sup angle & spine	Elevation Protraction / cervical spine Abd same side ↺ same side	Dorsal scapular n. C3 & C4 spinal nerves	Superficial cervical a. Transverse cervical a.
Rhomboideus Minor	Spinous process of C7 & T1	Med border scapula at level of the spine	Elevation Retraction ▼↺ glen fossa	Dorsal scapular n.	Descending scapular a.

Muscle	Origin	Insertion	Action	Nerve	Artery
Romboideus Major	Spinous process of T2-T5	Med border scapula between spine & inf angle	Elevation Retraction ▶○ glen fossa	Dorsal scapular n.	Descending scapular a.
Latissimus Dorsi	Lumbar aponeurosis; spinous processes of T6-T12, L1-L5 & sacral vertebrae	Distal part of intertubercular groove of humerus	/ shoulder Abd shoulder Med ○	Thoracodorsal n. C6-C8 spinal nerves	Subscapular a.
Pectoralis Major	Ant surface sternal 1/2 clavicle; ventral surface sternum; aponeurosis of obliquus externus abdominis	Crest of greater tubercle of humerus	Elevation Retraction ✓ shoulder Add shoulder Med ○ Protract; ▼▲	Med & lat pectoral n. C5-C8 spinal 1st thoracic n.	Thoraco-acromial a.
Pectoralis Minor	Ext surfaces of ribs three, four, & five near their cartilages	Caracoid process of scapula	Protraction Depression ▶○ glen fossa	Med pectoral n.	Thoraco-acromial a.
Subclavius	1st rib & its cartilage near their junction	Inf aspect of clavicle in the mid 3rd	Protraction Depression	Branch from brachial plexus (sup trunk)	Thoraco-acromial a.

Muscle	Origin	Insertion	Action	Nerve	Artery
Serratus Anterior	Ext surfaces of ribs one to nine	Ant aspect of med border of scapula from sup to inf angle	Protraction Depression ▲↻ glen fossa ✓ & /	Long thoracic n.	Lat thoracic a.
Subscapularis	Mid 2/3 subscapular fossa; inf 2/3 groove on axillary	Lesser tubercle of humerus	Med ✓ & / Abd & add	Subscapular n.	Circumflex scapular a.
Supraspinatus	Mid 2/3 supraspinatous fossa	Sub impression of greater tubercle of humerus	Abd Lat ↻ (weak) ✓ (weak)	Suprascapular n.	Suprascapular
Infraspinatus	Med 2/3 infraspinatus fossa	Mid impression of greater tubercle of humerus	Lat ↻ Abd & add	Suprascapular n.	Suprascapular
Teres Minor	Dorsal surface of axillary border of scapula	Inf impression of greater tubercle of humerus distal to inf impression	Lat ↻ Add	Branch of axillary n.	Post humeral circumflex a.
Teres Major	Oval area on dorsal surface of inf angle of scapula	Crest of lesser tubercle of humerus	Add / shoulder Med ↻	Lower subscapular n.	Circumflex scapular a.

Muscle	Origin	Insertion	Action	Nerve	Artery
Deltoideus	Ant border & sup surface of lat 3rd of clavicle; lat margin & sup surface of acromium; inf lip post border scapular spine	Deltoid prominence on mid of lat body of humerus	Abd shouler ✓ shouler / shoulder Med & lat ↻	Axillary n. from brachial plexus	Post humeral circumflex a.
Shoulder/Elbow					
Triceps Brachii	Long head: infraglenoid tuberosity of scapula; Lat head: post surface of humerus; Med head: post surface of humerus distal to radial groove	Post proximal surface of olecranon	/ elbow / shoulder Add shoulder	Branches radial n.	Profunda brachii a. Inf ulnar collateral a.
Brachialis	Distal 1/2 of ant aspect of humerus	Tuberosity of ulna; rough depression on ant surface of coronoid process	✓ elbow	Musculocutaneous n. Radial & med n.	Brachial a.
Biceps Brachii	Short head: apex of coracoid process; Long head: supraglenoid tuberosity at sup margin of glenoid	Rough post portion tuberosity of radius	✓ shoulder ✓ elbow Supination	Musculocutaneous n.	Brachial a.

Muscle	Origin	Insertion	Action	Nerve	Artery
Coracobrachialis	Apex of coracoid process	Impression at med surface & border of humerus	√ shoulder Add shoulder	Musculocutaneous n.	Brachial a.
Forearm/Wrist					
Pronator Teres	Humeral head: proximal to med epicondyle of humerus; Ulnar head: med side of coronoid process of ulna	Rough impression at mid of lat surface of radius	Pronation	Median n.	Inf ulnar collateral a.
Flexor Carpi Radialis	Med epicondyle of humerus	Base of 2nd metacarpal bone	√ wrist Radial √	Median n.	Radial a.
Palmaris Longus	Med epicondyle of humerus	Palmar aponeurosis	√ wrist	Median n.	Volar interosseous a.
Flexor Carpi Ulnaris	Humeral head: med epicondyle of humerus; Ulnar head: med margin olecranon; proximal 2/3 dorsal border of ulna	Pisiform bone	√ wrist Add wrist	Ulnar n.	Ulnar a.
Flexor Digitorum Superficialis	Humeral head: med epicondyle of humerus Ulnar head: med side of coronoid process Radial head: oblique line of radius	Divides into four tendons that are inserted into the sides of the 2nd phalanx	√ PIPs √ MCPs √ wrist	Median n.	Ulnar a.

Muscle	Origin	Insertion	Action	Nerve	Artery
Flexor Digitorum Profundus	Proximal 3/4 of volar & med surfaces of body of ulnar	Bases of last phalanges	✓ DIPs ✓ PIPs ✓ MCPs ✓ wrist	Palmar interosseous n. from median n. Branch of ulnar n.	Ulnar a. Volar interosseous a.
Flexor Pollicis Longus	Grooved volar surface of body of the radius	Base of distal phalanx of the thumb	✓ IP digit I ✓ MCP digit I ✓ & add wrist	Palmar interosseous n. from median n.	Radial a.
Pronator Quadratus	Pronator ridge on distal part of palmar surface of body of ulna; med part of palmar surface of distal 1/4 of ulna	Distal 1/4 of lat border & palmar surface of body of the radius	Pronation	Palmar interosseous n. from median n.	Ulnar & radial
Brachioradialis	Proximal 2/3 of lat supracondylar ridge of humerus	Lat side of base of styloid process of radius	✓ elbow	Branch of radial n.	Radial a.
Extensor Carpi Radialis Longus	Distal 1/3 lat supracondylar ridge of humerus	Dorsal surface of base of 2nd metacarpal bone—radial side	/ extension Abd wrist	Radial n.	Radial a.
Radialis Brevis	Lat epicondyle of humerus	Dorsal surface of base of 3rd metacarpal bone—radial side	/ wrist Abd wrist	Radial n.	Radial a.

Muscle	Origin	Insertion	Action	Nerve	Artery
Extensor Carpi Ulnaris	Lat epicondyle of humerus	Prominent tubercle on ulnar side of base of metacarpal V	/ wrist Add wrist	Deep radial n.	Ulnar a.
Extensor Digitorum	Lat epicondyle of humerus	2nd & 3rd phalanges of fingers; dorsal surface of distal phalanx	/ PIPs & DIPs / MCPs / wrist	Deep radial n.	Ulnar a.
Extensor Digiti Minimi	Common extensor tendon	Expansion of ext digitorum tendon on dorsum of 1st phalanx of little finger	/ PIPs, DIPs & MCP digit V	Deep radial n.	Ulnar a.
Anconeus	Separate tendon from dorsal part of lat epicondyle of humerus	Side of olecranon; proximal 1/4 of dorsal surface of body of ulna	/ elbow	Radial n.	Ulnar a.
Abductor Pollicis Longus	Lat part of dorsal surface of body of ulna	Radial side of base of 1st metacarpal bone	Abd IP, MCP of digit I Abd wrist	Deep radial n.	Radial a.
Extensor Pollicis Brevis	Dorsal surface of body of radius distal to that muscle & interosseous membrane	Base of 1st phalanx of thumb	/ IP, MCP of digit I / wrist	Deep radial n.	Radial a.

Muscle	Origin	Insertion	Action	Nerve	Artery
Extensor Pollicis Longus	Lat part of mid 1/3 of dorsal surface of body of ulna distal to origin of abductor pollicis longus	Base of last phalanx of thumb	/ IP, MCP of digit I / wrist	Deep radial n.	Radial a.
Extensor Indicis	Dorsal surface of body of ulna below origin of extensor pollicis longus	Joins ulnar side of tendon of extensor digitorum	/ & add of IP, MCP digit II	Deep radial n.	Radial a.
Supinator	Lat epicondyle of humerus from ridge of ulna	Lat edge of radial tuberosity & oblique line of radius & med surface of radius posteriorly	Supination	Deep radial n.	Radial a.
Hand					
Abductor Pollicis Brevis	Transverse carpal ligament, tuberosity of scaphoid, ridge of trapezium	Radial side of base of 1st phalanx thumb	Abd thumb	Median n.	Radial a.
Opponens Pollicis	Ridge of trapezium	Length of metacarpal bone of thumb on radial side	Abd thumb ⌄ thumb Med ↻	Median n.	Radial a.
Flexor Pollicis Brevis	Distal ridge of trapezium; ulnar side of 1st metacarpal	Radial side of base of proximal phalanx of thumb; ulnar side of base of 1st phalanx	⌄ thumb Add thumb	Median & ulnar n.	Radial a.

Muscle	Origin	Insertion	Action	Nerve	Artery
Adductor Pollicis	Capitale bone, bases of 2nd & 3rd metacarpals	Ulnar side of base of proximal phalanx of thumb	Add thumb	Deep palmar branch of ulnar n.	Ulnar n.
Palmaris Brevis	Tendinous fasciculi from palmar aponeurosis	Skin on ulnar border of palm of hand	Draws skin midpalm	Ulnar n.	Superficial ulnar a.
Abductor Digiti Minimi	Pisiform bone	Ulnar side of base of 1st phalanx of digit V	Abd digit V ✓ proximal phalanx	Ulnar n.	Ulnar a.
Flexor Digiti Minimi Brevis	Convex surface of hamulus of hamate bone	Ulnar side of base of 1st phalanx of digit V	✓ digit V	Ulnar n.	Ulnar a.
Opponens Digiti Minimi	Convexity of hamulus of hamate bone	Length of metacarpal bone of digit V along ulnar margin	Abd digit V ✓ digit V Med ↻ V	Ulnar n.	Ulnar a.
Lumbricals	Originate from the profundus tendons 1 & 2: radials sides & palmar surfaces of tendons of digits II & III; 3: contiguous sides of mid & ring fingers; 4: contiguous sides of tendons of ring & little finger	Tendinous expansion of extensor digitorum	✓ MCPs / PIPs & DIPs	1 & 2: median n. 3 & 4: ulnar n.	Median a. Ulnar a.

Muscle	Origin	Insertion	Action	Nerve	Artery
Interosseous Dorsales	Two heads from adjacent sides of metacarpal bone	Bases of 1st phalanx	Abd—midline (digit III)	Deep palmar branch n.	Ulnar a.
Interossei	All from entire length of metacarpal bones	Side of base of 1st phalanx	Add—midline (digit III) √ MCPs / PIPs & DIPs	Deep palmar branch n.	Ulnar a.
Hip					
Psoas Major (Iliopsoas)	Ventral surface of bases and caudal borders of transverse process of lumbar spine; sides and corresponding intervertebral discs of last thoracic and all lumbar vertebrae	Lesser trochanter of femur	√ of hip √ of spine in lumbar region	2nd & 3rd lumbar n.	Lumbar branch of iliolumbar a.
Psoas Minor (Iliopsoas)	Vertebral margins of T12 & L1 & corresponding discs	Pectineal line; iliopectineal eminence	√ of spine in lumbar region	1st & 2nd lumbar n.	Lumbar branch of iliolumbar a.
Iliacus (Iliopsoas)	Upper 2/3 of iliac fossa; iliac crest	Lesser trochanter of femur	√ at hip	Femoral n. (muscular branches)	Lumbar branch of iliolumbar a.

Muscle	Origin	Insertion	Action	Nerve	Artery
Tensor Fasciae Latae (TFL)	Ant part of outer lip of iliac crest; ant border of ilium	Lat part of fascia lata at junction of proximal & mid thirds of thigh (proximal end of ilio-tibial band)	Tenses TFL ✓ at hip Abd at hip Int ↻ at hip	Sup gluteal n.	Sup gluteal a.
Gluteus Maximus	Post gluteal line; dorsal surface of sacrum & coccyx	Gluteal tuberosity; lat part of TFL at junction of proximal and mid thirds of thigh (proximal end of iliotibial band)	/ at hip Add at hip Ext ↻ at hip / lower spine	Inf gluteal n.	Inf gluteal a.
Gluteus Medius	Outer surface of ilium from iliac crest & post gluteal line above to ant gluteal line below	Lat surface of greater trochanter	Abd at hip Int ↻ at hip	Sup gluteal n.	Sup gluteal a.
Piriformis	Pelvic surface of sacrum between ant sacral foramina & margin of greater sciatic foramen	Upper border of greater trochanter of femur	Ext ↻ at hip Abd at hip	1st & 2nd sacral n.	Sup gluteal a.
Obturator Internus	Margins of obturator foramen; pelvic surface of hip bone; post & sup obturator foramen	Med surface of greater trochanter	Ext ↻ at hip Abd at hip	Obturator n. to obturator internus & gemellus sup	Obturator a. Sup gluteal a.

Muscle	Origin	Insertion	Action	Nerve	Artery
Gemellus Superior	Outer surface of ischial spine	Med surface of greater trochanter	Ext ○ at hip	Obturator n. to obturator internus & gemellus sup	Obturator a. Sup gluteal a.
Gemellus Inferior	Upper part of ischial tuberosity	Med surface of greater trochanter	Ext ○ at hip	Obturator n. to quadratus femoris & gemellus inf	Sup gluteal a.
Quadratus Femoris	Lat margin of ischial tuberosity	Quadrate tubercle of femur; linea quadrata	Add at hip Ext ○ at hip	Obturator n. to quadratus femoris & gemellus inf	Sup gluteal a.
Obturator Externus	Outer margin of obturator foramen	Trochanteric fossa of femur	Add at hip Ext ○ at hip	Post branch of obturator n.	Obturator a.
Hip/Thigh					
Sartorius	Ant-sup iliac spine; upper half of iliac notch	Upper part of med surface of tibia	√ at hip Ext ○ at hip √ at knee Abd hip (weak)	Muscular branches of femoral n.	Femoral a.
Quadriceps Femoris					
Rectus Femoris	Ant-inf iliac spine	Patella by the patellar ligament to the tibial tuberosity	/ at knee √ at hip	Muscular branches of femoral n.	Femoral a.
Vastus Lateralis	Lat aspect of the shaft of the femur	Patella by the patellar ligament to the tibial tuberosity	/ at knee	Muscular branches of femoral n.	Femoral a.

Muscle	Origin	Insertion	Action	Nerve	Artery
Vastus Medialis	Med aspect of the shaft of the femur	Patella by the patellar ligament to the tibial tuberosity	/ at knee draws patella medially	Muscular branches of femoral n.	Femoral a.
Vastus Intermedius	Ant aspect of the shaft of the femur	Patella by the patellar ligament to the tibial tuberosity	/ at knee	Muscular branches of femoral n.	Femoral a.
Gracilis	Lower 1/2 of pubic symphysis; upper 1/2 of pubic arch	Proximal part of med surface of tibia	/ at knee Int ↻ at knee Add at hip	Ant branch of obturator n.	Med femoral circumflex a. (ascending)
Pectineus	Pubic pectineal line & an area of bone ant to it	Line leading from the lesser trochanter to the linea aspera	Add at hip / at hip Int ↻ hip	Muscular branches of femoral & obturator n.	Med femoral circumflex a.
Adductor Longus	Ant portion of pubis in angle between crest & symphysis	Mid part of linea aspera	Add at hip / at hip	Ant branch of obturator n.	Profunda femoris a.
Adductor Brevis	Ext surface of inf ramus of pubis	Proximal part of linea aspera	Add at hip / at hip	Ant branch of obturator n.	Mid femoral circumflex a.
Adductor Magnus	Pubic arch & ischial tuberosity	Oblique line along entire shaft of the femur	Add at hip / hip (upper) / hip (lower)	Post branch of obturator & sciatic n.	Profunda femoris & med femoris circumflex a.

Muscle	Origin	Insertion	Action	Nerve	Artery
Biceps Femoris	Long head: from ischial tuberosity; short head: lat lip of linea aspera, lat supracondylar line of femur	Head of fibula, lat condyle of tibia, deep fascia on lat side of leg	√ at knee / at hip; Ext ↻ knee (semiflexed)	Sciatic n. tibial branch to long head; peroneal branch to short head	Profunda femoris a.
Semitendinous	Upper & mid impression of ischial tuberosity (with tendon of the biceps femoris)	Proximal part of ant border & med surface of the tibia	√ at knee / at hip; Int ↻ knee (semiflexed)	Sciatic n.	Perforating branch profunda femoris a.
Semimembranous	Proximal & lat facet of ischial tuberosity	Med-post surface of med condyle of tibia	√ at knee / at hip; Int ↻ knee (semiflexed)	Sciatic n.	Perforating branch profunda femoris a.
Leg					
Tibialis Anterior	Lat surface of shaft of tibia; med aspect of fibula; ant interosseus membrane	Med & plantar surface of med cuneiform bone; base of 1st metatarsal bone	Dorsiflexion inversion	Deep peroneal n.	Ant tibial a.
Popliteus	Lat condyle of femur	Triangular area on post surface of tibia above soleal line	√ at knee; Int ↻ at knee	Tibial n. (med & int popliteal)	Post tibial a.

Muscle Leg/Foot	Origin	Insertion	Action	Nerve	Artery
Extensor Hallucis Longus	Lat surface of shaft of tibia; med aspect of fibula; ant interosseous membrane	Base of distal phalanx of great toe	/ MTP & IP dorsiflexion	Deep peroneal n. (ant tibial)	Ant tibial a.
Extensor Digitorum Longus (EDL)	Lat surface of shaft of tibia; med aspect of fibula; ant interosseous membrane	Dorsal surface of mid & distal phalanges of lat four digits	/ IPs digits II to V dorsiflexion	Deep peroneal n. (ant tibial)	Ant tibial a.
Extensor Digitorum Brevis (EDB)	Proximal & lat surface of calcaneus; lat talocalcaneal ligament	1st tendon dorsal surface of base of proximal phalanx of hallux; other 3 tendons lat sides of tendons of EDL	/ IPs	Deep peroneal n.	Ant tibial a.
Flexor Digitorum Longus	Post surface of shaft of tibia; post aspect of fibula; post interosseous membrane	Plantar surface of base of distal phalanx of lat four digits	√ digits II to V plantar-flexion	Tibial n. (med & int popliteal)	Post tibial a.
Flexor Hallucis Longus	Post surface of shaft of tibia; post aspect of fibula; post interosseous membrane	Base of distal phalanx of hallux	√ digit I plantar-flexion	Tibial n. (med & int popliteal)	Post tibial a.

Muscle	Origin	Insertion	Action	Nerve	Artery
Tibialis Posterior	Post surface of shaft of tibia; post aspect of fibula; post interosseous membrane	Tuberosity of navicular; plantar surface of cuneiform bones; plantar surface of base of 2nd-4th metatarsals, cuboid, sustentaculum tali	Plantar-flexion Inversion	Tibial n. (med & int popliteal)	Post tibial a.
Peroneus Tertius	Lat surface of shaft of tibia; med aspect of fibula; ant interosseous membrane	Dorsal surface of base of 5th metatarsal bone	Dorsiflexion Eversion	Deep peroneal n. (ant tibial)	Ant tibial a.
Peroneus Longus	Lat condyle of tibia; head & upper 2/3 of lat surface of fibula	Lat side of med cuneiform bone, base of 1st metatarsal bone	Plantar-flexion Eversion	Superficial peroneal n. (musculocutaneous)	Peroneal a.
Peroneus Brevis	Lower 2/3 of lat surface of fibula	Lat side of base of 5th metatarsal bone	Plantar-flexion Eversion	Superficial peroneal n. (musculocutaneous)	Peroneal a.
Gastrocnemius	Med head: med condyle & adjacent part of femur; capsule of knee; Long head: lat condyle & adjacent part of femur; capsule of knee	Calcaneus by the calcaneal tendon	Plantar-flexion √ at knee	Tibial n. (med popliteal)	Popliteal a.

Muscle	Origin	Insertion	Action	Nerve	Artery
Soleus	Post surface of head & proximal 1/3 of shaft of fibula; mid 1/3 of med border of tibia	Calcaneus by the calcaneal tendon	Plantar-flexion	Tibial n. (med popliteal)	Post tibial a.
Plantaris	Lat supracondylar line of femur	Med side of post part of calcaneus	Plantar-flexion	Tibial n. (med popliteal)	Post tibial a.
Foot					
Quadratus Plantae	Med head: med surface of calcaneus & med border of long plantar ligament; Lat head: lat border of plantar surface of calcaneus & lat border of long plantar ligament	Attached to tendons of flexor digitorum longus	√ last IP digits II to V	Lat plantar n.	Lat plantar a.
Lumbricals (4)	Tendons of flexor digitorum longus	Tendons of EDL & interossei into bases of last phalanges of digits II-V	√ MP joints / IP joints	Med plantar n. Deep lat plantar n.	Med plantar a.

Key

√ = flexion
/ = extension
↻ = rotation
▶ = depression, downward, caudal
◀ = elevation, upward, cephalic
▼ = outward, expand
n. = nerve
a. = artery
Add = adduction

Min = minimal
MTP = metatarsophalangeal
MCP = metacarpophalangeal
IP = interphalangeal
PIP = proximal interphalangeal
DIP = distal interphalangeal
Opp = opposite
Abd = abduction
Mid = middle

Lat = lateral
Med = medial
Ext = external
Int = internal
Sup = superior
Inf = inferior
Ant = anterior
Post = posterior

Nutrition

ChooseMyPlate is the "newest generation" program created by the USDA that gives recommendations for a healthy balanced diet that meets nutrition and calorie requirements. ChooseMyPlate.gov is based on the 2010 Dietary Guidelines for Americans and offers dietary assessment tools, resources for nutrition education, and simple, clear information about how to make positive eating choices.

10 Tips to Build a Healthier Meal

1. Make half your plate veggies and fruits: Vegetables and fruits are full of nutrients and may help to promote good health. Choose red, orange, and dark-green vegetables such as tomatoes, sweet potatoes, and broccoli.

2. Add lean protein: Choose protein foods, such as lean beef and pork, or chicken, turkey, beans, or tofu. Twice a week, make seafood the protein on your plate.

3. Include whole grains: Aim to make at least half your grains whole grains. Look for the words "100% whole grain" or "100% whole wheat" on the food label. Whole grains provide more nutrients, like fiber, than refined grains.

Jacobs, K., & Simon, L. (Eds.). *Quick Reference Dictionary for Occupational Therapy, Sixth Edition* (pp. 635-638). © 2015 SLACK Incorporated.

4. Don't forget the dairy: Pair your meal with a cup of fat-free or low-fat milk. They provide the same amount of calcium and other essential nutrients as whole milk, but less fat and calories. Don't drink milk? Try soymilk (soy beverage) as your beverage or include fat-free or low-fat yogurt in your meal.

5. Avoid extra fat: Using heavy gravies or sauces will add fat and calories to otherwise healthy choices. For example, steamed broccoli is great, but avoid topping it with cheese sauce. Try other options, like a sprinkling of low-fat parmesan cheese or a squeeze of lemon.

6. Take your time: Savor your food. Eat slowly, enjoy the taste and textures, and pay attention to how you feel. Be mindful. Eating very quickly may cause you to eat too much.

7. Use a smaller plate: Use a smaller plate at meals to help with portion control. That way you can finish your entire plate and feel satisfied without overeating.

8. Take control of your food: Eat at home more often so you know exactly what you are eating. If you eat out, check and compare the nutrition information. Choose healthier options such as baked instead of fried.

9. Try new foods: Keep it interesting by picking out new foods you've never tried before, like mango, lentils, or kale. You may find a new favorite! Trade fun and tasty recipes with friends or find them online.

10. Satisfy your sweet tooth in a healthy way: Indulge in a naturally sweet dessert dish—fruit! Serve a fresh fruit cocktail or a fruit parfait made with yogurt. For a hot dessert, bake apples and top with cinnamon.

INFORMATION ABOUT FOOD GROUPS

Fruit Group: Any fruit or 100% fruit juice counts as part of the Fruit Group. Fruits may be fresh, canned, frozen, or dried and may be whole, cut-up, or puréed.

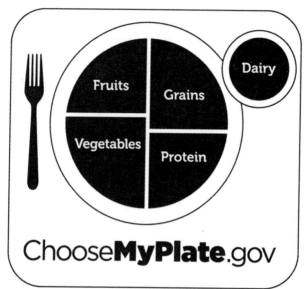

A full-size version is located at www.choosemyplate.gov/images/MyPlateImages/JPG/myplate_bw.jpg

Vegetable Group: Any vegetable or 100% vegetable juice counts as a member of the Vegetable Group. Vegetables may be raw or cooked; fresh, frozen, canned, or dried/dehydrated; and may be whole, cut-up, or mashed.

Grains Group: Any food made from wheat, rice, oats, cornmeal, barley, or another cereal grain is a grain product. Bread, pasta, oatmeal, breakfast cereals, tortillas, and grits are examples of grain products. Grains are divided into 2 subgroups: whole grains and refined grains. Whole grains contain the entire grain kernel—the bran, germ, and endosperm.

Protein Foods Group: All foods made from meat, poultry, seafood, beans and peas, eggs, processed soy products, nuts, and seeds are considered part of the Protein Foods Group. Beans and peas are also part of the Vegetable Group.

Dairy Foods Group: All fluid milk products and many foods made from milk are considered part of the Dairy Foods Group. Most Dairy Group choices should be fat-free or low-fat. Foods made from milk that retain their calcium content are part of the group. Foods made from milk that have little to no calcium, such as cream cheese, cream, and butter, are not. Calcium-fortified soymilk (soy beverage) is also part of the Dairy Group.

Oils: Oils are fats that are liquid at room temperature, such as the vegetable oils used in cooking. Oils come from many different plants and from fish. Oils are not a food group, but they provide essential nutrients. Therefore, oils are included in USDA food patterns.

For information about the amounts of grains and protein you should be eating based on your age, check the ChooseMyPlate.gov website at www.choosemyplate.gov/food-groups

Source: United States Department of Agriculture. www.choosemyplate.gov/

Pharmacology

Compiled by Jaime C. McNeil, MS, PA-C

Note: This is a list of brand name (denoted by uppercase first letter) and generic drugs (all lowercase letters). Please consult each drug's literature for further information. Mention of specific products is not intended as an endorsement by the author or publisher.

Alcohol Withdrawal
diazepam (Valium)
lorazepam (Ativan)
oxazepam (Serax)
chlordiazepoxide (Librium)

Alzheimer's Disease/Dementia
donepezil (Aricept)
rivastigmine (Exelon Patch)
memantine HCL (Namenda)
galantamine (Razadyne)

Anxiety Disorders
lorazepam (Ativan)
clonazepam (Klonopin)
diazepam (Valium)
alprazolam (Xanax)
± antidepressants

Jacobs, K., & Simon, L. (Eds.). *Quick Reference Dictionary for Occupational Therapy, Sixth Edition* (pp. 639-649).
© 2015 SLACK Incorporated.

Arthritis, All Types
acetaminophen
ibuprofen
naproxen
celecoxib (Celebrex)
meloxicam (Mobic)

Arthritis, Gout
indomethacin (Indocin)
colchicine (Colcrys)
prednisone
probenecid
allopurinol
febuxostat (Uloric)

Arthritis, Rheumatoid
hydroxychloroquine (Plaquenil)
sulfasalazine
methotrexate
prednisone
adalimumab (Humira)
etanercept (Enbrel)
infliximab (Remicade)
abatacept (Orencia)

Asthma/Chronic Obstructive Pulmonary Disease
albuterol (Ventolin, Proair, Proventil)
levalbuterol(Xopenex)
pirbuterol (Maxair)
albuterol and ipratropium (Combivent)
tiotropium (Spiriva)
fluticasone/salmeterol (Advair)
mometasone/formoterol (Dulera)
budesonide/formoterol (Symbicort)
fluticasone (Flovent)
budesonide (Pulmicort)
beclomethasone dipropionate (Qvar)

mometasone furoate (Asmanex)
ciclesonide (Alvesco)
ipratropium, albuterol (DuoNeb)
montelukast (Singulair)
theophylline (Choledyl)

Atrial Fibrillation
warfarin (Coumadin)
dabigatran etexilate mesylate (Pradaxa)
rivaroxaban (Xarelto)
dronedarone (Multaq)
diltiazem
amiodarone

Attention Deficit Hyperactivity Disorder
methylphenidate (Ritalin)
methylphenidate (Concerta)
dextroamphetamine (Dexedrine)
amphetamine and dextroamphetamine (Adderall)
dexmethylphenidate (Focalin)
lisdexamfetamine (Vyvanse)
atomoxetine (Strattera)

Bipolar Disorder
lithium (Eskalith)
aripiprazole (Abilify)
lamotrigine (Lamictal)
divalproex sodium (Depakote)
quetiapine (Seroquel)

Cancer
anastrozole (Arimidex)
letrozole (Femara)
exemestane (Aromasin)
tamoxifen
trastuzumab (Herceptin)
epirubicin (Ellence)

docetaxel (Taxotere)
paclitaxel (Taxol)
cyclophosphamide (Cytoxan)
carboplatin (Paraplatin)
cisplatin (Platinol)
vincristine
doxorubicin
bleomycin

Coronary Artery Disease
hypertension medications (*see* **Hypertension**)
dyslipidemia medications (*see* **Hyperlipidemia**)
warfarin (Coumadin)
aspirin
clopidogrel (Plavix)
nitroglycerin
isosorbide mononitrate (Imdur)

Depression
Serotonin–Norepinephrine Reuptake Inhibitors
venlafaxine (Effexor)
duloxetine (Cymbalta)
desvenlafaxine (Pristiq)

Selective Serotonin Reuptake Inhibitors
paroxetine (Paxil)
fluoxetine (Prozac)
sertraline (Zoloft)
escitalopram (Lexapro)
citalopram (Celexa)
vilazodone hydrochloride (Viibryd)

Tricyclic Antidepressants
amitriptyline (Elavil)
imipramine (Tofranil)

Others
bupropion (Wellbutrin)
mirtazapine (Remeron)

Diabetes
Oral Agents
metformin (Glucophage)
glipizide (Glucotrol)
glyburide (Micronase)
pioglitazone (Actos)
sitagliptin phosphate (Januvia)
saxagliptin (Onglyza)

Non-Insulin Injections
exenatide (Byetta)
pramlintide acetate (Symlin)
liraglutide (Victoza)

Insulin—Long Acting
insulin glargine (Lantus)
insulin detemir (Levemir)

Insulin—Short Acting
insulin regular (Humulin)
insulin lispro (Humalog)
insulin regular (Novolin)
insulin aspart (Novolog)

Edema
spironolactone (Aldactone)
furosemide (Lasix)
hydrochlorothiazide (HCTZ)
bumetanide (Bumex)
torsemide (Demadex)

Gastroesophageal Reflux Disease

cimetadine (Tagamet)
ranitidine (Zantac)
omeprazole (Prilosec)
lansoprazole (Prevacid)
esomeprazole (Nexium)
pantoprazole (Protonix)
rabeprazole (Aciphex)
dexlansoprazole (Kapidex)

Headache, Cluster

oxygen
sumatriptan (Imitrex)
divalproex (Depakote)
topiramate (Topamax)
verapamil
prednisone
gabapentin
ergotamine

Headache, Migraine

Acute Treatment
ibuprofen
naproxen
acetaminophen
sumatriptan (Imitrex)
zolmitriptan (Zomig)
rizatriptan (Maxalt)
eletriptan (Relpax)
dihydroergotamine (DHE 45)
metoclopramide (Reglan)

Preventive Treatment
propranolol (Inderal)
verapamil
amitriptyline (Elavil)
valproic acid (Depakote)

topiramate (Topamax)
gabapentin (Neurontin)

Headache, Tension
ibuprofen
naproxen
aspirin, butalbital, and caffeine (Fiorinal)
acetaminophen, butalbital, and caffeine (Fioricet)

HIV
lamivudine and zidovudine (Combivir)
emtricitabine and tenofovir (Truvada)
abacavir and lamivudine (Epzicom)
efavirenz (Sustiva)
nevirapine (Viramune)
lopinavir and ritonavir (Kaletra)
atazanavir sulfate (Reyataz)
ritonavir (Norvir)
fosamprenavir calcium (Lexiva)
emtricitabine (Emtriva)
rilpivirine (Edurant)

Hyperlipidemia
simvastatin (Zocor)
pravastatin (Pravachol)
atorvastatin (Lipitor)
rosuvastatin (Crestor)
gemfibrozil
fenofibric acid
fenofibrate (Tricor)
omega-3-acid ethyl esters (Lovaza)
niacin (Niaspan)
ezetimibe (Zetia)

Hypertension
metoprolol (Lopressor)
atenolol (Tenormin)
lisinopril (Zestril)
enalapril (Vasotec)
captopril (Capten)
atorvastatin (Lipitor)
diltiazem (Cardizem)
hydrochlorothiazide (HCTZ)
chlorthalidone (Thalitone)
amlodipine (Norvasc)
benazepril (Lotensin)
atenolol (Tenormin)
enalapril (Vasotec)
losartan (Cozaar)
valsartan (Diovan)
verapamil (Calan)
bisoprolol (Zabeta)

Inflammatory Diseases (Asthma, Crohn's Disease, Rheumatoid Arthritis)
budesonide (Entocort)
betamethasone
dexamethasone (Decadron)
fludrocortisone (Florinef)
hydrocortisone (Cortef)
methylprednisolone (Solu-Medrol, Medrol)
prednisone
prednisolone

Insomnia
benadryl
temazepam (Restoril)
zolpidem (Ambien)
eszopiclone (Lunesta)
ramelteon (Rozeram)
zaleplon (Sonata)

quetiapine (Seroquel)
trazodone

Muscle Relaxant
baclofen
carisoprodol (Soma)
metaxalone (Skelaxin)
tizanidine (Zanaflex)
orphenadrine (Norflex)
cyclobenzaprine (Flexeril)
diazepam (Valium)

Obsessive-Compulsive Disorders
antidepressants (*see* **Selective Serotonin Reuptake Inhibitors** and **Serotonin–Norepinephrine Reuptake Inhibitors**)

Osteoporosis
alendronate (Fosamax)
risedronate (Actonel)
ibandronate (Boniva)
raloxifene (Evista)
zoledronic acid (Reclast)
calcitonin salmon nasal (Miacalcin)

Pain
acetaminophen (Tylenol)
ibuprofen (Motrin)
naproxen (Aleve)
ketorolac (Toradol)
fentanyl (Duragesic)
hydromorphone (Dilaudid)
meperidine (Demerol)
methadone (Dolophine)
morphine (Avinza)
oxycodone (OxyContin, Percocet, Roxicet)
hydrocodone (Vicodin, Lortab, Norco)
tramadol (Ultram)

pregabalin (Lyrica)
duloxetine (Cymbalta)
gabapentin (Neurontin)

Parkinson's Disease

carbidopa-levodopa (Sinemet)
selegiline (Eldepryl)
rasagiline (Azilect)
pramipexole (Mirapex)
ropinirole (Requip)
tolcapone (Tasmar)
entacapone (Comtan)
trihexyphenidyl (Artane)
amantadine (Symmetrel)

Pneumonia, Aspiration

clindamycin
ampicillin-sulbactam (Unasyn)
amoxicillin/clavulanate (Augmentin) + metronidazole

Pneumonia, Community Acquired

penicillin
ampicillin
ampicillin-sulbactam (Unasyn)
cefotaxime
ceftriaxone
amoxicillin/clavulanate (Augmentin)
amoxicillin
azithromycin
erythromycin
doxycycline
clarithromycin (Biaxin)
cefurixime (Ceftin)
levofloxacin (Levaquin)
moxifloxacin (Avelox)

Schizophrenia

olanzapine (Zyprexa)
ziprasidone (Geodon)
risperidone (Risperdal)
aripiprazole (Abilify)
paliperidone (Invega)
quetiapine (Seroquel)
haloperidol (Haldol)
± antidepressants and anxiolytics

Seizure Disorders

carbamazepine (Tegretol)
gabapentin (Neurontin)
lamotrigine (Lamictal)
phenobarbital
phenytoin (Dilantin)
topiramate (Topamax)
valproic acid (Depakote)

BIBLIOGRAPHY

Epocrates. (2013). *Epocrates [Mobile application software].* Retrieved from www.epocrates.com/mobile/android/essentials

Gold Standard Inc. (2008). *Clinical pharmacology.* Retrieved from www.goldstandard.com

Rugo, H. (2006). Cancer. In L. M. Tierney, S. J. McPhee, & M. A. Papadakis (Eds.), *2006 Current medical diagnosis & treatment* (45th ed., pp. 1639-1702). New York, NY: Lange Medical Books/McGraw-Hill.

Tarsy, D. (2008). Pharmacologic treatment of Parkinson's disease. In D. S. Basow (Ed.), *UpToDate.* Waltham, MA: UpToDate.

United States Department of Health and Human Services. (2008). *Guidelines for the use of antiretroviral agents in HIV-1-infected adults and adolescents.* Retrieved from http://aidsinfo.nih.gov/contentfiles/lvguidelines/AdultandAdolescentGL.pdf

Positive Language

It is important to use positive language in all your communications. This appendix provides phrases/words to use and those to avoid.

Phrases/Words to Use	Phrase/Words to Avoid
Person with a disability	The disabled, handicapped
Physically disabled	Crippled, lame, deformed
Says he/she has a disability	Admits he/she has a disability
Person who has/is affected	Afflicted
Has	Suffers from
Condition	Disease
Person who is blind, person who is visually impaired	The blind
Person who is deaf, person who is hard of hearing	The deaf, suffers a hearing loss
Unable to speak, nonverbal	Dumb, mute
Person who uses a wheelchair	Wheelchair-bound, confined to a wheelchair
Person with an intellectual disability	Retarded, mentally defective
Person with psychiatric disability	Crazy, nuts

Jacobs, K., & Simon, L. (Eds.). *Quick Reference Dictionary for Occupational Therapy, Sixth Edition* (pp. 650-651).
© 2015 SLACK Incorporated.

Phrases/Words to Use	Phrase/Words to Avoid
Person who has multiple sclerosis	Afflicted by multiple sclerosis
Person with cerebral palsy	Cerebral palsy victim, cerebral palsied
Person with epilepsy, person with seizure disorder	Epileptic
Seizure	Fit
Person who has muscular dystrophy	Stricken by muscular dystrophy
Person who has Down syndrome	Person with Down's
Person with autism	Autistic person
Children with special needs	Special needs children, victim, poor
Person without a disability	Normal
Successful, productive	Drain, burden, poor, unfortunate, courageous

Reprinted with permission from United Cerebral Palsy, Incorporated.

Rancho Los Amigos Scales of Cognitive Functioning

ORIGINAL SCALE

Cognitive Functioning

Level I	No response to touch, pain, sound, or sight.
Level II	Generalized reflex response to pain.
Level III	Localized response. Blinks to strong light, turns toward/away from sound, responds to physical discomfort, inconsistent response to commands.
Level IV	Confused/agitated. Alert, very active, aggressive or bizarre behaviors, performs motor activities but behavior is non-purposeful, extremely short attention span.
Level V	Confused/non-agitated. Gross attention to environment, highly distractible, requires continual redirection, difficulty learning new tasks, agitated by too much stimulation. May engage in social conversation but with inappropriate verbalizations.
Level VI	Confused/appropriate. Inconsistent orientation to time and place, retention span/recent memory impaired, begins to recall past, consistently follows simple directions, goal-directed behavior with assistance.
Level VII	Automatic/appropriate. Performs daily routines in a highly familiar environment in a non-confused but automatic robot-like manner. Skills noticeably deteriorate in unfamiliar environment. Lacks realistic planning for own future.

Jacobs, K., & Simon, L. (Eds.). *Quick Reference Dictionary for Occupational Therapy, Sixth Edition* (pp. 652-659).
© 2015 SLACK Incorporated.

Cognitive Functioning

Level VIII   Purposeful/appropriate.

Level IX   Purposeful, appropriate: Stand-by assistance on request.

Level X   Purposeful, appropriate: Modified independent.

REVISED SCALE

Level I—No Response: Total Assistance

- Complete absence of observable change in behavior when presented visual, auditory, tactile, proprioceptive, vestibular, or painful stimuli.

Level II—Generalized Response: Total Assistance

- Demonstrates generalized reflex response to painful stimuli.

- Responds to repeated auditory stimuli with increased or decreased activity.

- Responds to external stimuli with physiological changes generalized, gross body movement, and/or not purposeful vocalization.

- Responses noted above may be the same regardless of type and location of stimulation.

- Responses may be significantly delayed.

Level III—Localized Response: Total Assistance

- Demonstrates withdrawal or vocalization to painful stimuli.

- Turns toward or away from auditory stimuli.

- Blinks when strong light crosses visual field.

- Follows moving object passed within visual field.

- Responds to discomfort by pulling tubes or restraints.

- Responds inconsistently to simple commands.

- Responses directly related to type of stimulus.

- May respond to some persons (especially family and friends) but not to others.

Level IV—Confused/Agitated: Maximal Assistance

- Alert and in heightened state of activity.

- Purposeful attempts to remove restraints or tubes or crawl out of bed.

- May perform motor activities such as sitting, reaching, and walking but without any apparent purpose or upon another's request.

- Very brief and usually non-purposeful moments of sustained alternatives and divided attention.

- Absent short-term memory.

- May cry out or scream out of proportion to stimulus even after its removal.

- May exhibit aggressive or flight behavior.

- Mood may swing from euphoric to hostile with no apparent relationship to environmental events.

- Unable to cooperate with treatment efforts.

- Verbalizations are frequently incoherent and/or inappropriate to activity or environment.

Level V—Confused, Inappropriate Non-Agitated: Maximal Assistance

- Alert, not agitated but may wander randomly or with a vague intention of going home.

- May become agitated in response to external stimulation, and/or lack of environmental structure.

- Not oriented to person, place, or time.

- Frequent brief periods, non-purposeful sustained attention.

- Severely impaired recent memory, with confusion of past and present in reaction to ongoing activity.

- Absent goal-directed, problem-solving, self-monitoring behavior.

- Often demonstrates inappropriate use of objects without external direction.

- May be able to perform previously learned tasks when structured and cues provided.

- Unable to learn new information.

- Able to respond appropriately to simple commands fairly consistently with external structures and cues.

- Responses to simple commands without external structure are random and non-purposeful in relation to command.

- Able to converse on a social, automatic level for brief periods of time when provided external structure and cues.

- Verbalizations about present events become inappropriate and confabulatory when external structure and cues are not provided.

Level VI—Confused, Appropriate: Moderate Assistance

- Inconsistently oriented to person, time, and place.

- Able to attend to highly familiar tasks in non-distracting environment for 30 minutes with moderate redirection.

- Remote memory has more depth and detail than recent memory.

- Vague recognition of some staff.

- Able to use assistive memory aide with maximum assistance.

- Emerging awareness of appropriate response to self, family, and basic needs.

- Moderate assist to problem solve barriers to task completion.

- Supervised for old learning (e.g., self-care).

- Shows carry over for relearned familiar tasks (e.g., self-care).

- Maximum assistance for new learning with little or no carry over.

- Unaware of impairments, disabilities, and safety risks.

- Consistently follows simple directions.

- Verbal expressions are appropriate in highly familiar and structured situations.

Level VII—Automatic, Appropriate: Minimal Assistance for Daily Living Skills

- Consistently oriented to person and place, within highly familiar environments. Moderate assistance for orientation to time.

- Able to attend to highly familiar tasks in a non-distraction environment for at least 30 minutes with minimal assist to complete tasks.

- Minimal supervision for new learning.

- Demonstrates carryover of new learning.

- Initiates and carries out steps to complete familiar personal and household routine but has shallow recall of what he/ she has been doing.

- Able to monitor accuracy and completeness of each step in routine personal and household ADL and modify plan with minimal assistance.

- Superficial awareness of his/her condition but unaware of specific impairments and disabilities and the limits they place on his/her ability to safely, accurately and completely carry out his/her household, community, work and leisure ADL.

- Minimal supervision for safety in routine home and community activities.

- Unrealistic planning for the future.

- Unable to think about consequences of a decision or action.

- Overestimates abilities.

- Unaware of others' needs and feelings.

- Oppositional/uncooperative.

- Unable to recognize inappropriate social interaction behavior.

Level VIII—Purposeful, Appropriate: Stand-By Assistance

- Consistently oriented to person, place, and time.

- Independently attends to and completes familiar tasks for 1 hour in distracting environments.

- Able to recall and integrate past and recent events.

- Uses assistive memory devices to recall daily schedule and "to do" lists and to record critical information for later use with stand-by assistance.

- Initiates and carries out steps to complete familiar personal, household, community, work, and leisure routines with stand-by assistance and can modify the plan when needed with minimal assistance.

- Requires no assistance once new tasks/activities are learned.

- Aware of and acknowledges impairments and disabilities when they interfere with task completion but requires stand-by assistance to take appropriate corrective action.

- Thinks about consequences of a decision or action with minimal assistance.

- Overestimates or underestimates abilities.

- Acknowledges others' needs and feelings and responds appropriately with minimal assistance.

- Depressed.

- Irritable.

- Low frustration tolerance/easily angered.

- Argumentative.

- Self-centered.

- Uncharacteristically dependent/independent.

- Able to recognize and acknowledge inappropriate social interaction behavior while it is occurring and takes corrective action with minimal assistance.

Level IX—Purposeful, Appropriate: Stand-By Assistance on Request

- Independently shifts back and forth between tasks and completes them accurately for at least 2 consecutive hours.

- Uses assistive memory devices to recall daily schedule and "to do" lists and to record critical information for later use with assistance when requested.

- Initiates and carries out steps to complete familiar personal, household, work and leisure tasks independently and unfamiliar personal, household, work, and leisure tasks with assistance when requested.

- Aware of and acknowledges impairments and disabilities when they interfere with task completion and takes appropriate corrective action but requires stand-by assist to anticipate a problem before it occurs and take action to avoid it.

- Able to think about consequences of decisions or actions with assistance when requested.

- Accurately estimates abilities but requires stand-by assistance to adjust to task demands.

- Acknowledges others' needs and feelings and responds appropriately with stand-by assistance.

- Depression may continue.

- May be easily irritable.

- May have low frustration tolerance.

- Able to self-monitor appropriateness of social interaction with stand-by assistance.

Level X—Purposeful, Appropriate: Modified Independent

- Able to handle multiple tasks simultaneously in all environments but may require periodic breaks.

- Able to independently procure, create, and maintain own assistive memory devices.

- Independently initiates and carries out steps to complete familiar and unfamiliar personal, household, community, work, and leisure tasks but may require more than usual amount of time and/or compensatory strategies to complete them.

- Anticipates impact of impairments and disabilities on ability to complete daily living tasks and takes action to avoid problems before they occur but may require more than usual amount of time and/or compensatory strategies.

- Able to independently think about consequences of decisions or actions but may require more than usual amount of time and/or compensatory strategies to select the appropriate decision or action.

- Accurately estimates abilities and independently adjusts to task demands.

- Able to recognize the needs and feelings of others and automatically respond in appropriate manner.

- Periodic periods of depression may occur.

- Irritability and low frustration tolerance when sick, fatigued and/or under emotional stress.

- Social interaction behavior is consistently appropriate.

Reprinted with permission from Hagen, C., Malkmus, D., & Durham, P. (1979). *Rancho levels of cognitive functioning. Rehabilitation of the head injured adult: Comprehensive physical management.* Downey, CA: Professional Staff Association of Rancho Los Amigos National Rehabilitation Center.

Range of Motion

UPPER EXTREMITY RANGE OF MOTION

Cervical Spine

Flexion	0 to 45 degrees
Extension	0 to 45 degrees
Lateral flexion	0 to 45 degrees
Rotation	0 to 60 degrees

Shoulder

Flexion	0 to 170 degrees
Extension	0 to 60 degrees
Abduction	0 to 170 degrees
Adduction	0 degrees
Horizontal abduction	0 to 40 degrees
Horizontal adduction	0 to 130 degrees
Internal rotation	0 to 60-70 degrees
External rotation	0 to 90 degrees

Elbow and Forearm

Extension-flexion	0 to 150 degrees
Supination	0 to 80-90 degrees
Pronation	0 to 80-90 degrees

Jacobs, K., & Simon, L. (Eds.). *Quick Reference Dictionary for Occupational Therapy, Sixth Edition* (pp. 660-662). © 2015 SLACK Incorporated.

Wrist

Flexion	0 to 80-90 degrees
Extension	0 to 70 degrees
Ulnar deviation	0 to 30-35 degrees
Radial deviation	0 to 20 degrees

Thumb (1st Digit)

MP flexion	0 to 50-90 degrees
MCP hyperextension	0 to 15-45 degrees
IP flexion	0 to 80-90 degrees
Abduction	0 to 50 degrees
Opposition	0 (cm)

Fingers

MP flexion	0 to 90 degrees
PIP flexion	0 to 100-110 degrees
DIP flexion	0 to 80 degrees
Abduction	0 to 25 degrees

LOWER EXTREMITY RANGE OF MOTION

Hip

Flexion	0 to 120 degrees
Extension	0 to 30 degrees
Abduction	0 to 40 degrees
Adduction	0 to 35 degrees
Internal rotation	0 to 45 degrees
External rotation	0 to 45 degrees

Knee

Extension-flexion	0 to 135 degrees

Ankle-Foot

Dorsiflexion	0 to 15 degrees
Plantarflexion	0 to 50 degrees
Inversion	0 to 35 degrees
Eversion	0 to 20 degrees

Adapted from Trombly, C. A. (1995). Evaluation of biomechanical and physiological aspects of motor performance. In C. A. Trombly (Ed.), *Occupational therapy for physical dysfunction* (4th ed., pp. 73-156). Baltimore, MD: Williams & Wilkins and from Duesterhaus Minor, M. A., & Duesterhaus Minor, S. (1985). *Patient evaluation methods for the health professional.* Reston, VA: Reston Publishing Co., Inc.

Range of Motion: Illustrations

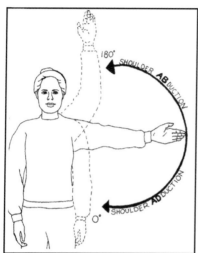

Figure 48-1. Shoulder abduction and adduction.

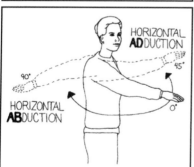

Figure 48-2. Horizontal abduction and adduction.

Jacobs, K., & Simon, L. (Eds.). *Quick Reference Dictionary for Occupational Therapy, Sixth Edition* (pp. 663-667). © 2015 SLACK Incorporated.

Figure 48-3. Shoulder flexion and extension.

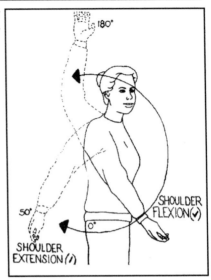

Figure 48-4. External rotation and internal rotation.

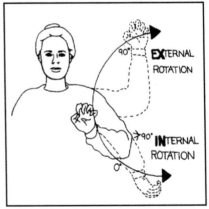

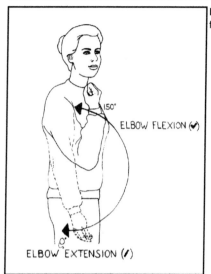

Figure 48-5. Elbow flexion and extension.

150°

ELBOW FLEXION (✔)

0°

ELBOW EXTENSION (✓)

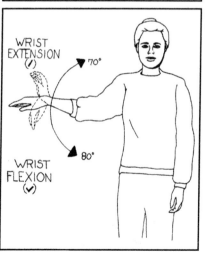

Figure 48-6. Wrist extension and flexion.

WRIST EXTENSION (✓)

70°

80°

WRIST FLEXION (✔)

Figure 48-7. Supination and pronation.

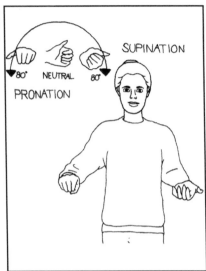

Figure 48-8. Knee flexion and extension.

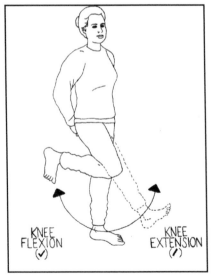

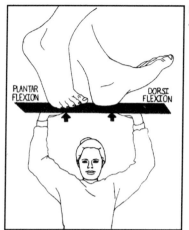

Figure 48-9. Plantarflexion and dorsiflexion.

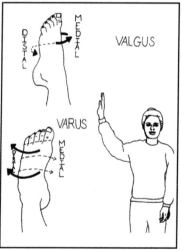

Figure 48-10. Valgus (eversion) and varus (inversion).

Illustrations by Barbara Revilla.

Reflex/Reaction

Reflex/ Reaction	Reaction Type	Age Range	Stimulus/Response
Associated reactions	Brainstem reflex	Normal throughout life when attempting strenuous activity	When a client exerts against resistance with one upper extremity, the other upper extremity will mimic the motion
Asymmetrical tonic neck reflex	Brainstem reflex	Birth to 4-6 mos	When the client's head is actively or passively turned 90 degrees to one side, the extensor tone of the limbs on the face side increases and the flexor tone of the limbs on the skull side increases

Jacobs, K., & Simon, L. (Eds.). *Quick Reference Dictionary for Occupational Therapy, Sixth Edition* (pp. 668-674). © 2015 SLACK Incorporated.

Reflex/ Reaction	Reaction Type	Age Range	Stimulus/Response
Body righting acting on the head	Midbrain reaction	6 mos to 5 yrs	When the client is blindfolded in prone or supine and has asymmetrical pressure applied to the sense organs on the anterior body surface, the client will bring the head into a face-vertical position. This orients the head to the surface with which the client is in contact.
Body righting on the body	Midbrain reaction	6 to 18 mos	When the client's head is actively or passively turned to one side, the body rotates in segments around the body axis toward the direction of the head
Crossed extension reflex	Spinal level	Birth to 2 mos	When the client is in supine with one leg flexed and the other extended, passive flexion of the extended leg will cause the flexed leg to extend and the hip to internally rotate and adduct

Reflex/Reaction	Reaction Type	Age Range	Stimulus/Response
Equilibrium reaction	Cortical reaction	6 mos to throughout life	When a client is rocked enough to disturb balance, there are automatic protective movements and movements to maintain balance and right the head and body
Extensor thrust	Spinal level reflex	Birth to 2 mos	When the client is in supine with one leg flexed and the other extended, pressure applied to the ball of the flexed foot will cause it to extend uncontrollably
Flexor withdrawal	Spinal level reflex	Birth to 2 mos	When stimulation is applied to the sole of the foot, the leg flexes uncontrollably
Grasp reflex	Innate primary reaction	Birth to 3-4 mos	When pressure is applied to the palm or ulnar side of the hand, the fingers flex, grasping the stimulus object
Labyrinthine righting acting on the head	Midbrain reaction	2 mos to throughout life	When vision is occluded, the client's head will seek a vertical position when the body is placed in a prone, supine, or vertical position

Reflex/Reaction	Reaction Type	Age Range	Stimulus/Response
Landau reflex	Automatic movement reflex	4 to 12-24 mos	With the client prone and suspended in space with a support under the chest, passive or active neck extension will cause the back and legs to extend
Moro reflex	Automatic movement reflex	Birth to 5 mos	When the client is startled, either by a loud noise or by allowing the head to drop backward, he or she will extend or flex and abduct the arms as well as spread the fingers
Neck righting	Midbrain reaction	Birth to 6 mos	When the head is passively turned to one side, the body rotates as a whole in the direction of the face
Optic righting	Cortical reaction	2 mos to throughout life	With the head laterally flexed, the client will vertically orientate the head in relation to landmarks observed in space
Placing reaction	Innate primary reaction	Birth to 2 mos	When the dorsum of the client's hand is brushed against the underside of a table, the client will flex the arm and place the hand on the tabletop

Reflex/Reaction	Reaction Type	Age Range	Stimulus/Response
Positive supporting reaction	Brainstem reflex	Birth to 6 mos	When the ball of a dorsiflexed foot is placed firmly on the floor, the lower extremity will extend rigidly due to co-contraction of the flexors and extensors of the knee and hip joints
Protective extensor thrust	Automatic movement reflex	6 mos to throughout life	When the client's body is displaced forward, backward, or laterally, the client will extend the limbs to protect the head
Reflex stepping	Innate primary reaction	Birth to 3 mos	If the client is supported in an upright position and leaned forward so that pressure is applied to the feet, rhythmic, alternate stepping will occur
Rooting reflex	Innate primary reaction	Birth to 4 mos	When the outer corner of the lips or the cheek is touched or stroked, the client will move the lower lip, tongue, and head toward the stimulus

Reflex/Reaction	Reaction Type	Age Range	Stimulus/Response
Sucking reflex	Innate primary reaction	Birth to 2 mos	When the lips, gums, or front of tongue is stimulated, the client will suck and make swallowing motions
Symmetrical tonic neck reflex	Brainstem reflex	Birth to 4-6 mos	When the client is sitting or in quadruped, flexing the client's head will cause the upper extremities to flex and the lower extremities to extend; conversely, extending the client's head will cause the upper extremities to extend and the lower extremities to flex
Tonic labyrinthine reflex: Extremities	Brainstem reflex	Birth to 4 mos	When the client is prone with the head at midline, will flex or have increased flexor tone
Tonic labyrinthine reflex: Supine	Brainstem reflex	Birth to 4 mos	When the client is supine with the head at midline the extremities will extend or have increased extensor tone

GRADING OF REFLEXES

By convention the deep tendon reflexes are graded as follows:

0 = no response; always abnormal

1+ = a slight but definitely present response; may or may not be normal

2+ = a brisk response; normal

3+ = a very brisk response; may or may not be normal

4+ = a tap elicits a repeating reflex (clonus); always abnormal

Whether the 1+ and 3+ responses are normal depends on what they were previously (i.e., the patient's reflex history), what the other reflexes are, and analysis of associated findings, such as muscle tone, muscle strength, or other evidence of disease. Asymmetry of reflexes suggests abnormality.

Source: National Center for Biotechnology Information, U.S. National Library of Medicine. www.ncbi.nlm.nih.gov/books/NBK396/

Safe Patient Handling and Movement Skills for Occupational Therapy Practitioners and Students

Theta Grimaud, OTD, BS, OTR/L, CEAS

Researchers report that at least 12% of occupational therapy practitioners are injured during the use of manual transfer and mobility skills (Campo & Darragh, 2010; Darragh, Huddleston, & King, 2009; Rice, Dusseau, & Miller, 2011). The use of Safe Patient Handling and Movement (SPHM) devices and techniques can improve safety and enhance client outcomes. The following are examples of possible device and technique applications.

Jacobs, K., & Simon, L. (Eds.). *Quick Reference Dictionary for Occupational Therapy, Sixth Edition* (pp. 675-679).
© 2015 SLACK Incorporated.

Task/Problem	Devices Needed	Staff Requirements	Benefit to Client	Benefit to Staff
Pull up in bed	Z-Slider, Pink Slip, or similar device used as directed with open side horizontal on the bed	At least 2 staff depending on the client's weight and ability to assist.	Client can use feet and arms to assist with the transfer. Builds strength, endurance, and confidence.	Decreased force to staff to pull client up becomes a part of ADL treatment.
Move to edge of bed	Z-Slider, Pink Slip, or similar device used as directed with open side vertical on the bed but positioned on the opposite half of the bed only to prevent a fall	At least 1 or 2 staff depending on the client's weight and ability to assist.	Client can help slide to edge of bed using arms legs and trunk to assist the lateral move.	Decreased force to assist client to edge of bed for next step to sit at edge of bed as part of the ADL treatment.

The next set requires either a ceiling or floor lift that has a "T" bar design for maximum flexibility for therapeutic use.

Task/Problem	Devices Needed	Staff Requirements	Benefit to Client	Benefit to Staff
Client is unable to roll in bed or get up from side lying	Turning straps	2 staff; place straps under shoulders and hips to assist the roll. The strap under the shoulders can be used to assist the push up to sit.	Assists in learning how to roll/get up from side lying.	Staff is able to teach client how to roll/get up from side lying as part of the therapeutic process.
A limb needs to be held for wound care or splinting type needs	Turning straps	1 or 2 staff depending on the size of the limb and task to be completed.	Limb can be held for splinting, wound care type needs.	Staff is able to keep limb in proper position for task.

Task/Problem	Devices Needed	Staff Requirements	Benefit to Client	Benefit to Staff
Client is unable to assist with bed mobility for a variety of diagnostic reasons	Full sling	2 staff; place sling and lift client to a position seated at bedside or in a chair as needed for support.	Ability to get into an upright, seated posture to improve strength and endurance and engage in activity.	Staff is able to have client in an upright position for pre-ADL/ADL therapeutic treatment.
Client has trouble with sitting balance during ADL	Walking vest	1 or 2 staff; place walking vest on client while in seated position.	Client is able to test and challenge sitting balance during ADL activity.	Staff has hands free to assist with balance activity, both in midline and off center.
Client has trouble with standing/walking balance during ADL	Walking vest	2 staff; placing walking vest on client while in a seated position and lift to standing position (a scale on the lift can help modulate weight bearing).	Client is able to test and challenge standing and walking balance during ADL activity.	Staff has their hands free to assist with balance activity in both midline and off center.

The previous uses for SPHM devices do not currently have evidence-based research to support their efficacy. Each skill should be practiced with the facility's available equipment before use on a client. If there are questions about the appropriate use of the facility's equipment, contact the lift company vendor.

REFERENCES

Campo, M., & Darragh, A. (2010). Impact of work-related pain on physical and occupational therapists. *Physical Therapy, 90,* 905-920.

Darragh, A., Huddleston, W., & King, P. (2009). Work-related musculoskeletal injuries and disorders among occupational and physical therapists. *American Journal of Occupational Therapy, 63,* 351-362.

Rice, M., Dusseau, J., & Miller, B. (2011). A questionnaire of musculoskeletal injuries associated with manual patient lifting in occupational therapy in the state of Ohio. *Occupational Therapy in Health Care, 25,* 95-107. doi: 10.3109/07380577.2011.566308

Splints

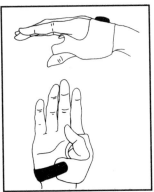

Figure 51-1. C-splint.

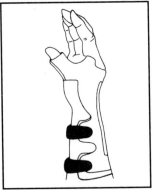

Figure 51-2. Dorsal long opponens.

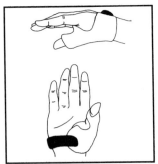

Figure 51-3. Short opponens.

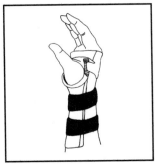

Figure 51-4. Volar wrist cock-up.

Jacobs, K., & Simon, L. (Eds.). *Quick Reference Dictionary for Occupational Therapy, Sixth Edition* (pp. 680-681). © 2015 SLACK Incorporated.

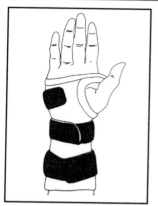

Figure 51-5. Volar wrist cock-up.

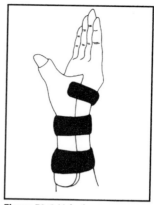

Figure 51-6. Volar long opponens splint.

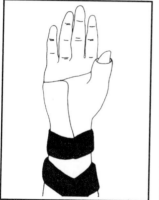

Figure 51-7. Volar long opponens splint.

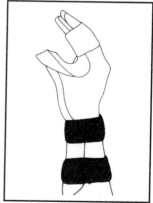

Figure 51-8. Resting hand.

Illustrations by Barbara Revilla.

Stages of Alzheimer's Disease

Early stage 1	Forgetfulness (forget recent conversations, appointments, ordinary words, special dates) Fatigue Mild memory deficits Difficulty with novel and complex tasks Apathy and social withdrawal
Moderate stage 2	Moderate to severe objective memory deficits (may lose ability to count and spell) Disorientation to time and place Language disturbance (may mismatch units of measurement with nouns) Personality and behavioral changes (may show aggressive behavior in response to frustration and resist offers for help) Requires supervision
Severe stage 3	Intellectual functions are commonly untestable Severely limited verbal communication Maximal to total assistance with self-care Usually do not recognize caregivers Incontinent of bowel and bladder

Jacobs, K., & Simon, L. (Eds.). *Quick Reference Dictionary for Occupational Therapy, Sixth Edition* (pp. 682-683). © 2015 SLACK Incorporated.

Final stage 4	Terminal stage
	Lose almost all motor control, memory
	Unaware of environment
	Near or total loss of speech
	Repetitive humming or groaning
	Bedridden
	Joint contractures
	Pathological reflexes
	Clonus
	This is the final step for many families where the parent/child role reverses forever

Because of the incurable and progressive nature of this disease, treatment must focus on maintaining and maximizing the quality of life through enabling the person to maintain as much independence as possible.

Stages of Alzheimer's Disease: Seven Stages From the Alzheimer's Foundation

Alzheimer's symptoms vary. The stages below provide a general idea of how abilities change during the course of the disease.

Stage 1   No impairment
Stage 2   Very mild decline
Stage 3   Mild decline
Stage 4   Moderate decline
Stage 5   Moderately severe decline
Stage 6   Severe decline
Stage 7   Very severe decline

Not everyone will experience the same symptoms or progress at the same rate. This seven-stage framework is based on a system developed by Barry Reisberg, MD, clinical director of the New York University School of Medicine's Silberstein Aging and Dementia Research Center.

Remember: It is difficult to place a person with Alzheimer's in a specific stage as stages may overlap.

Stage 1   No impairment (normal function):
          The person does not experience any memory problems. An interview with a medical professional does not show any evidence of symptoms of dementia.

Stage 2   Very mild cognitive decline (may be normal age-related changes or earliest signs of Alzheimer's disease):
          The person may feel as if he or she is having memory lapses—forgetting familiar words or the location of

Jacobs, K., & Simon, L. (Eds.). *Quick Reference Dictionary for Occupational Therapy, Sixth Edition* (pp. 684-687).
© 2015 SLACK Incorporated.

everyday objects—but no symptoms of dementia can be detected during a medical examination or by friends, family, or coworkers.

Stage 3   Mild cognitive decline (early-stage Alzheimer's can be diagnosed in some, but not all, individuals with these symptoms):

Friends, family, or coworkers begin to notice difficulties. During a detailed medical interview, doctors may be able to detect problems in memory or concentration. Common Stage 3 difficulties include:

- Noticeable problems coming up with the right word or name

- Trouble remembering names when introduced to new people

- Having noticeably greater difficulty performing tasks in social or work settings

- Forgetting material that one has just read

- Losing or misplacing a valuable object

- Increasing trouble with planning or organizing

Stage 4   Moderate cognitive decline (mild or early-stage Alzheimer's disease):

At this point, a careful medical interview should be able to detect clear-cut symptoms in several areas:

- Forgetfulness of recent events.

- Impaired ability to perform challenging mental arithmetic—for example, counting backward from 100 by 7s.

- Greater difficulty performing complex tasks, such as planning dinner for guests, paying bills, or managing finances.

- Forgetfulness about one's own personal history.

- Becoming moody or withdrawn, especially in socially or mentally challenging situations.

Stage 5   Moderately severe cognitive decline (moderate or mid-stage Alzheimer's disease):

Gaps in memory and thinking are noticeable, and individuals begin to need help with day-to-day activities. At this stage, those with Alzheimer's may:

- Be unable to recall their own address or telephone number or the high school or college from which they graduated.

- Become confused about where they are or what day it is.

- Have trouble with less challenging mental arithmetic; such as counting backward from 40 by subtracting 4s or from 20 by 2s.

- Need help choosing proper clothing for the season or the occasion.

- Still remember significant details about themselves and their family.

- Still require no assistance with eating or using the toilet.

Stage 6   Severe cognitive decline (moderately severe or mid-stage Alzheimer's disease):

Memory continues to worsen, personality changes may take place, and individuals need extensive help with daily activities. At this stage, individuals may:

- Lose awareness of recent experiences, as well as of their surroundings.

- Remember their own name but have difficulty with their personal history.

- Distinguish familiar and unfamiliar faces but have trouble remembering the name of a spouse or caregiver.

- Need help dressing properly and may, without supervision, make mistakes such as putting pajamas over daytime clothes or shoes on the wrong feet.

- Experience major changes in sleep patterns—sleeping during the day and becoming restless at night.

- Need help handling details of toileting (for example, flushing the toilet, wiping or disposing of tissue properly).

- Have increasingly frequent trouble controlling their bladder or bowels.

- Experience major personality and behavioral changes, including suspiciousness and delusions (such as believing that their caregiver is an impostor), or compulsive, repetitive behavior such as hand-wringing or tissue shredding.

- Tend to wander or become lost.

Stage 7   Very severe cognitive decline (Severe or late-stage Alzheimer's disease):

In the final stage of this disease, individuals lose the ability to respond to their environment, to carry on a conversation, and, eventually, to control movement. They may still say words or phrases.

At this stage, individuals need help with much of their daily personal care, including eating or using the toilet. They may also lose the ability to smile, to sit without support, and to hold their heads up. Reflexes become abnormal, muscles grow rigid, and swallowing is impaired.

Stages of Decubitus Ulcers

NATIONAL PRESSURE ULCER ADVISORY PANEL/ EUROPEAN PRESSURE ULCER ADVISORY PANEL PRESSURE ULCER DEFINITION

A pressure ulcer is a localized injury to the skin and/or underlying tissue usually over a bony prominence, as a result of pressure or pressure in combination with shear. A number of contributing or confounding factors are also associated with pressure ulcers; the significance of these factors is yet to be elucidated.

PRESSURE ULCER STAGES/CATEGORIES

Category/Stage I: Nonblanchable Erythema

Intact skin with nonblanchable redness of a localized area usually over a bony prominence. Darkly pigmented skin may not have visible blanching; its color may differ from the surrounding area. The area may be painful, firm, soft, warmer, or cooler as compared with adjacent tissue. Category/Stage I may be difficult to detect in individuals with dark skin tones. May indicate "at risk" persons.

Jacobs, K., & Simon, L. (Eds.). *Quick Reference Dictionary for Occupational Therapy, Sixth Edition* (pp. 688-690).
© 2015 SLACK Incorporated.

Category/Stage II: Partial Thickness

Partial thickness loss of dermis presenting as a shallow open ulcer with a red pink wound bed, without slough. May also present as an intact or open/ruptured serum-filled or sero-sanginous filled blister. Presents as a shiny or dry shallow ulcer without slough or bruising, which indicates a deep tissue injury. This category should not be used to describe skin tears, tape burns, incontinence associated dermatitis, maceration, or excoriation.

Category/Stage III: Full Thickness Skin Loss

Full thickness tissue loss. Subcutaneous fat may be visible but bone, tendon, and muscle are not exposed. Slough may be present but does not obscure the depth of tissue loss. May include undermining and tunneling. The depth of a Category/Stage III pressure ulcer varies by anatomical location. The bridge of the nose, ear, occiput, and malleolus do not have (adipose) subcutaneous tissue, and Category/Stage III ulcers can be shallow. In contrast, areas of significant adiposity can develop extremely deep Category/Stage III pressure ulcers. Bone/tendon is not visible or directly palpable.

Category/Stage IV: Full Thickness Tissue Loss

Full thickness tissue loss with exposed bone, tendon, or muscle. Slough or eschar may be present. Often includes undermining and tunneling. The depth of a Category/Stage IV pressure ulcer varies by anatomical location. The bridge of the nose, ear, occiput, and malleolus do not have (adipose) subcutaneous tissue, and these ulcers can be shallow. Category/Stage IV ulcers can extend into muscle and/or supporting structures (e.g., fascia, tendon or joint capsule), making osteomyelitis or osteitis likely to occur. Exposed bone/muscle is visible or directly palpable.

Additional Categories/Stages for the United States

Unstageable/Unclassified: Full Thickness Skin or Tissue Loss—Depth Unknown

Full thickness tissue loss in which actual depth of the ulcer is completely obscured by slough (yellow, tan, gray, green or brown) and/or eschar (tan, brown or black) in the wound bed. Until enough slough and/or eschar are removed to expose the base of the wound, the true depth cannot be determined, but it will be either a Category/Stage III or IV. Stable (dry, adherent, intact without erythema or fluctuance) eschar on the heels serves as "the body's natural (biological) cover" and should not be removed.

Suspected Deep Tissue Injury—Depth Unknown

Purple or maroon localized area of discolored intact skin or blood-filled blister due to damage of underlying soft tissue from pressure and/or shear. The area may be preceded by tissue that is painful, firm, mushy, boggy, warmer, or cooler compared with the adjacent tissue. Deep tissue injury may be difficult to detect in individuals with dark skin tones. Evolution may include a thin blister over a dark wound bed. The wound may further evolve and become covered by thin eschar. Evolution may be rapid exposing additional layers of tissue even with optimal treatment.

Statistics: Basic

Compiled by Wendy Coster, PhD

MEASURES OF CENTRAL TENDENCY

Measures of central tendency are measures of the "average" or "most typical" and are the most widely used statistical description of data. Measures of central tendency include:

1. **Mean:** The arithmetic average—the mean of a set of observations is simply their sum, divided by the number of observations.

2. **Median:** The median is the 50th percentile of a distribution—the point below which half of the observations fall.

3. **Mode:** The mode is the most frequently occurring observation—the most popular score of a class of scores.

MEASURES OF VARIABILITY OR DISPERSION

Measures of variability reflect the degree of spread or dispersion that characterizes a group of scores and the degree to which a set of scores differs from some measure of central tendency.

1. **Range:** The difference between the highest and lowest scores in a distribution.

Jacobs, K., & Simon, L. (Eds.). *Quick Reference Dictionary for Occupational Therapy, Sixth Edition* (pp. 691-696).
© 2015 SLACK Incorporated.

2. **Standard deviation:** The most commonly used measure of variability. The standard deviation is (roughly) the average amount that the individual scores vary from the mean of the set of scores.

THE MOST COMMONLY USED STATISTICAL PROCEDURES

1. **Chi-square (χ^2):** A statistic that can be used to analyze nominal (categorical) data. It compares the observed frequency of a particular category to the expected frequency of that category.

   Example: Is left-handedness more common among architects than accountants? (Handedness and profession are both nominal data.)

   Result is written as: χ^2 (df) = 289.3, p < .05

   Result is reported as: A chi-square analysis found that left-handedness occurred significantly more frequently among architects than among accountants (χ^2 [150] = 289.3, p < .05).

2. **t-test:** A statistical analysis that is used to compare the means of two groups.

   Example: Do left- and right-handers differ in speed of writing?

   Result is written as: t(df) = 3.86, p < .05

   Result is reported as: The mean speed of writing in the two groups was compared with a t-test and found to be significantly different (t[df] = 3.86, p < .05).

   Note: You must look at the descriptive statistics (means) to tell which group had the higher score.

3. **Analysis of variance (ANOVA):** A more complex statistical procedure that can be used to compare more than two groups on a dependent variable. ANOVA can also be used when the design has more than one independent variable. (There are several different "types" of ANOVA.)

Example: Does weekly participation in an occupation-focused group result in significantly increased community participation by frail elders compared to a social group or no intervention at all?

IV = intervention/group;   DV = community participation score

Result is written as: F (df, df) = 9.82, p < .01

Result is reported as: Differences in community participation were examined using analysis of variance. There was a significant difference between groups (F [df, df] = 9.82, p < .01).

Note: The "F" value only tells you that there is a difference between groups. It does not necessarily mean that each pairwise comparison between groups will be significant. You will need to look at the means (and sometimes conduct further tests, referred to as post-hoc analyses) to determine which groups performed significantly higher (or lower) than the others.

4. **Correlation:** A measure of the extent to which two variables tend to change together (i.e., a measure of the degree of association between them). Because correlational designs do not involve manipulation, they do not have an IV or DV.

An "r" may vary between –1.0 and +1.0:

Negative correlation: As one measure increases, the other decreases (e.g., air temperature and amount of clothing worn are negatively correlated).

Positive correlation: The measures tend to increase or decrease together (e.g., age and height are positively correlated through childhood).

Result is written as: r = .42, p < .05

Result is reported as: The two tests of hand function were only moderately correlated (r = .42, p < .05), suggesting that they do not measure the exact same skills.

Note: Correlations are particularly sensitive to variations in sample size. When interpreting a correlation, the size of the correlation should be considered as well, not just the "p" level. When samples are in the hundreds, even a correlation of $r = .10$ may be "significant." However $r = .10$ is still quite small, and an association of this magnitude may not have particular "real life" value.

5. **Regression:** Regression is a type of analysis in which one or more variables is used to try to predict (statistically) levels of another variable. There are several different types of regression, but they all have essentially the same goal of prediction.

Example: In a set of variables that includes age, measures of mobility limitation, general health, and a measure of self-efficacy (IVs), which variables best predict an elderly person's degree of social involvement (DV)?

Results are written in a variety of ways, depending on the study. One general approach is to report the overall amount of variance "accounted for" (predicted) by the regression model (e.g., $R^2 = .27$), and to provide additional statistics (referred to as Beta-weights) in a table.

Result is reported as: Only general health and self-efficacy were significant predictors, accounting for 27% of the variance in social involvement.

Note: A "significant" regression analysis only tells you that the set of selected variables can statistically predict an individual's score on the outcome variable (DV) to some degree better than chance. The closer the R^2 is to 1, the better the prediction (so in the example above, the prediction was not terrific). It does not tell you (1) that there is a causal relationship between the IVs and DV or (2) that variables that were not "significant" had no relation to the DV, rather it just tells you that the variables selected could create a good predictive model without them.

FURTHER NOTES ON THE INTERPRETATION OF STATISTICAL RESULTS

1. **Degrees of freedom:** The (df) in parentheses following χ^2, t, or F reflect the size of your sample and the number of variables in your analyses. Each statistical test has a formula for calculating the appropriate degrees of freedom (e.g., for t, $df = n - 2$). The df are important because they determine the "p" level of a given value obtained for χ^2, t, or F (using tables found in the back of all statistics texts).

   Example: Using the appropriate formula, I calculated $t = 2.20$. When I look this number up in the table, I find that if my df were 10, this result would not be significant at $p < .05$. However, if I had a large sample, and my $df = 30$, the result would be significant.

   A note on "p": As seen above, all of these statistical analyses yield a "p level." The "p" is a measure of the probability that the particular result obtained could have occurred by chance. Some examples of the correct way to interpret "$p < .05$" are:

   a. There is less than a 5% likelihood that a difference of this size between the means of the two groups occurred by chance (i.e., because of random events or by fluke rather than due to the effect you are examining).

   b. There is less than a 5% likelihood that a correlation of this size would have occurred by chance (i.e., occurred randomly rather than because there is some solid or true basis for the association).

CHECKING INTERPRETATIONS FOR ACCURACY

1. When interpreting statistical results in a research report, it is not appropriate to say that statistically significant results prove a hypothesis was correct or prove that two groups were really different. "Statistically significant" results mean that the results are "not very likely" to be due to chance alone

(but there is always a small chance that one could be wrong). Significant results "lend support" to a hypothesis or "provide evidence" that a hypothesis may be correct, but (except in very extraordinary circumstances) a single study never proves anything.

2. When interpreting results from a study that uses "t" or "ANOVA," you cannot assume that simply because groups are being compared that this is a true experimental design from which causal implications can be drawn. The study design must meet other requirements (e.g., random selection and assignment to groups) in order for causal interpretations to be appropriate.

3. Correlational designs do not establish causality, so interpretations of "r" should not use language that implies a causal relation between the two variables, regardless of what the author's favorite theory suggests. A "statistically significant" correlation means that the variables change together in a predictable way more than would be likely because of chance (but there is always a small possibility that one could be wrong). A significant correlation does not demonstrate "the effect of A on B" or the "impact of intensity of treatment A on functional assessment score B." Similarly, results of regression analyses (which are a variation of correlational design) show "the extent to which variance in outcome A can be predicted by cognitive status measure B," not "the effect of cognitive status on outcome."

Symbols

↑	increase
↓	decrease
→	follow
↔	to and from
1°	primary/first degree
2°	secondary/due to/second degree
3°	tertiary/third degree
@	at
α	alpha
β	beta
Δ	delta, change
n	total sample size
N	total population size
μ	micron (former term for micrometer)
Π	pi, 3.1416, ratio of circumference of a circle to its diameter
√	root, square root, radical
+	plus, excess, positive
−	minus, deficiency, negative
±	plus or minus, indefinite
~	approximately
≈	approximately equal
=	equals
>	greater than
<	less than

Jacobs, K., & Simon, L. (Eds.). *Quick Reference Dictionary for Occupational Therapy, Sixth Edition* (pp. 697-698). © 2015 SLACK Incorporated.

$\geq$	greater than or equal to
$\leq$	less than or equal to
Σ	sum
:	ratio, "is to"
::	equality between ratios, "as"
...	therefore
$\overline{c}$	with
$\overline{s}$	without
#	number, pound
/	per
♂	male
♀	female

Thoracic Outlet Syndrome

Dana Emery, OT/L

Thoracic outlet syndrome is characterized by compression of any or all of the neurovascular structures in the area known as the scalene triangle and the thoracic outlet. Structures included are the anterior and middle scalene muscles, the first rib, the clavicle, the brachial plexus, and the pectoralis minor muscle.

CAUSE

- The scalene muscle may become inflamed or hypertrophied; as the muscle size increases, the nerves, artery, or vein becomes compressed causing pain, swelling, weakness, numbness, and/or tingling.

- If a cervical rib is present, a fibrous band may grow, causing the space for the above structures to shrink, creating pressure on the nerves, artery, or vein.

- The pectoral minor muscle may be inflamed or fibrosed, causing pressure on the veins, arteries, or nerves.

- The clavicle may also be involved if it is calloused or misshapen.

- A blood clot in the artery or vein may cause swelling in the arm, leading to weakness and pressure on the nerves.

- Mechanical causes, see Aggravating Factors.

Jacobs, K., & Simon, L. (Eds.). *Quick Reference Dictionary for Occupational Therapy, Sixth Edition* (pp. 699-702).
© 2015 SLACK Incorporated.

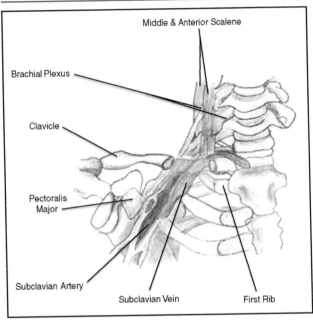

Illustration by Christopher Emery.

TESTING

- Cervical causes should be ruled out first.

- Electromyography studies of the distal extremity are usually normal.

- Nerve conduction velocity test of the median or ulnar nerves across the thoracic outlet of < 85 m/s confirms diagnosis.

- Sudden withdrawal from pressure to the lateral neck over the scalene muscles, the medial aspect of the supraclavicular fossa, and/or the area just medial to the pectoralis insertion.

- Positive venogram or upper extremity ultrasound of an edematous extremity.

- Elevated Arm Stress Test exhibits weakness, color changes of the extremity, or changes in sensation.

- All other peripheral nerve provocative testing is normal.

SYMPTOMS

- Paresthesias of the upper extremity may also be present in lateral neck and face.

- Weakness and decreased endurance of the upper extremity.

- Pain in the upper trapezius, chest near pectoralis insertion, chest wall, upper extremity; occipital headache.

- Sudden onset edema of the upper extremity.

- Color changes: bright red usually indicates venous compression, white or blue indicates arterial compression.

- May have associated splinter hemorrhages in the fingernails of the affected extremity with arterial compression.

- Temperature changes of the affected extremity.

- Band-like sensation of the upper arm around the humerus.

AGGRAVATING FACTORS

- With increased movement of the upper extremity these symptoms are amplified.

- During repetitive or sustained motion overhead or at shoulder height, these nerves, arteries, or veins may become pinched off and ultimately cause symptoms.

- Pulling, straining, or sudden unexpected motion, such as in whiplash or a fall while hanging from the affected upper extremity, may cause symptoms.

- Repetitive positioning or use in high-velocity sports may cause symptoms.

BIBLIOGRAPHY

Urschel, H. C., Jr., & Kourlis, H. (2007). Thoracic outlet syndrome: A 50-year experience at Baylor University Medical Center. *Baylor University Medical Center Proceedings, 20,* 125-135.

Total Hip Precautions

1. No flexion of the operated hip greater than 90 degrees.
How to explain to the patient:
   a. Do not bend your body forward more than 90 degrees.
   b. Do not raise the operated leg more than 90 degrees.

2. Do not cross the operated leg beyond midline of the body.
How to explain to the patient:
   a. Do not cross your knees.

3. Do not allow the operated leg to turn or twist inward, no internal rotation.
How to explain to the patient:
   a. Do not turn the operated foot inward (no walking like a pigeon).

Jacobs, K., & Simon, L. (Eds.). *Quick Reference Dictionary for Occupational Therapy, Sixth Edition* (pp. 703-704).
© 2015 SLACK Incorporated.

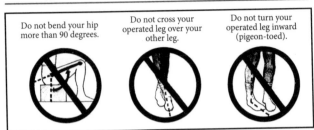

Do not bend your hip more than 90 degrees.

Do not cross your operated leg over your other leg.

Do not turn your operated leg inward (pigeon-toed).

To care for your new hip and keep it from sliding out of position, you will need to follow a few general restrictions at first. Your surgeon may recommend some additional restrictions based on your condition and type of surgery.

COMMON ADAPTIVE EQUIPMENT USED TO INCREASE INDEPENDENCE WITH ACTIVITIES OF DAILY LIVING

- Long-handled sponge
- Dressing stick
- Reachers
- Sock aid
- Long-handled shoehorn
- Elastic shoelaces
- Raised commode
- Tub transfer bench

Useful Spanish Phrases

Translated by Yvette Méré

1. Good morning. Please come in and sit down.
   Buenos dias. Por favor, pase y tome asiento.

2. What is your name?
   Cual es su nombre? Como se llama usted?

3. Pleased to meet you.
   Mucho gusto en conocerle.

4. My name is _____ and I will be your occupational therapist.
   Mi nombre es _____ y yo sere su terapeuta profesional.

5. Dr. _____ referred you to me to help you return to your job.
   El doctor _____ me sugirio le ayudara a reanudar su trabajo.

6. What are your goals?
   Cuales son sus objetivos?

7. What day is it? What time is it? Where are you?
   Qué dia es hoy? Qué hora es? Donde esta usted?

Jacobs, K., & Simon, L. (Eds.). *Quick Reference Dictionary for Occupational Therapy, Sixth Edition* (pp. 705-707).
© 2015 SLACK Incorporated.

8. Where do you live?
    Donde vive usted?

9. With whom do you live?
    Con quien vive usted?

10. How old are you?
    Qué edad tiene usted?

11. Are you taking any medications?
    Esta usted tomando algun medicamento?

12. Do you have any allergies?
    Padece usted de alguna alergia?

13. Have you ever had any surgeries and/or been admitted to
    the hospital?
    Ha sido usted operada en alguna ocasion o ingresada en el
    hospitale?

14. Describe the activities you do in a typical day.
    Describa sus actividades diarias normales.

15. Does anyone help you bathe, dress, or cook meals?
    Le ayuda alguien a banarse, vestirse, o preparar y cocinar
    sus alimentos?

16. Do you drive?
    Guia o maneja un vehiculo usted?

17. How physically active are you?
    Cuan fisicamente activa es usted?

18. When did you notice a change in your ability to complete
    your daily activities?
    Cuando se dio usted cuenta de un cambio en su habilidad
    para realizar sus actividades diarias?

19. Besides this problem, have you had any other health-related
    problems?
    Aparte de este problema, ha tenido usted otro problema rela-
    cionado con su salud?

20. Are your exercises helping you?
    Le estan ayudando los ejercicios?

21. Are you feeling better since beginning your treatment program?
    Se siente usted mejor desde qué empezo su tratamiento.

22. What is your occupation? What do you do for a living?
    Cual es su profesion? Qué hace para mantenerse?

23. What are the physical demands of your job?
    Qué exigencias fisicas requiere su trabajo?

24. Is there an activity where the pain feels worse or better?
    Existe una actividad en la cual empeore o mejore su dolencia?

25. Does your home have a staircase? Is it difficult for you to walk up the stairs?
    Tiene su casa escaleras? Se le dificulta subir las escaleras?

26. Is it difficult for you to use your hands during everyday activities?
    Se le dificulta el uso de sus manos en sus actividades diarias?

27. Do you mind if I touch your [arm] while I do my evaluation?
    Le molesta si le toco su [brazo] mientras hago mi evaluacion?

28. This home exercise program will help to strengthen your muscles so you can complete your tasks more easily.
    Este programa de ejercicios para hacer en su casa le fortalecera sus musculos de manera qué pueda realizar sus tareas mas facilmente.

29. What type of insurance do you have?
    Qué clase de seguro tiene usted?

Useful Spanish Words

Translated by Yvette Méré

Terms to Develop Rapport

1. please: por favor
2. thank you: gracias

General Terms

1. disorder: una condicion anormal fisica o mental
2. therapeutic: tratamiento de enfermedades o condiciones anormales a tranes de melodos reparadones o correctivos
3. medications: medicamento
4. occupational therapist: terapeuta profesional
5. evaluation: evalacion
6. pain/painful: dolor/doloroso
7. job: empleo/ocupacion
8. activities: actividades
9. active: activo
10. therapy: terapeuta
11. health/to be in good health: salud/estar bien de salud
12. insurance: seguro

Jacobs, K., & Simon, L. (Eds.). *Quick Reference Dictionary for Occupational Therapy, Sixth Edition* (pp. 708-711). © 2015 SLACK Incorporated.

ANATOMICAL TERMS

1. right: derecho
2. left: izquierdo
3. hand: mano
4. thumb (#1): pulgar
5. index finger (#2): indice
6. middle finger (#3): dedo medio/dedo del carazon
7. ring finger (#4): anular
8. little finger (#5): menique
9. wrist: muneca
10. arm: brazo
11. forearm: antebrazo
12. knee: rodilla
13. leg: pierna
14. foot: pie
15. ankle: tobillo
16. toes: dedo del pie
17. hip: cadera
18. joints: conjuntura/articulacion
19. muscle: musculo

HOME-RELATED TERMS

1. home/house: casa
2. staircase/stair: escalera/escalon
3. kitchen: cocina
4. bathroom: bano
5. bedroom: alcoba

6. bed: cama

7. stove/oven: horno

8. clock: reloj

DRESSING-RELATED TERMS

1. clothes: ropa

2. shirt: camisa

3. sweater: sueter

4. coat: abrigo

5. pants: pantalones

6. socks: calcetines

7. shoes: sapatos

8. to dress: vestir

9. hairbrush: cepillo para el pelo

10. toothbrush/toothpaste: cepillo de dientes/pasta dentifrica

11. towel: toalla

VERBS AND NOUNS RELEVANT DURING TREATMENT SESSIONS

1. to strengthen: fortalecer

2. to stretch: estirar

3. to walk: caminar

4. to limp: cojear

5. to sit/to sit down: sentar/sentarse

6. to reach for: alcanzar

7. to reach out one's hand: extender la mano

8. to help: ayudar

9. helpful: util

10. to succeed/to turn out well: tener buen exito

11. success: exito

12. effort/stress: esfuerzo

13. once more: una vez mas

14. little by little: poco a poco

TERMS RELATED TO DATES

1. week: semana

2. tomorrow: manana

3. today: hoy

Visual Impairment

Jennifer Kaldenberg, MSA, OTR/L, SCLV, CLVT and Karen Huefner, OTS

The following charts provide information on common visual impairments, assessments, and intervention strategies. The common interventions on pages 715 through 717 apply to all visual impairment categories unless otherwise noted.

Visual Impairment	Assessment and Specific Interventions for the General Occupational Therapy Visual Impairment Practitioner*
Visual acuity (VA) or refractive error caused by conditions such as hyperopia, myopia, or presbyopia (a normative aging change)	*Assessments:* Visual acuity testing for distance and near (i.e., Feinbloom Chart, biVABA, Lighthouse Near Acuity Card) Reading acuity measurement/continuous text (i.e., Pepper test or MNRead) *Specific Intervention:* Refer to optometry/ophthalmology for refraction and prescription

Jacobs, K., & Simon, L. (Eds.). *Quick Reference Dictionary for Occupational Therapy, Sixth Edition* (pp. 712-718).
© 2015 SLACK Incorporated.

Visual Impairment	Assessment and Specific Interventions for the General Occupational Therapy Visual Impairment Practitioner*
Central visual field loss caused by conditions such as macular degeneration or diabetic retinopathy	*Assessments:* Visual acuity testing for distance and near (i.e., Feinbloom Chart, biVABA, Lighthouse Near Acuity Card) Amsler grid (available online) Color vision (functional assessment or use of color chips) Contrast sensitivity testing (see CS assessments below) Visual field testing (confrontation fields for peripheral field; macular perimetry such as tangent screen for mapping central scotoma) *Specific Interventions:* Eccentric viewing (Freeman & Jose, 1997; Lane, 2005; Warren, 1996; Wright & Watson, 1995)
Peripheral visual field loss caused by such conditions as glaucoma or retinitis pigmentosa	*Assessment:* Visual field testing (confrontation fields or tangent screen) *Specific Interventions:* Optical remediation (i.e., prism, reverse telescopes)
Visual field impairments such as homonymous or heteronymous hemianopsias caused by stroke or traumatic brain injury	*Assessments:* Visual field testing (confrontation fields or tangent screen) Line bisection Figure drawing *Specific Interventions:* Optical remediation (i.e., prism)

Visual Impairment	**Assessment and Specific Interventions for the General Occupational Therapy Visual Impairment Practitioner***
Contrast sensitivity impairment caused by such conditions as cataracts and diabetic retinopathy	*Assessments:* Pelli-Robson Mars Lea symbols charts *Specific Interventions:* See Common Interventions chart
Glare and photophobia caused by such conditions as cataracts and diabetic retinopathy	*Assessments:* Glare test/Brightness Acuity Tester (BAT) Functional assessment/client report of complaints Compare results of testing (i.e., VA testing) with and without glare source *Specific Interventions:* Optical remediation (i.e., filters)
Diplopia (double vision)	*Assessments* (Gillen, 2009; Zoltan, 2007): Test monocularly and binocularly Test at distance and at near Test in all positions of gaze Ocular motility Ocular alignment *Specific Interventions* (Gillen, 2009): Binasal taping Prisms (fresnel and drilled) Eye exercises Vision therapy Patching

Visual Impairment	Assessment and Specific Interventions for the General Occupational Therapy Visual Impairment Practitioner*
Visuospatial deficits	*Assessments* (Gillen, 2009; Zoltan, 2007): Ocular motility Pursuits Saccades Convergence/divergence Assessment tools such as biVABA, MVPT, figure drawing or line bisection, and AMPS *Specific Interventions* (Gillen, 2009): Eye exercises Vision therapy Functional activities Cueing strategies

*Optimal practice is to collaborate with the OD/MD before initiation of intervention strategies. Many recommendations are made with this assumed.

COMMON INTERVENTIONS TO SUPPORT OCCUPATIONAL PERFORMANCE OF CLIENTS WITH LOW VISION

Magnification	Nonoptical or large-print items (i.e., large-button telephone, clock, address book) to support decline in visual acuity or central vision loss. Optical devices (i.e., prescribed magnifier) are utilized to enlarge the image, allowing the individual to more easily perceive a word or item.
Minification	Use of reverse telescope or minus lens can help individuals with reduced or constricted peripheral visual fields. Minimizing the size of an object in the distance creates greater available visual field.

Scanning	Organized viewing strategy to improve awareness of the environment (i.e., for reading tasks begin at top left of page, orient to general layout and then to left column).
Contrast enhancements	Improve visibility of items by increasing contrast of objects and their backgrounds. Black and white is optimal for contrast sensitivity impairment (i.e., place high-contrast tape on edge of stairs, lip of tub, grab bars, bath bench; use 20/20 pens and signature guides).
Organizational strategies	Develop organizational system to compensate for vision loss (i.e., place all articles of clothing for an outfit together, keep magnifier in designated reading area).
Lighting	Increase ambient (overhead) and task lighting. Use gooseneck table and floor lamps to best direct light at or near (to reduce glare) the task. Minimum suggested light level (using light meter) is 300 lux for ambient and 1000 lux for task (Figueiro, 2001).
Glare	For all clients, especially with photophobia or problems with glare, use sheer curtains or shades to filter natural light while decreasing glare. Use glare screens on computer monitors. Wear hat and sunglasses outside. Cover exposed light bulbs.
Filters	Clients wear filters over glasses. For contrast sensitivity impairment, try yellow filters when indoors to improve perception of contrast. To minimize glare or for photophobia, try dark amber or Polaroid gray filters when outdoors.
Tactile strategies	For all clients, try tactile strategies to help compensate for vision loss (i.e., bump dots on common buttons of stove or telephone, non-rust safety pins in navy vs. black clothes).

Auditory strategies	For all clients, try auditory strategies to help compensate for vision loss (i.e., talking products such as watches, Say-when device for pouring hot liquids).
Client education	Share information on eye conditions, normative aging changes, resources for services, role of the environment in supporting vision loss, and genetic and modifiable risk factors for eye disease. Educate on importance of maintaining overall health to support vision (i.e., maintaining blood sugar levels helps protect individual with diabetes from developing eye disease).

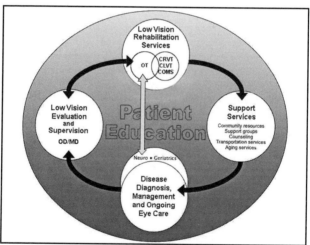

Optimal Practice Model in Low Vision Rehabilitation. Developed by the A-Team: A Coalition of the American Occupational Therapy Association, Association for Education and Rehabilitation of the Blind and Visually Impaired, American Academy of Optometry Study Group, and American Optometric Association. Reprinted with permission from the American Occupational Therapy Association.

FUNCTIONAL DIAGNOSTIC CODES:
CODES SPECIFIC TO LOW VISION REHABILITATION

	Total	Near Total	Profound	Severe	Moderate
Total	369.1	369.03	369.06	369.12	369.16
Near Total		369.04	369.07	369.13	369.17
Profound			369.08	369.14	369.18
Severe				369.22	369.24
Moderate					369.25

Homonymous bilateral field defect	368.46
Heteronymous bilateral field defect	368.47
Central scotoma	368.41

Total impairment=NLP, near total impairment=<20/1000=<5 degrees, profound impairment=20/500 to 20/1000=<10 degrees, severe impairment=<20/160 to 20/400=<20 degrees, moderate impairment=<20/60 to 20/160. Adapted from Colenbrander (2002) and International Classification of Disease (2008).

REFERENCES

Colenbrander, A. (2002). *Visual standards: Aspects and ranges of vision loss.* Retrieved from www.ski.org/Colenbrander/Images/Vis_Standards_ICO_2002.pdf

Figueiro, M. G. (2001). Lighting the way: A key to independence. *Lighting Research Center.* Retrieved from www.lrc.rpi.edu/publicationDetails.asp?id=210

Freeman, P. B., & Jose, R. T. (1997). *The art and practice of low vision.* Boston, MA: Butterworth-Heinemann.

Gillen, G. (2009). *Cognitive and perceptual rehabilitation: Optimizing function.* St. Louis, MO: Mosby, Inc.

International Classification of Disease. (9th rev.). *Clinical modifications.* Retrieved from http://icd9cm.chrisendres.com/

Lane, K. (2005). *Developing ocular motor and visual perceptual skills: An activity workbook.* Thorofare, NJ: SLACK Incorporated.

Warren, M. (1996). *Pre-reading and writing exercises for persons with macular scotomas.* Birmingham, AL: visABILITIES Rehab Services.

Wright, V., & Watson, G. R. (1995). *Learn to use your vision for reading* (LUV reading series). Lilburn, GA: Bear Consultants.

Zoltan, B. (2007). *Vision, perception, and cognition: A manual for the evaluation and treatment of the adult with acquired brain injury* (4th ed.). Thorofare, NJ: SLACK Incorporated.

Wheelchair Measurement Procedures

1. Seat width
   a. Measure the individual across the widest part of either the hips or thighs
   b. Add 2 inches to the individual's measurement for seat width

2. Seat depth
   a. Measure the individual from the rear of the buttocks to the inside of the bent knee
   b. Subtract 1 to 2 inches from the measurement for seat depth

3. Seat height
   a. Measure the leg from the bottom of the heel to just under the thigh (popliteal fossa)
   b. Add 2 inches to the leg length for the seat height

4. Arm rest height
   a. Measure from the wheelchair seat to the individual's bent elbow
   b. Add 1 inch to the measurement for the arm rest height

Jacobs, K., & Simon, L. (Eds.). *Quick Reference Dictionary for Occupational Therapy, Sixth Edition* (pp. 719-720). © 2015 SLACK Incorporated.

5. Back rest height
   a. Measure from the seat platform to the axilla of the individual
   b. Add 4 inches to the measurement for back rest height

STANDARD DIMENSIONS (INCHES)

Chair Style	Width	Depth	Seat Height	Arm Height	Back Height
Adult	18	16	20	10	20
Narrow Adult	16	16	20	10	20
Junior	16	16	18.5	10	18
Low Seat	18	16	17	10	16

APPENDIX 63

Workstation Checklist

Using this checklist is one way an employer or employees can identify, analyze, and control musculoskeletal disorder hazards in computer workstation tasks.

WORKING CONDITIONS

The workstation is designed or arranged for doing video-display terminal (VDT) tasks so it allows the employee's. . .

A. **Head** and **neck** to be about upright (not bent down/back).   Y   N

B. **Head, neck** and **trunk** to face forward (not twisted).   Y   N

C. **Trunk** to be about perpendicular to floor (not leaning forward/backward).   Y   N

D. **Shoulders** and **upper arms** to be about perpendicular to floor (not stretched forward) and relaxed (not elevated).   Y   N

E. **Upper arms** and **elbows** to be close to body (not extended outward).   Y   N

F. **Forearms, wrists,** and **hands** to be straight and parallel to floor (not pointing up/down).   Y   N

G. **Wrists** and **hands** to be straight (not bent up/down or sideways toward little finger).   Y   N

Jacobs, K., & Simon, L. (Eds.). *Quick Reference Dictionary for Occupational Therapy, Sixth Edition* (pp. 721-724). © 2015 SLACK Incorporated.

H. **Thighs** to be about parallel to floor and lower legs to be about perpendicular to floor.   Y   N

I. **Feet** to rest flat on floor or be supported by a stable footrest.   Y   N

J. **VDT tasks** to be organized in a way that allows employee to vary VDT tasks with other work activities, or to take micro-breaks or recovery pauses while at the VDT workstation.   Y   N

SEATING

The chair

1. **Backrest** provides support for employee's lower back (lumbar area).   Y   N

2. **Seat width** and **depth** accommodate specific employee (seat pan not too big/small).   Y   N

3. **Seat front** does not press against the back of employee's knees and lower legs (seat pan not too long).   Y   N

4. **Seat** has cushioning and is rounded/has "waterfall" front (no sharp edge).   Y   N

5. **Armrests** support both forearms while employee performs VDT tasks and do not interfere with movement.   Y   N

KEYBOARD/INPUT DEVICE

The keyboard/input device is designed or arranged for doing VDT tasks so that...

6. **Keyboard/input device platform(s)** is stable and large enough to hold keyboard and input to keyboard so it can be operated without reaching   Y   N

7. **Input device** (mouse or trackball) is located right next to keyboard so it can be operated without reaching.   Y   N

8. **Input device** is easy to activate and shape/size fits hand of specific employee (not too big/small).   Y   N

9. **Wrists** and **hands** do not rest on sharp or hard edge.   Y   N

MONITOR

The monitor is designed or arranged for VDT tasks so that . . .

10. **Top line** of screen is at or below eye level so employee is able to read it without bending head or neck down/back. (For employees with bifocals/trifocals, see next item.)   Y   N

11. **Employee with bifocals/trifocals** is able to read screen without bending head or neck backward.   Y   N

12. **Monitor distance** allows employee to read screen without leaning head, neck or trunk forward/backward.   Y   N

13. **Monitor position** is directly in front of employee so employee does not have to twist head or neck.   Y   N

14. **No glare** (e.g., from windows, lights) is present on the screen which might cause employee to assume an awkward posture to read screen.   Y   N

WORK AREA

The work area is designed or arranged for doing VDT tasks so that. . .

15. **Thighs** have clearance space between chair and VDT table/keyboard platform (thighs not trapped).   Y   N

16. **Legs** and **feet** have clearance space under VDT table so employee is able to get close enough to keyboard/input device.   Y   N

ACCESSORIES

17. **Document holder,** if provided, is stable and large enough to hold documents that are used.   Y   N

18. **Document holder,** if provided, is placed at about the same height and distance as monitor screen so there is little head movement when employee looks from document to screen.   Y   N

19. **Wrist rest,** if provided, is padded and free of sharp and square edges.   Y   N

20. **Wrist rest,** if provided, allows employee to keep forearms, wrists and hands straight and parallel to ground when using keyboard/input device.   Y   N

21. **Telephone** can be used with head upright (not bent) and shoulders relaxed (not elevated) if employee does VDT tasks at the same time.   Y   N

GENERAL

22. Workstation and equipment have sufficient adjustability so that the employee is able to be in a safe working posture and to make occasional changes in posture while performing VDT tasks.   Y   N

23. VDT Workstation, equipment and accessories are maintained in serviceable condition and function properly.
    Y   N

Passing Score = "YES" answer on all "working postures" items (A-J) and no more than two "NO" answers on remainder of checklist (1-23).

Source: Occupational Safety and Health Administration.

Additional appendices are available at
www.healio.com/books/qrdappendices6th